Medical Eldering *for* Physicians

Co-creating a Living Future

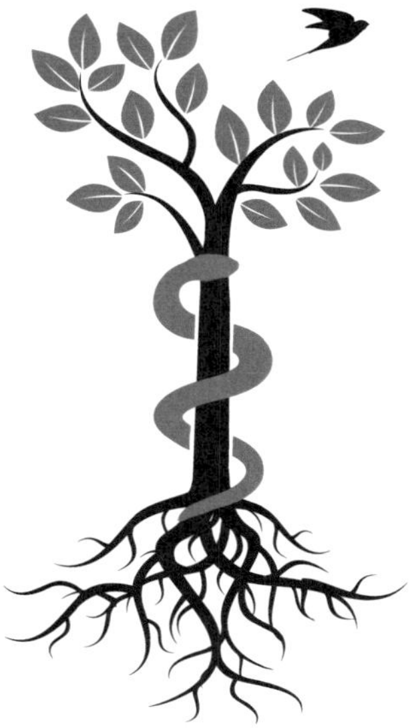

A Year to Envision Your Living Legacy

Beth W. Alderman, MD, MPH

PUBLISHED BY FUTURE MEDICINE, LLC

Medical Eldering for Physicians:
Co-creating a Living Future

by Beth W. Alderman, MD, MPH

www.FutureMedicine.us

For related online courses visit www.EvolveMedicine.us

Book Design: BookSavvyStudio.com

Library of Congress Control Number: 2020906407
ISBN: 978-1-7332849-0-5

First Edition
Printed in the United States of America

Human life [is] a quest, a work in progress on every level, in which individual integrity and initiative are critically needed.

Roger Lipsey
in *Hammarsjöld: A Life*, 2016

To Eva and Bryan for a Living Future

and

To Berton Roueché and Dr. Oliver Sacks
for advancing the art of the
medical narrative

Contents

WINTER

SPRING

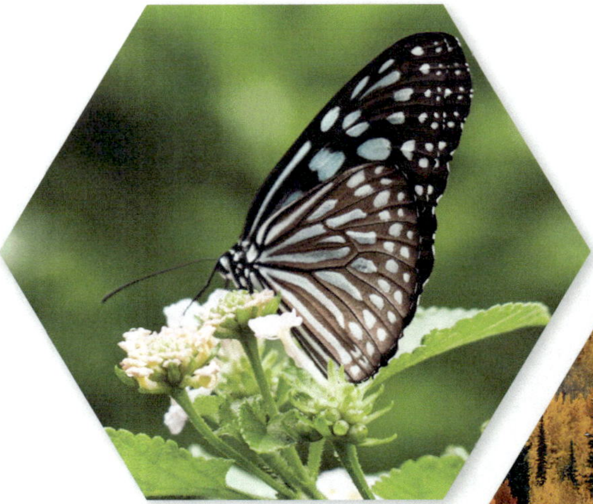
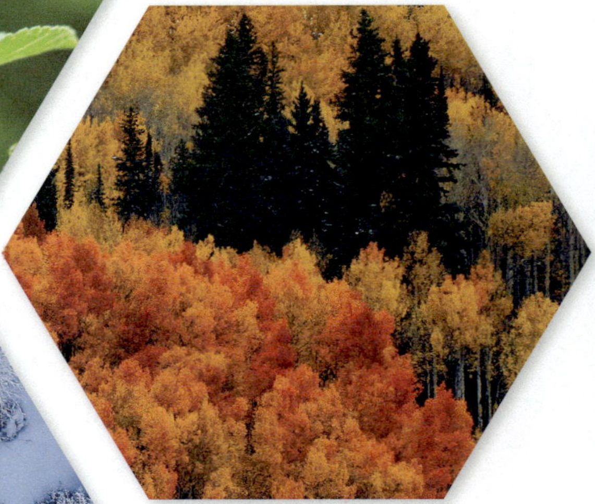
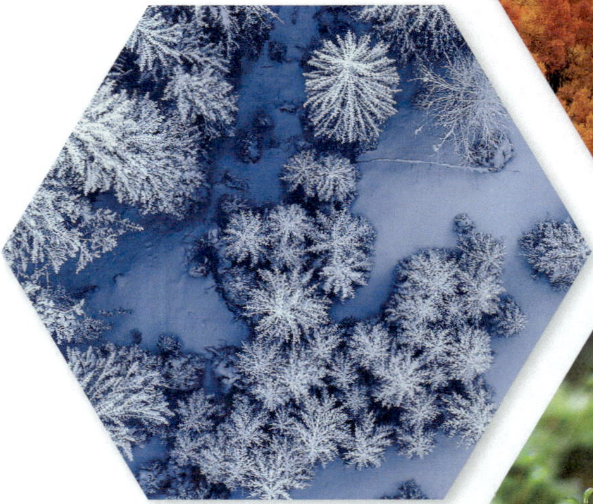
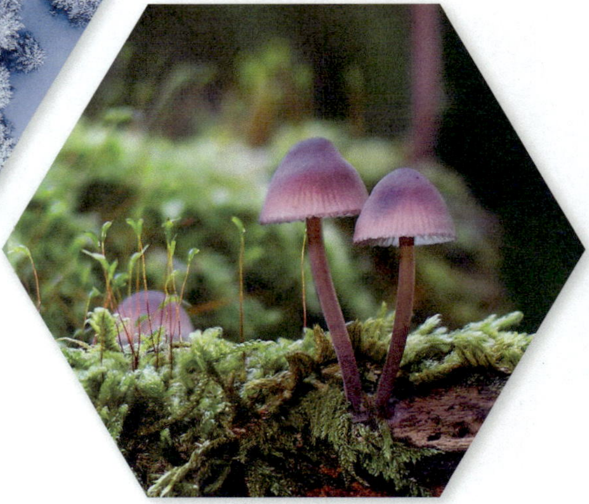

Preparation

EXPECTATIONS

Over the course of a year of transition to:

- Reorient to deep time and evolved context
- Optimize freedom of time and time use for eldering
- Form your personal narrative and vital purpose
- Harness your unspent or new passions
- Review your present direction and reset it as needed
- Add to your knowledge base to suit your direction
- Release embodied experiences to form new wisdom
- Repattern your habits to realize the items above
- Galvanize your personal and interpersonal agency by engaging your embodied wisdom with gusto
- Have—and prepare for—the time of your life

Over the next several years

- Use tools such as this book and its ideas and methods to guide your personal evolution as an elder, to focus and enhance your personal efficacy, and to effect your unique destiny.

Supplemental Material

For every season, a supplemental month is included for your use. Feel free to choose any three months or to use all four, and to pick and choose from the recommended exercises and extra reading. However, be sure to study all constructs and to do related exercises and working questions that look 'juicy' to you—that is, that are not 'old hat' and thus offer new possibilities. If you like, you can also take the courses available online at www.EvolveMedicine.us. and join the Doctors of Life International discussion group. Be aware that there will be some overlap, especially certain anecdotes included in materials destined for various audiences.

Journaling

Make sure that you have a blank journal for your individual use, taking appropriate measures to ensure privacy. The habit of journaling—when not overdone—engages expressive as well as receptive speech centers, and catalyzes insight and perspective.

To learn more about modern journaling for change, see Eve LaPlante's book *Samuel Sewall: Salem Witch Judge*, or Roger Lipsey's 2016 biography, *Dag Hammarsjöld: A Life*. Books and articles on cognitive behavioral therapy, a recent repackaging of the perennial practice of journaling, may also be of use.

Instructions for Monthly Progress

Feel free to start the book at the chapter corresponding to the month in which you take it up, or to wait until summer to engage it as designed. The materials provided for you in this book are not prescriptions: they are tools that you can choose, use, and hone to augment your humanity, wisdom, and efficacy in rescuing life on earth, including your species. They are offered with well-wishes for forming a biocentric, unitive view of the ailments of the body of life, of habitats, of species, and of you as an individual. In other words, they support you in emboding care and cure for evolved life. To orient yourself now, you can take the looming sixth extinction as your impetus and the emergence of the medical paradigm to avert extinction as your vision, and elaborate those over the course of your year of transition.

Other

Further instructions are offered with specific elements of the text.

May these tools serve you well.

MEDICAL ELDERING *for* PHYSICIANS

Co-creating a Living Legacy

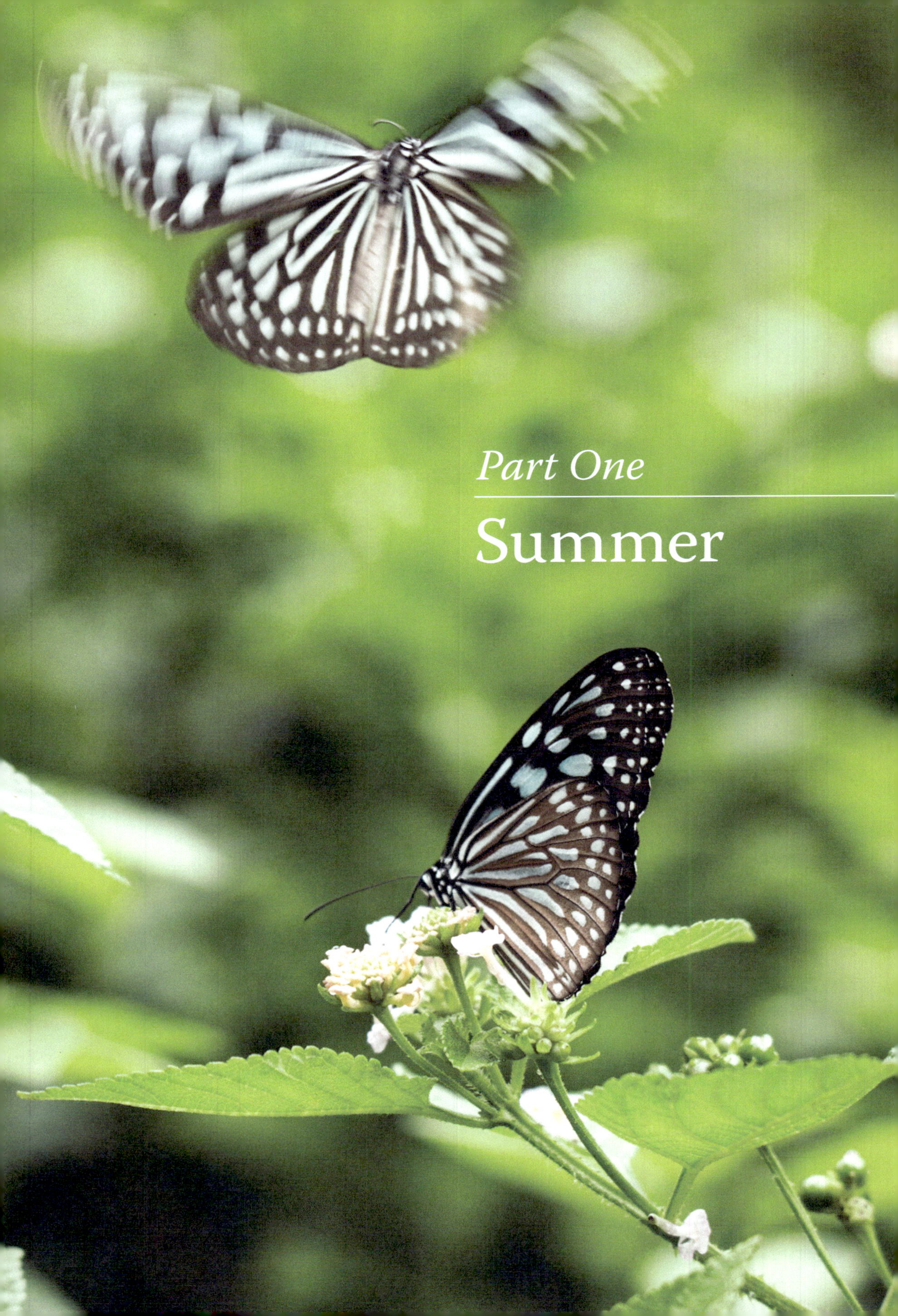

Part One
Summer

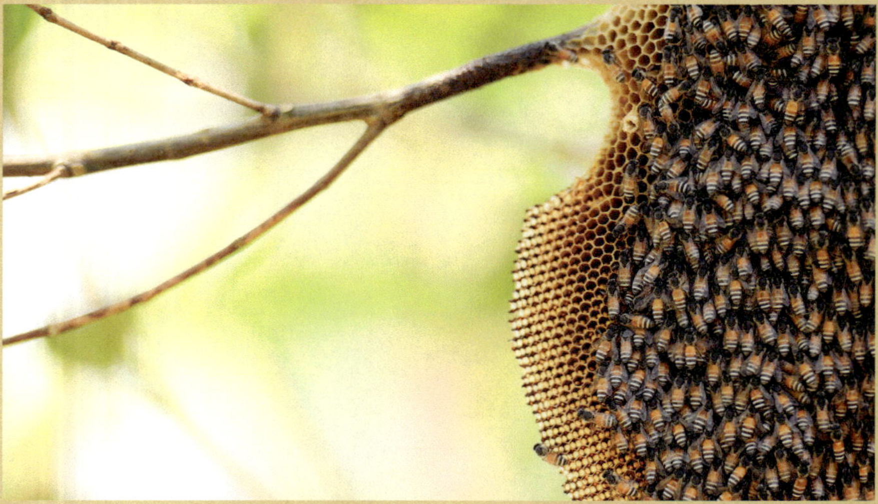

ELDERING IS ALL ABOUT TIME. TIME WITHOUT HURRY. TIME DEFINED BY BIOLOGY RATHER THAN BY HUMAN FOLLY. THIS GUIDE THEREFORE BEGINS WITH THREE MONTHS OF LETTING GO OF THE CLOCKS, DEVICES, AND CALENDARS THAT WOULD DISTRACT YOU FROM THE PACE AND RHYTHM OF YOUR NEWLY WELL-CARED-FOR BODY AND YOUR REBIRTH INTO THE WISDOM YEARS.

Pondering Biological Time

SUMMER

...Graves at my command Have waked their sleepers, oped, and let 'em forth By my so potent art. But this rough magic I here abjure ; and when I have required Some heavenly music (which even now I do) To work mine end upon their senses that This airy charm is for, I'll break my staff, Bury it certain fathoms in the earth, And deeper than did ever plummet sound I'll drown my book.

—Shakespeare as Prospero in *The Tempest*

As life expectancy increases, and more people pursue active aging, authors such as President Jimmy Carter and counselors Richard Rohr, Joan Chittester, Jack Kornfield, and Reb Zalman Schachter-Shalomi are writing books that reveal the virtues of the wisdom years and encourage others to make the last phase of their lives the best and most rewarding. These encourage elders to live an examined life—that is, to process, reconcile, and harness a lifetime of learning. For example, in Zalman's book *Age-ing to Sage-ing*, he describes a path to spiritual eldering that entails celebrating past gains; releasing troubling events and maladaptive responses to them; and gathering and sharing a lifetime of experiential learning. This mindful maturing of the past yields the wisdom to be a wise elder.

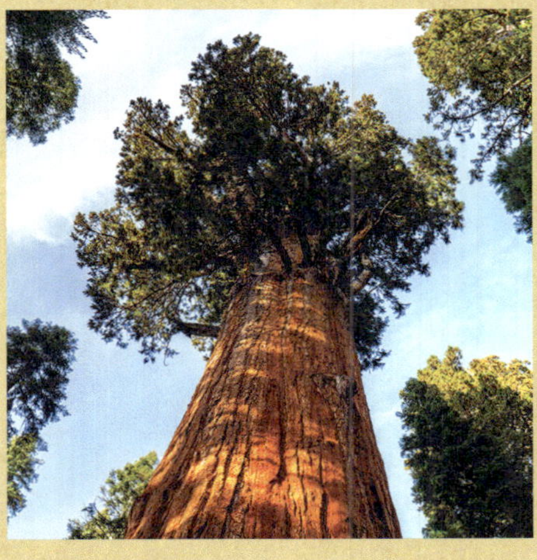

This guide takes you through one method for combining the personal work of processing your lifetime with the professional processing of a life in medicine at a time of profound change. Although it is outside the scope of this book, I recommend that you begin by celebrating your personal and professional accomplishments to date. Include obstacles overcome and intentions realized that matter to you and to your kith and kin. Reflect on hands well-played, quagmires escaped, and pitfalls eluded. Then, after you have used this material as a tool in your transition to the wisdom years, celebrate the beginning of the completion of your lifework and the creation of your living legacy. During your transition year, keep a journal and record in it your new insights and perspectives as well as your encounters with the emerging paradigm. As you do this, allow the questions and exercises to expand and enhance your knowledge base and your toolkit of skills, as that will inform the wisdom years that you have earned.

Eldering is all about time. Time without hurry. Time defined by biology rather than by human folly. This guide therefore begins with three months of letting go of the clocks, devices, and calendars that would distract you from the pace and rhythm of your newly well-cared-for body and your rebirth into the wisdom years. During this month you can leave behind your domination by late modern social mores steeped in algorithms of industrial engineering and information technology that devalue life and living. You can also take time to allow your flesh and all that it generates to separate from the tools of your day to day employment, and to stew your further maturation in the fruits of millennia of evolution. As you allow your most precious gifts of time and attention to read and respond to your embodied experience, and engage your receptive and expressive language skills in discerning your developing existence, you open the door to becoming more fully human, more alive to possibility, and better equipped to guide epochal changes in your profession.

Medical eldering is all about making the best of life as it has come down to you from your antecedents and from the miracles of generative biological processes that moderns barely grasp and yet presume to control. As a medical elder, you free yourself to solve complex, species-scale problems in their living context. This requires letting go of the modern ways of care and cure that have been formed by thinking that is antithetical to living systems and, as described in Rachel Carson's *Silent Spring* and Elisabeth Kolbert's T*he Sixth Extinction*, is hurtling all life toward extinction within the near future.

Our juniors are faced with the rescue of life on earth, a feat that no amount of adrenaline can effect—but that contemplation and loving care can. There is no point in saving the patient and losing the species. Medical elders who can exit the system are in a position to recognize the blind spots of modern medicine and to mentor juniors who are embedded in it. You can gather the wisdom of prior periods of change by consulting the writings of Hippocrates, Avicenna, Maimonides, Vesalius, and the doctors of the Scottish Enlightenment. As recently as pediatrician Dr. Benjamin Spock, nature was appreciated by doctors of all eras as integral to care. As an elder, you can allow life to renew you as you renew it, beginning herein with leaving behind any addiction to 'busy' and making room in your new life for the future of life on earth.

Taking a Breather

That awful fever of overwork which we feel especially in the United States—he had it. A trembling in the arms and thighs, a tightness of the neck and in the head above the eyes—fast breath, vague pains in the muscles and in the feet. Followed by an orgasm, crashing the job through, putting it over in a fever heat. The looseness afterward. Not pleasant. But there it is.

— William Carlos Williams in *Old Doc Rivers*

YOU BEGIN AT THE START OF SUMMER, when you may have the chance to enjoy the simple pleasures of life: sunshine on closed eyelids, the sound of a mountain rill, rests that renew, friends that inspire or content, and the scents of trees in their glory. The idea behind such enjoyment is to reconnect with the natural world and thereby with your deepest self, the one that modern medicine often replaces with addiction to adrenal overload. This addiction may disconnect you from the original motivations that spurred you to delve into the mysteries and miracles of the body with a passionate desire to free it from disease or early death, and so allow it to support the precious gift of a life rich in meaning and moment.

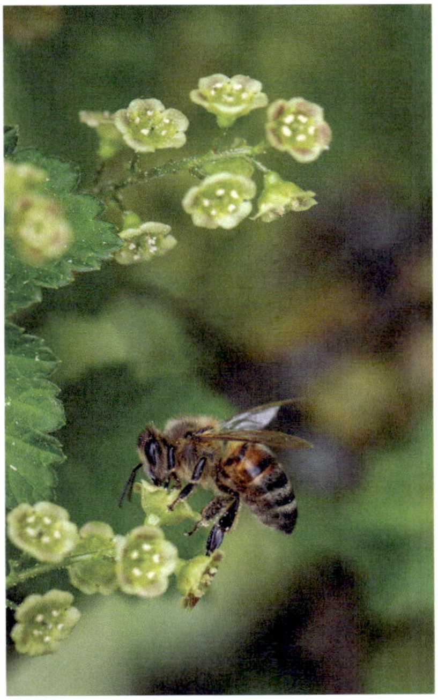

In most ancient traditions—your Hippocratic lineage included—seasons defined the art of medicine through the body of life as well as through doctors' parent communities and new initiates. Even if you have dissociated from nature as a result of modern urban living, you will have remained aware of changes in the duration of daylight and can become aware of your bodily responses to them, and through them engage the perennial rhythms of the earth's seasons.

For the purposes of this book, you regard summer as the time to step out of your routines and to return to the natural world; fall as the time when you

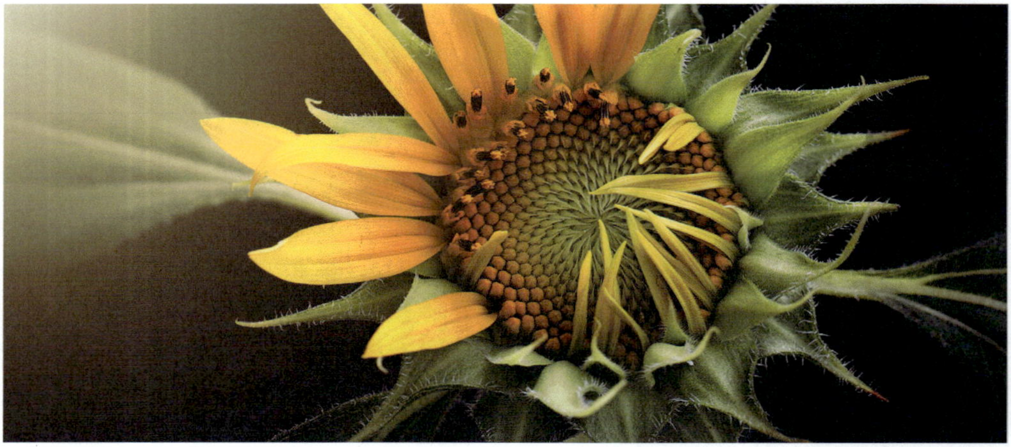

look back on and study your life so far; winter as the time you do the hard work of seeing and solving any lingering problems that you have created in your hurry through life; and spring as the time when you refresh yourself and look forward to becoming a part of the solution to medical mistakes that are too big to see. In other words, you anticipate paying your debts to life forward for the sake of all evolved life that is facing the sixth extinction of the Anthropocene era, a topic to which we will return.

This sequence is designed to support you in taking up the challenge to see and be the change that you want to see in the world for the sake of a living future. You therefore begin by learning the self-care that is essential to changing your life from the core of your body. This way, you will not perpetuate into your elder years any habits of responding to emergencies without stepping back to see the big picture, will not lose the chance to care for and cure life in context, and will not realize on your deathbed that you never created a living legacy to help rejuvenate and sustain life in the aggregate. You may even find that you have in the past been a party to the modern illusion of control that has enchanted humanity with spiral nebulae and myriads of molecules at the cost of obscuring our species' imperilment of itself and all evolved life on earth. You may see that your heroic efforts to save individual lives have inadvertently enabled the loss of the species.

And so you begin to become more than you have been by sustaining your body now, at the time of life when you are, according to ancient traditions, entering your wisdom years. You make time to enjoy life so as to remind yourself of what is at stake and of how much you have loved life and still love it. Then you will be able to draw from the deep well of everyday miracles and the resolve to relish your role in the save of the millennium—the save that rescues the body of life from human abuse and neglect. Life needs care and cure now and—if you and others succeed—will continue to need it into the indefinite future.

And so you approach the summer of your elderhood by freeing space and time to engage and enjoy life, as do painters who express nature in delicate nuances of light and shade and in broad strokes of vibrant color; as do musicians who listen for the rhythms of other creatures; and as do poets who take rays of late, slanting sunlight as seeds for rhymes. You suspend outmoded cares and habits, take pleasure in the fragile web of life on earth that is not yet beyond your aid, and refresh the body that Maimonides saw as flesh with a five-part soul and that the emerging paradigm in this book frames as comprised of seven parts: flesh, energy, sensations, perceptions, understanding, awareness, and interbeing.

If you have been conditioned to take your flesh or being for granted, or to neglect it or place it last, or to punish it for taking leisure time, this may be the hardest season of this fellowship in eldering. You may be hit by guilt, regret, shame, or angry blame. You may feel an urge to continue trying to outrun the future you have been creating. If so, feel free to start with any season or chapter that suits you better at this time. For example, you may wish to begin with the work of winter, when you face the dragons of your past and—to paraphrase Rilke—re-cast them as princes or princesses waiting to be kissed. Now—or whenever you come to your summer—take time to stop, look, listen, and engage the present moment, and so to prepare for the adventure of creating the capstone of your life in medicine.

ANECDOTES FROM MEDICAL LIVES

If you think adventure is dangerous, try routine; it is lethal.

—Paulo Coelho, author of *The Alchemist*

In times past, doctors who had the opportunity took locums, and professor doctors took sabbaticals. Those who were not too hard-pressed developed avocations, second lives that could refresh them when routine became oppressive, exhausting, or confining. Many today hike or climb, play a musical instrument, provide medical aid in other parts of the world, or follow a favorite sports team. If you have been—as the apt phrase has it—keeping your nose to the grindstone instead of engaging the full scope of life, one of the anecdotes below may inspire you in learning to re-engage with life.

Daniel and Marie: The Weekend Holiday

During Daniel's fellowship, he and his wife Marie—a nurse specializing in conflict resolution and later in communications—were already outdoor sports enthusiasts. Like my then-husband and me, they were using their free time to explore the Cascadia bioregion, which held some of the last wild places on earth. One weekend, the four of us drove north for a weekend at a cross-country ski area in a provincial park in British Columbia, where we stayed at an inexpensive lodge. The park was beautiful then, and continues to support traditional winter skiing now. The lodge went defunct long ago—for good reasons that our weekend outing would soon reveal.

When we arrived, we had trouble finding a place to park. The parking area had, at some time in the past, subsided into the ground below, which had once been the septic field. Efforts to turn it into a skating rink by pouring water on it only added to the subsidence. When we went inside the lodge—which was, to our relief, toasty warm—we saw that all the decorative plants were dead from lack of water. When we entered the café, the bright-faced, athletic-looking waiter apologized and informed us that we couldn't have espresso because if he turned on the machine, the electrical system would fail. When we came back from skiing, there was no water for showers. We spent a ripe night in a shared room. We were used to being on call; nothing in the experience posed a real hardship.

In fact, the lodge presented an opportunity for non-stop hilarity. We got to the point where we couldn't wait to see what else was wrong with the place so that we could laugh heartily and think back on our good fortune at home. No comedy entertainment could have given us so many laughs to take with us and enjoy. We still laugh about it to this day. Daniel and Marie have backpacked the Pacific Crest Trail since, and all four of us still enjoy the outdoors.

Joel and Aliya: Crafting a Sustainable Medical Life

Joel's father died young of a heart attack, after which the doctor told Joel that he had inherited a predisposition to high cholesterol and must lead a very healthy life to avoid a similar result. Joel traveled the world and came to enjoy sports like hiking and skiing, then went on to medical school. Even before entering medical school, he had decided to choose a specialty that he loved and that was relatively low in stress. When the time came, he specialized in psychiatry. During his fellowship, his loving and capable girlfriend Aliya, who was soon to become his wife, made a complementary decision: she would take a business degree and be ready to act as the primary or sole wage-earner of the family in case of need. And so Joel and Aliya incorporated self-care and sustainability into their family lives from the start of his medical life.

Many years later, when his mother died, Joel committed to doing a full year of saying the mourner's Kaddish daily with a local congregation. This was complicated in his town; there were many Jewish congregations, but none offered daily opportunity for this prayer, which meant going from one congregation to the next all week long. He recognized, though, that his self-care was inclusive of the ethereal as well as the material aspects of the body, and determined that his religion offered the best practice for sustaining his spiritual health as he grieved his mother's loss.

In other words, Joel recognized that his religion—and his continuing close relation to the natural world in his home city and the nearby mountains—were integral to his ongoing self-care as a man, a doctor, a husband, and a father. As the year drew to a close, he looked back with gratitude on the congregations that had welcomed him and on the ancient practice of mourning that had honored his mother and—at the same time—sustained his well-being, and indirectly the well-being of his family.

Quartet: a Hobby for Fun and Refreshment

By the time my daughter entered primary school, teachers were ready for complex families—more ready than the parents. I had heard from my daughter that in addition to classmates who were children of divorce, she made a new friend who had two moms. Being physicians—one of whom studied reproductive outcomes—her father and I tended to take such families for granted, and to assume that we would be able to answer any questions that might come up.

It wasn't until our daughter said that this new friend also had two dads and asked exactly how that had worked, and I had already opened my mouth to explain, that I realized that our first conversation about conception might involve a technological narrative. That would bury the thread of the family story. As I paused, my daughter suggested that each mom had been married to one of the dads. I finally filled in the blank by saying that two loving moms and two loving dads had decided to have a family. She didn't ask how they went about it; that part of the story didn't matter to her.

Not long after, my daughter received an invitation to go to the house of her new friend. We learned then that one mom was a doctor and the other a nurse. When we came to pick up our daughter, we learned that the moms, in addition to holding down two jobs and having a child, had taken on a legendary hobby: they had joined the circus. They were practical about it; they helped found a circus school and that way were able to refresh their lives by enjoying the development of new circus skills while keeping their day jobs and living near their daughter's school. My daughter said that the play date at their home consisted of playing acrobalancing in the living room. When I asked what it was, she did her best to explain it, and the family once again opened our eyes to new ways of living.

BETH LOOKS BACK: You Have to Stop Running to Stretch

In comparing the certainty of things spiritual and things temporal, let us not forget this—Mind is the first and most direct thing in experience; all else is remote inference.

—Sir Arthur Stanley Eddington in *Science and the Unseen World*

When I left the University of Colorado, where I was an Assistant Professor of Preventive Medicine and Biometrics, I took a research position at the University of Washington in the Department of Epidemiology School of Public Health and Community Medicine. Most faculty there depended entirely on federal grant support and had great success in winning funding. This meant that space was tight, that faculty were judged on their ability to gain money and status, and that investigations were closely overseen by managers dedicated to economic, regulatory, and legal values.

My new job felt corporate. My salary was still well below those of medical school classmates who had opted for conventional career paths, but my fancy new office was a perk they might have envied. It was in a downtown high-rise that presumed to energy efficiency by virtue of being air-tight. The University got a good deal on the rent as occupancy rates were low then and the owner, who had a reputation of threatening bankruptcy, apparently saw my working group—the Epidemiology Research Unit of the Fred Hutchinson Cancer Research Center—as a good bet.

The office was convenient for me. My husband and I, striving to meet all of

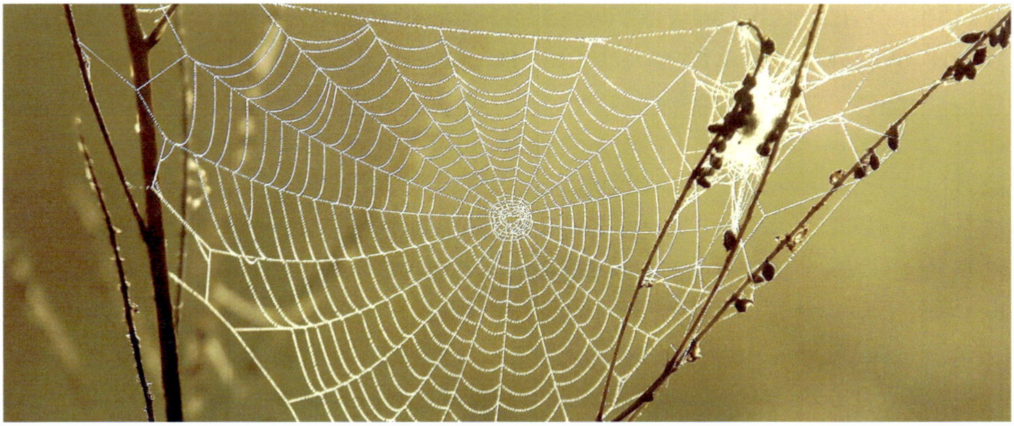

the expectations that weighed on our generation, were attempting to sustain two careers, two small children, a large damp house, and a long commute; I was commuting from a nearby island where the cost of living was lower. I had often been reminded that I had 'taken' a medical school position from a man, and was determined to pull my weight. In that context, my job, which allowed me to telecommute and work flexible hours, seemed like a good one for a wife and mother. The relative ease of the commute felt like a bonus.

Even so, things weren't going well for me. I was having trouble keeping up. I blamed it on being a member of the so-called sandwich generation and on my tendency to take risks. I had chosen an area of research that was unusual, that required travel and an entrepreneurial spirit, and that was based in part at a state registry from which the funding was soon yanked. I could have bowed out gracefully when the funding went, but it was against my lifetime habits of hard work, faith in prevention as the best route to cure, and stubborn conscientiousness. I refused to take no for an answer. I kept at it.

I started to fail. I had one health problem after the next—and I wasn't alone. The female peers whom I consulted about my problems were on antidepressants, and thought that I might need them too. Many of the people who worked in my office suite suspected the building of poisoning them, and refused to come to work on days when the smell of carpet glue filled the indoor air. Some avoided the building and whispered that it was sick. Others developed illnesses—a large number for a small unit. There was early onset breast cancer, multiple sclerosis, fibromyalgia, rare synovial cancer, and so on and so on.

One day, I cornered a colleague. She was unique in that her face turned red like an indicator light whenever she entered the building. She seemed ashamed of it and didn't like to talk about it. Both of us knew that the accepted view in our field of research, the one that we had to take in order to be funded, was that the ailments cropping up around us were distinct anatomically and therefore unlike in cause and consequence. But we also knew from prospective studies of drinking and smoking that one exposure might relate to many outcomes, and one outcome to many exposures. We knew that biology was complicated and that we should view cause and consequence as forming an ecological web. We also knew that even the best of our present methods of study suited few real-life problems.

Having figuratively grabbed her collar and kept her from bolting, I observed that her response to the building and the illnesses around us revealed a problem that we should take as a gold opportunity for furthering medical knowledge about health and disease. She replied sotto voce and with a rueful laugh that we couldn't do that with our methods. We would lose our funding. We would undermine our own salaries. Then, as now, I was the only person I knew who had studied a real problem after it appeared in news headlines—a cluster of birth defects in Colorado. I had learned by doing just how impotent our methods were. We had too fanciful a faith in the magic of statistics and the forms of estimation that policy makers and legislators accepted as the lingua franca of population research. We assessed exposures crudely, defined outcomes arbitrarily, and constructed causal models simplistically. The 'happy' few with the courage to point this out soon chose income over integrity. She and I, standing in the impressive lobby of our sick building, saw no choice but to place our faith in the system and to wait for it to work.

I resolved to form a viable strategy by which to get funded to do the right thing, but was unable to follow through. My health failed. I developed a brain fog that seemed to short-circuit the computer in my brain, which had been absorbing and processing the raw data and multifactorial models that we relied on to simulate comprehension. On my last day of employment, I sat all day at my home computer and in all that time was unable to write a single line of code. I accepted defeat. I gave up my career.

I spent the next few months in bed and in constant pain. I discovered that there were states worse than death, and resolved to end my life if the symptoms didn't ease. I already knew that no doctor could help me, and soon confirmed that they would treat me as a head case, refuse to see me, or advise that I accept my fate. And so I dove into the wild and woolly world of alternative medicine. I found help, first from doctors of Oriental medicine, counselors, bodyworkers, and clergy, and much later from rare maverick colleagues who acknowledged realities that our peers were eager to deny.

During that time, I was almost overwhelmed by unprocessed memories and consequently found my way into the world of spirituality and religion. My time in the figurative wilderness was a long one, unexpectedly and paradoxically filled with adventures both great and small as well as with broad experiential learning. Eventually I became well enough to see that the system was programmed to fail and that it would be up to me to construct my own care and cure. This was not a popular choice with my new, likewise-sick friends who themselves placed all of their faith in their personal physicians, nor with social media monitors who deleted posts on cure for fear of charlatanry.

Finally, I found my way to Dr. Fernando Vega, who prescribed an elimination diet that worked for me. My baseline health improved so much that I could begin to experiment on myself, to investigate and discover the causes of my own disease. This required me to accept the particular as a source of the general and to rely on multiple observations on one case rather than a few observations on many. There was only one study method available to me, but it was a time-honored one—an N-of-1 study based on trial and error.

I was fortunate in being able to rely on my formal education: firstly, on my liberal education at the University of Chicago, which engaged students with primary sources and allowed faculty like Joachim Weintraub a safe haven and academic freedom; on my clinical education, especially the skills of pre-tomogram neurologists like Dr. Louis Kaplan and the anecdotes of emeritus professors like Dr. Buchanan who sustained the storytelling traditions of nineteenth-century Scottish medicine; and on the course from the Centers for Disease Control for Epidemic Intelligence Service officers offered to a small group of medical students by Dr. Pierce Gardner.

By synthesizing these valuable resources, I was able to discern and confirm that I was suffering from chronic poisoning related to conventional foods—poisoning complicated by many other causes and consequences. This finding enabled me to limit the continuing damage caused by neurotoxic poisons and the immune responses caused by adjuvants, and to be free of pain and suffering most of the time. I later learned to avoid inhaled toxic chemicals mixed with pollens (Seattle outdoor air) as well as non-ionizing radiation. (For more, see *Medical Detective: Chronic Ambient Poisoning.*) It took me another decade to formulate Alderman Syndrome and a cure of the species: habitat restoration and integration to avert the sixth extinction.

So what? So, like everyone who reaches the crossroads that leads to the wisdom years, I had to—in the words of theologians—die before I died. I had to let go of the group mind of my peers, and of all of my expectations, and then to see afresh what was right in front of me. And then I had to engage the unknown by holding questions open in the face of every obstacle and by taking urgent necessity as the source of new meaning and purpose. I could not have found my problems or solved them in the 'safe' places where I—and all my colleagues—had been was looking. So what? So, now I have the chance to do my part to protect my children and the future of life. Now I can experience and express the full spectrum of life—from its harrowing lows to its joyous highs—and I invite you to do the same.

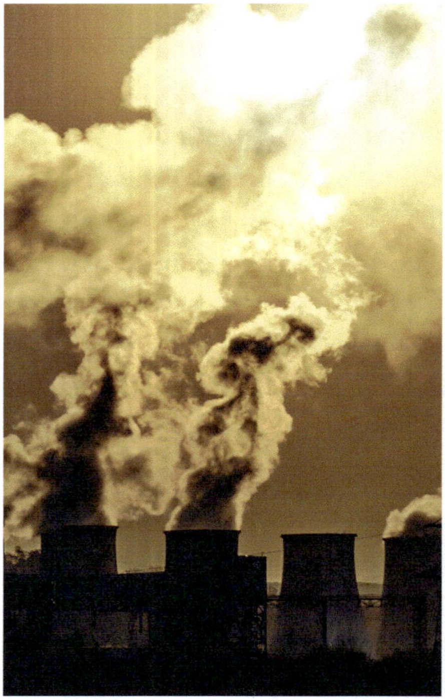

Comment on Taking a Breather

A majority of our late modern patients experience overweight and obesity. After doctors advise them to lose weight, and they put in what they imagine to be a good-faith effort, they express genuine surprise when they learn that they have not lost weight—or have even gained it. They may say they have changed their diet, but do not try to regulate portion size or calorie counts, nor to check their weight on a home scale. They do not judge their efforts against their experience—and may be eating cheap, poison-laden foods that make it excruciatingly difficult to lose weight.

We, too, may believe that we are making changes and yet become dimly aware of engaging in wishful or ineffective thinking. We may imagine that we can effect change by believing in it rather than by paying careful attention to what we are doing and whether it is enabling us to reach our goal. For example, academic physicians who must produce curricula or publications in order to keep their positions often find that they cannot make the time to actually do so. One reason is that academic positions provide no time for thought. Likewise, many non-academic physicians who must or who wish to pause long enough to think, to effect a change, or to refresh themselves feel helpless to do so. They may be afraid to sample alternative career paths or to re-evaluate the direction of their career. Or, they may become aware of locum positions or a possibility for extended leave, but become too fatalistic or passive to take the chance.

Changing the outcome of the medical life therefore requires changing the processes that lead to it. We can help this fundamental change along by keeping in mind the definition of insanity that some attribute to Confucius, Franklin, or Einstein and that Rita Mae Brown wrote in *Sudden Death*: insanity is doing the same thing over and over and expecting different results. People use the same language in reference to stupidity, and could use it in reference to the helplessness engendered by the complex systems that so many doctors and patients know all too well, which limit authority and diffuse responsibility.

We humans cope with complexity by developing habits that resist change. This includes the constellation of conditioned responses that we call 'ego.' If you let your habits remain as they are, you cannot take hold of your ways of life and change them for the better. You cannot become the author of your own life. If you wish to contribute to rescuing the future of life, you therefore need to observe this phenomenon and to spend patience and wiles examining it and devising ways to change. As a physician, you provide ideas, reassurance, and encouragement to patients who attempt such changes. By exploring these yourself, and by improvising and mastering the art of change, you can succeed in transitioning to elderhood and model a new and essential way of practicing your profession.

To begin, immerse yourself in the emerging views and constructs in this book. Play with them as you choose and adopt new ways of thinking. Note that this year, you have the chance to celebrate the past, to bring forward what promotes life, to leave behind what doesn't, and to try self-patterning for elderhood. This begins with becoming aware of your body, observing your inner Dr. Jekyll and Mr. Hyde—that is, your professional expert self and all that you have disregarded or disowned—and deciding what you need to be and become in order to accomplish what you choose to do. The formulation of this process used here is intended to return you to the historical template for maturing gracefully as a doctor, and to bring that template up to date by expressing it as an open-frame multipurpose algorithm that you can use to enhance your individual personhood—including owning your role in society as a medical elder.

Before you go on, prepare yourself by studying the following constructs that support the transition of your comprehension.

Nested Bodies

In this biocentric view of your body, it is easy to see the living context of which you are a unique and essential part. You may also be able to appreciate that you are—literally—nothing without it. When the body of life that comprises all living entities in the oceans of air and water is harmed by modernism, so are you. When pollinators and other lynchpin species are poisoned, so are you. When life on earth is threatened—as reflected in the loss of 60% of vertebrate species since the 1970s—so are you. Therefore, it is best to care for yourself biocentrically—that is, for your body as integral to the bodies in which it nests.

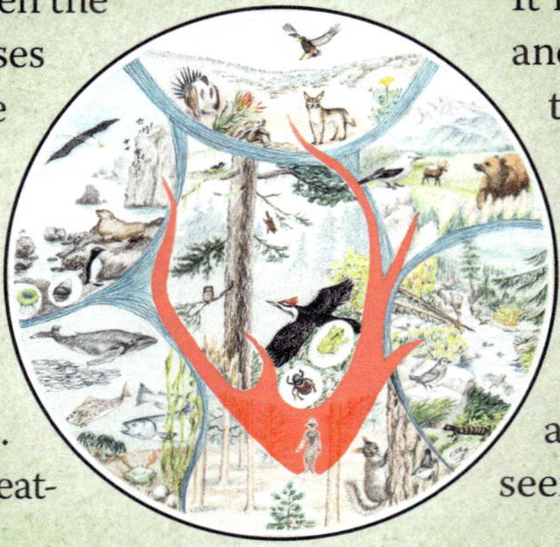

This illustration represents your body and the aggregated bodies that give you life.

While it may seem that your body is contained by your skin, and that you can, as it were, see its boundary, this is a modern misperception that clergy and doctors have never reconciled. The sevenfold model of the body, which is inclusive of the material and non-material, shows that your interbeing interfaces with shared interbeing; your awareness, understanding, and perceptions range far and wide in life, place, and time; and your sensations and energy interface with life in place and time. Only your flesh is bounded by your skin, and that is continually exchanging matter and energies with your milieu.

It is therefore key in care and cure to think biocentrically and to remain aware of your living context as aggregated bodies of which you form an integral part. The construct of the aggregated body may seem strange at first, but when you stop to consider it you will be able to recall or recognize many historical uses of this idea. Examples include the body politic, the body of Christ, the body of the guru in large form (Hindu), and the body corporate.

All humans and aggregated living bodies care for you directly or indirectly as members of habitats and/or the biome. You in turn are there to care for them, including those from whom you must protect your body because they pose an immediate threat, such as pathogens and predators. This may require ingenuity as they may also be essential to you through the larger bodies that give you life.

Individual

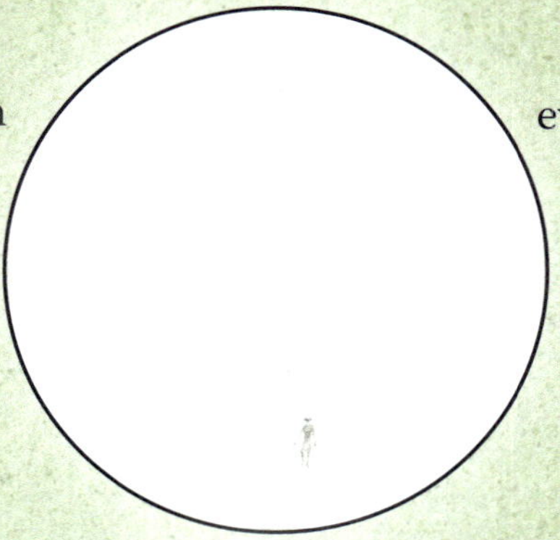

As you begin to own the ideal of nested bodies, in your mind's eye replace the individual in this drawing with an image of your own body.

Species

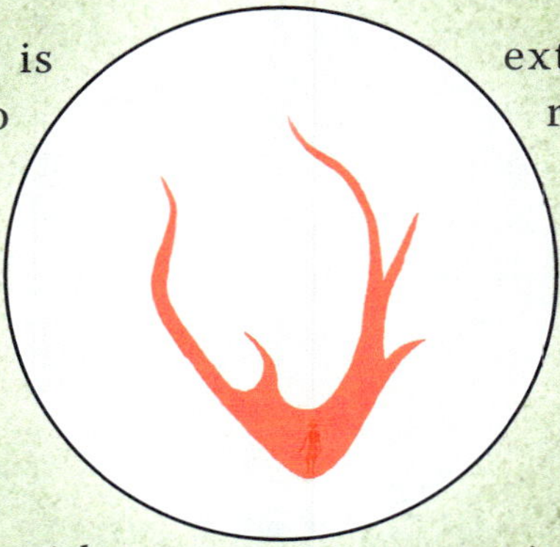

Here your species is shown entering into habitats. While the habitat in which you were born may be extinct, many habitat reservoirs exist from which the body of life could be restored enough to survive and to thrive.

Habitat

Habitats interface with weather, watercourses, soils, and other aspects of the physical environment. They also combine to create life on earth, herein referred to as the body of life. The International Union for Conservation of Nature and Natural Resources recognizes thirteen major categories of wild habitats: forest, savanna, shrubland, grassland, wetlands (inland), rocky areas, caves and subterranean (non-aquatic), desert, marine neritic, marine oceanic, marine deep ocean floor, marine intertidal, and marine coast/supratidal. Within each major category are many minor ones that contain each unique instance of the habitat. Many such are disappearing rapidly, leaving less and less biomass and fewer and fewer sources of oxygen. Before Thoreau and Darwin, when the Anthropocene—the human-created era—began, moderns took habitats as sources of free or raw materials that could be owned and consumed. John Muir, George Bird Grinnell, Teddy Roosevelt, and others made efforts to turn the tide of habitat destruction, and emergence can support your care and cure by effecting the transformation from destruction to restoration.

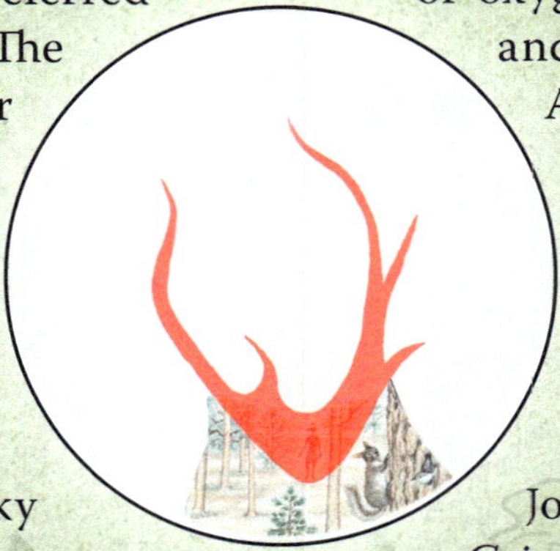

Bioregion

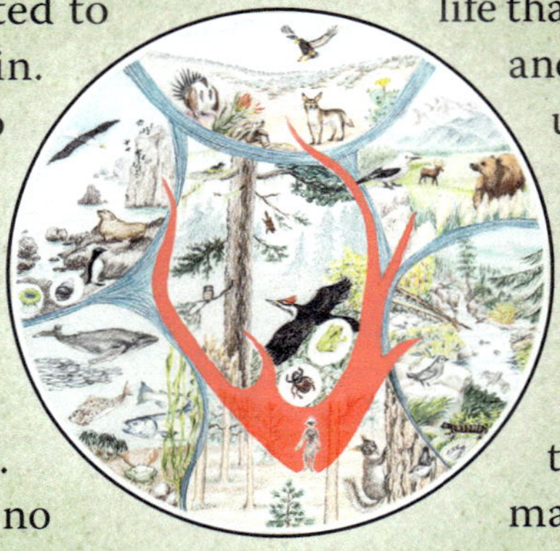

During your infancy, your immune system adapted to your habitat(s) of origin. Later adaptations to habitat may be less satisfactory—perhaps more so if you have moved out of your bioregion *and* into a more allergenic habitat. Though there is as yet no consensus as to how to define bioregions, if you have the chance, identify your bioregion and its watersheds, and any areas of abundant life that may, spa-like, ease pain and suffering. The example used here is the region of Cascadia, where many remnants of healthy wild habitats have been preserved. Cascadia is home to patches of temperate rainforest that manifest the abundant life that was once plentiful in the New World and that is still taken for granted.

Biome

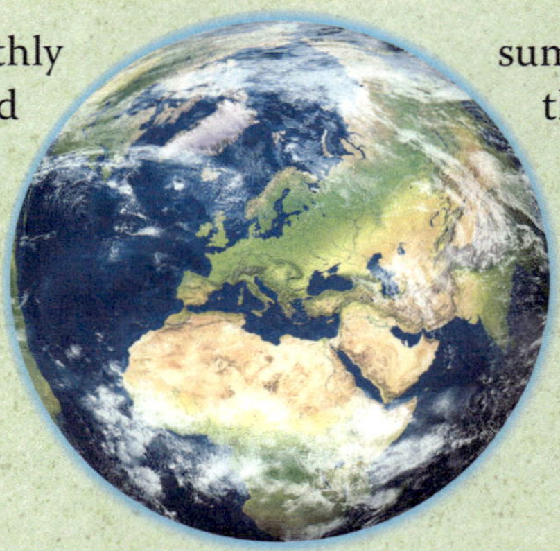

The sum of all earthly life past, present, and future, and thus the sum of a set of bioregions that is mutually exclusive, comprehensive, and dynamic.

The Sevenfold Body

FLESH WITH ITS BEING

The body is represented by an image that evokes the sacred as an angel and that appropriates modern stained glass images of angels as well as late modern images of the body that depict its intangible aspects. The image is comprised of seven layers that will be considered individually below.

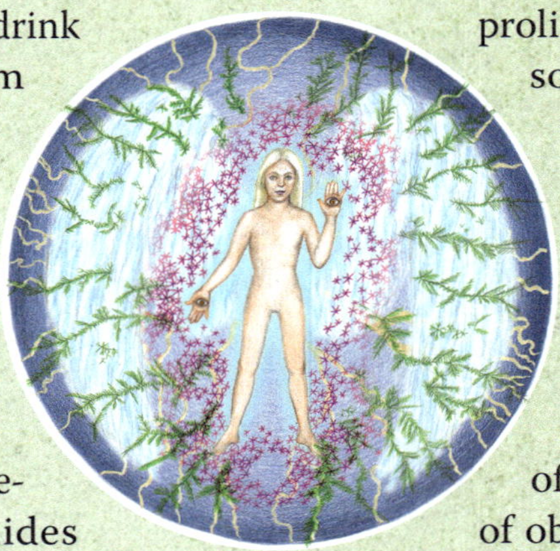

In ancient times, humans thought of the body as composed of four to five elements such as earth, air, fire, water, and metal. This view is useful today when the thirsty drink and the chilled warm themselves. Over two and a half millennia ago, Hippocrates, a Greek physician, noticed that the body contained its own fluids, which he called humors. In medieval times, Maimonides considered the activities of organ systems to be the vegetative soul, which embodied ethics. A syncretic thinker, he combined medicine with ideas and practices from around the globe. In the Renaissance, European physicians broke the centuries-old prohibition against autopsy, and began once again to study the flesh and its diseases objectively. During the Scottish Enlightenment, doctors who were too far from Rome to be suppressed by the papacy decided to try and cure disease and save lives. Their discoveries of anesthesia, antisepsis, and other breakthroughs gave birth to late modern interventionist medicine that was centralized after World War II. It has since proliferated interventions, some highly advanced technologically.

In the heady days after the discovery of penicillin, the development of polio vaccines, and the eradication of smallpox, the power of objectivity eclipsed the subjective felt experience and the ideas and methods of self-care by which the sick could help themselves. These began in the Himalayas in the time of the Buddha, who viewed the body as comprised of five heaps (*skandhas*): form, feeling, perceptions, impulses, and consciousness. Later, during the classical period of Indian civilization, the energy body was discovered, mapped in great detail, and used to catalyze inner meditative work. While these methods are the most detailed and require mastery by the patient, every living religious and spiritual tradition has kept practices of self-care and personal healing transformation. You may have practiced some already.

The emerging method of self-care presented by Evolve Medicine uses ideas and practices from around the globe to support self-care as well as the development of skills that support care-seeking all types of practitioners. Key abilities that you can choose to master include:

- enhancing well-being by entering into care states and by shifting your baseline state toward care
- owning your own placebo for relief of pain
- strengthening your energy body to bypass fleshly obstacles
- countering the toxicity and negative placebos of mainstream care (and modern life)
- countering social isolation through grounding in life and time
- release of deep tension and energy wastage by embodied trauma and past distress

This is facilitated by a seven-fold model of the body that allows you to care for up to seven aspects of the body at one time. Two of these, flesh and interbeing, are comprised of matter—at least in part. The other five represent aspects of being generated by those two.

Flesh

This depiction of the flesh, being angelic, is pre-gendered. It represents the generative matter of an individual with its symbiotic microbiome. The flesh is viewed on the human scale and above. For the purposes of medical care, in this method, it can be analyzed down to the level of organ systems.

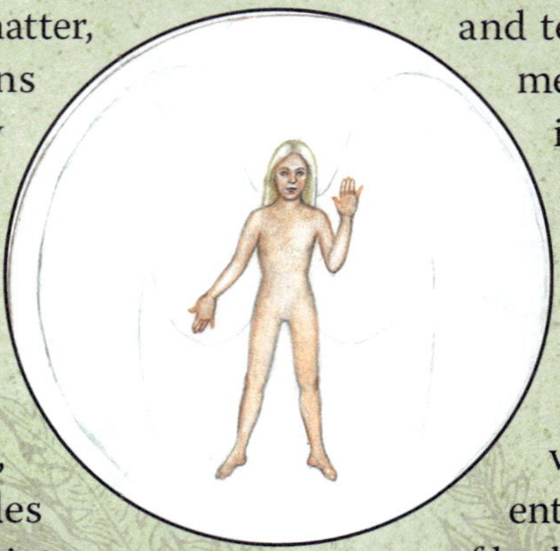

The flesh aspect of the seven-fold body includes all matter, structures, and actions comprehended by modern medicine. That is, in addition to the matter that is subject to histological and anatomical analysis by biopsy, surgery, and autopsy, it includes physiology, biochemistry, and cellular and molecular actions subject to physical examination and technological measurements. It does not include intangible derivatives of the body, which can be regarded from a spiritual or subjective standpoint as being, or from a quantitative viewpoint as like differential or integral measures of bodily actions.

Chronic illness due to ongoing exposure to poisons of the flesh or to irreversible alterations in the flesh has material consequences that are not amenable to spiritual treatments. For this reason, medical assessment is a must so that harmful exposures can be pinpointed and reversed, and organ functions recovered. In other words, material problems call for material solutions if and when such exist.

Energy

The energy body is depicted as the late modern aura. This depiction fits infrared and other energies well in that they decay rapidly—that is, they diminish with $1/r^2$*, with r being the distance from the body. In this method, energy is not identical to fitness or vitality, which belong to the flesh. It is the resultant electromagnetic field produced by the entirety of the body, with the conductive tissues predominating.*

Each tissue of the human body generates electrical currents and electromagnetism that reflects its actions. The sum total of this, called the subtle body, is the construct of all of these. The trained mind may perceive the intangible structure of the subtle body as centers and channels. While the central channel in front of the spine parallels the spinal cord and autonomic trunks, and the centers arise near ganglia, the subtle body has no single anatomic correlate. It can, however, influence the function of the anatomical structures with electromagnetic activity.

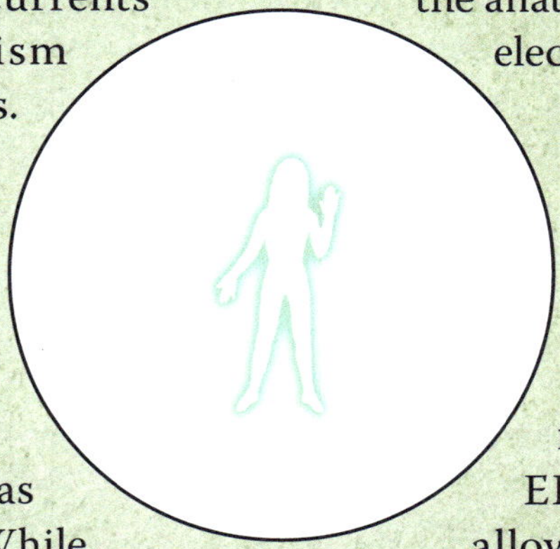

While the aura remains elusive to objective forms of measurement, some aspects of the subtle body produce strong fields (e.g. the EKG, EEG, and EMG) that allow diagnosis of cardiac and neuromuscular diseases. For the patient who is able to subjectively detect and skillfully harness the energy body, it is a powerful aid in enhancing relief and wellbeing.

Sensations

Sensations and sensory skills are represented by the ancient symbols called hamsas that depict the sensitivity of the palms of the hands.

From shortly after your moment of conception and continuously until your death, your sensory systems are collecting data on your body and its surroundings in the way that your body has been evolving since life on earth began. The material mediator of these data comprises the neural pathways that you formed in response to your experience. These pathways change as your experience—and your interpretation of it—changes. In other words, your sensory systems—like your energy—interface with all other aspects of body and being. These mediate your living ability to create your subjective existence.

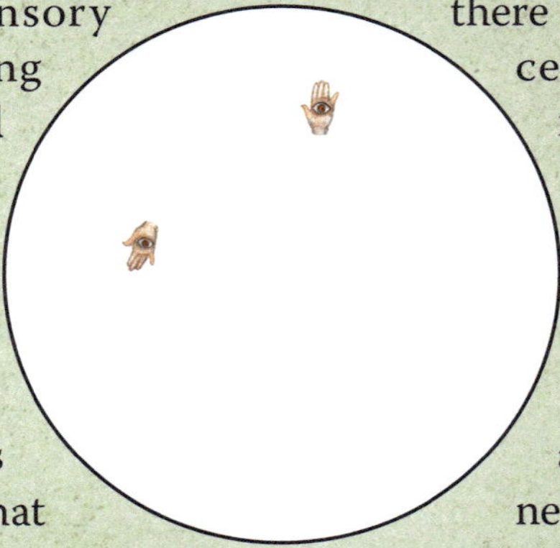

In addition to the five senses (hearing, sight, taste, touch, and smell) there are others like proprioception (position), the inner ear (acceleration), and pain. Pleasure—like the appreciation of music, art, cuisine, and happiness—is a skill. Like energy, sensations are closely related to the nervous system.

Clergy continue to constuct historically recognized means of constructing sensations that you can share with others as part of care, such as the eyes of the palms, that is hamsas, depicted here as well as the eye of the heart, that is the *horus*, that was important to Jews in the time of Jesus as per the *Gospel of Mary.*

Perceptions

Perceptions are represented by an image of what some cognitive psychologists have called the perceptual filter. This filter screens out data that you have the habit of ignoring to free your flesh and being for other tasks. It is a living barrier that may be like an intense, orotective forcefield which, when opened slowly and with deliberation, can admit a far greater range of experience (such as that which Dr. Carl Jung called the shadow).

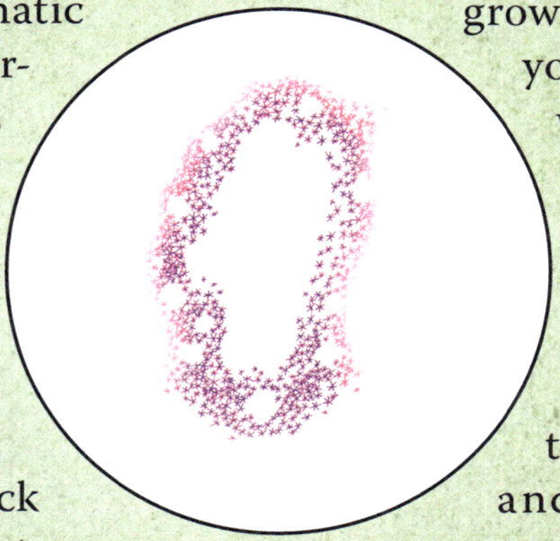

Perceptions form your detector of cues for the responses of daily life. These are automatic and preserve your understanding and awareness to which you choose to devote your attention and reason. They filter out stimuli that you have at one time disliked or disregarded, and that you now block out or ignore. Those that you let in cue routine responses that you at one time found useful and accepted as a pattern—that is, a habit or conditioned response. In other words, perceptions are your preset expectations and reactions, and are apt to become fixed and dated.

When perceptions cause trouble, you may become angry with your context or circumstances. Then you can become aware of them, own them, and repattern them. This may require that you see things that you would rather not and learn from experience or education how to grow and adapt to manage your life as it is in the world as it changes.

Perceptions comprise the least familiar aspect of the body. One reason for this is that moderns tend to ignore context, and your perceptions respond to your dynamic context. Repatterning them is critical in care and cure, when many of your expectations and reactions and habits may become dysfunctional all at once. Perceptions may then be both invisible and troublesome. One reason for this is that you are a social being whose basic patterns were set long ago in the womb and in childhood, and are now covered over by subsequent perceptions that may take time and ingenuity to penetrate.

Understanding

Understanding, inclusive of apprehension (recognition), comprehension, and reasoning, is here represented by ice crystals that are accreting on an abstract plane. Like Platonic solids, these are idealized visions of our imaginings that are useful insofar as they pattern successful problem-solving.

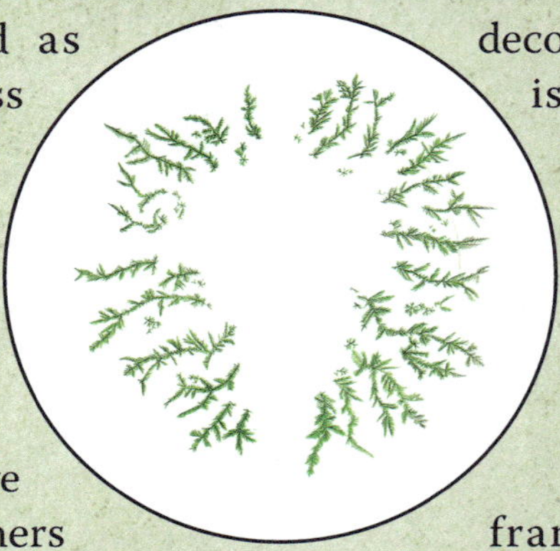

Understanding is a human creation that has been handed down and modified as needed over countless generations since before recorded history. Your embodied understanding may include new views, frames, and constructs, but it is more likely that you have rediscovered what others have discovered and rediscovered before you, or that you learned from others through interaction or education. This is especially true of human inventions such as language and perennial tools such as hearthfires and bowls.

From archaeology, we learn that tangible goods found in burials may be easy to recognize and understand, but the intangible meaning may be simple to speculate on yet remain forever impossible to recover. Within recorded history, the basis of human understanding has come apart of its own weight at the end of every era. This time it is our taking for granted the life on which all life depends—i.e. the biome—that is accelerating deconstruction of modernism and emergence of the new. As with the bubonic plagues that heralded modernity, it is chronic ambient poisoning that is heralding emergence.

Emerging views, frames, and constructs that structure our largely three-dimensional thinking aim to have traction on the human scale and above, for the continuation of the evolved living context, with integration of all existing human wisdom, in biological time, free of human exceptionalism and other errors destructive to the body of life. The fundamental view is biocentrism, that is, valuing and protecting and restoring the body of life by resacralizing it in a panentheistic manner and recognizing it as having greater value than anything created by the human species.

Awareness

Awareness is here represented by an image of wings that reminds us of the human fascination with flight, from Icarus to angels to Da Vinci and air and space flight. These wings allow your body to encounter the unknown mysteries of ailments and to make sense of them.

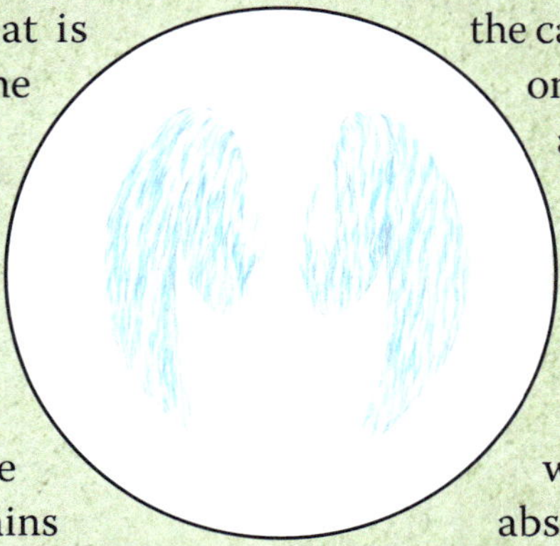

Awareness is the aspect of the sevenfold body that is capable of flight from the beginning of time to the distant future, and from the depths of the ocean and the core of the planet to the stars in the firmament. Awareness is expansive and boundless, and contains your greatest gifts: the ability to pay attention to a chosen object and the capability of concentrating on it. A relaxed, spacious, and unobstructed awareness supports you in bringing all aspects of the body to bear on your self-care. Without awareness, we live in a world of matter without abstractions necessary for grasping the illness experience or discovering actionable causes.

Interbeing

Interbeing is represented here as roots that ground you in life and place and time. It orients you and gives your life as your umbilical cord gave you life when you were in your mother's womb.

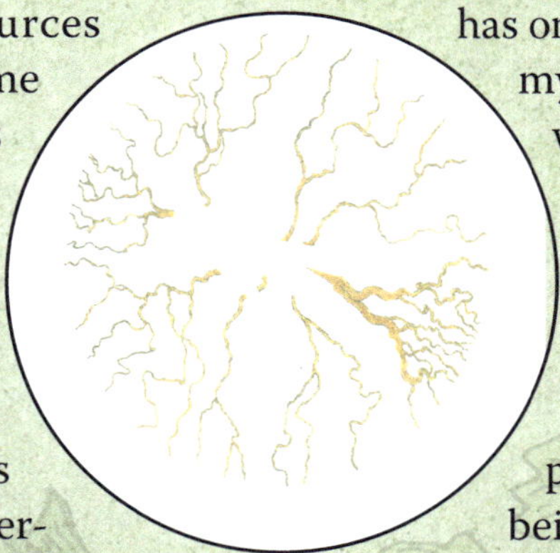

Your sevenfold body is continually exchanging resources with your milieu. Some of these are tangible, as when you breathe in oxygen or drink water produced or purified by your habitat. Others are intangible, as when the sun's rays or a friend's smile warms you. Interbeing is a new word coined by Thich Nhat Hanh to acknowledge that we are all one. In this method of self-care, we mean this biologically (ecologically) as well as spiritually. The fact that the language for human unity has only been preserved by the mystical traditions of the world reflects the degree to which moderns ignore cooperation and overdo competition. The process of self-care that becomes more available through paying attention to interbeing can thus serve as a particularly precious blessing. Even in loneliness and isolation, you are never alone or abandoned by society; it is not in anyone's power to divide aspects of life that evolved as one.

CONSTRUCT 3

Self-Patterning

Historically, doctors matured through emulation of mentors on several time scales. From the time of the first sacred clinical encounter to the last, doctors progressed from doing a methodological and complete history and physical, search for information, and assessment and plan to relying more and more on automatic recognition and response. With experience, they developed respect for the unknown and unforeseeable, all with a religious construct that supported reconciliation with any errors and shortcomings. With a reading of medical history, all of this experience would be turned to wisdom of use to juniors. The learning curve during training was very steep; that during the junior role in a practice was less steep; and that of a lifetime in medicine might be limited to scholar mentors. Now, with institutionalization and automation of care, the horizon of expert judgment may extend no farther than following given algorithms. It may be arrested by complex systems that learn nothing from your experience.

How do you mature as a doctor now, when managers may not allow you to take time for thought for fear of inefficiency? How do you know your mind and accomplish what you recognize to be the most important thing to leave behind when you die? That is up to you. Keep these larger questions in the back of your mind as you bring forth the fertility of old age for forming new habits of being, becoming, and doing. On the pages that follow, you will find a pattern for doing—including becoming—that will provide a pedagogic paradigm and a place for you to start.

Embodiable Process for Action

Here is an embodiable process that may become a useful tool as you move forward. I took it from the process I used to create a new and better life rich in care and cure. I hope that it may serve you and inspire you to create habits that serve your future.

Let's take a closer look at that:

PRIMING ▸	STANCE ▸	STATE ▸	STRATEGY ▸	SKILLS ▸	VISION ▸
(push)	(direction)	(care or cure)	(you are already rich in these and can add more)		(pull)

Priming & Vision

Priming is the point A where you are now, and vision is the point B that you would like to reach. Both are alive in you and therefore change with you as you gain experience, inspiration, and responsiveness to your ever-changing living context. Both are sources of motivation: priming is the passion for change that your life has instilled through your sense of wrong, and vision is the possible world that you conceive of that would right what you see as wrong. Put differently, priming is the potential energy that drives you toward what draws you.

Stance

Your stance is the primal direction that you set to align your personal resources with your process of moving from point A to point B. It joins your past with your contextualized future, and allows each step of the journey to hone your direction and vision. Passionate or coolly understated, it suits your abilities and resources as you become fully human and fully engaged in mentoring those who will live on after you.

State

The lynchpin of the process leading from where you are now to where you will end up is the state of being in which you abide. In medicine, two are key: care and cure. You already know these and need only become aware of them. The care state—the optimal baseline state for moving toward abundant life—is kind, equanimous, and shares something of the joys and sorrows of your patients and mentees. It is altruistic and protective while remaining relaxed and responsive. The cure state is determined, focused, and potentially aggressive, like the state of an investigative researcher or detective. Care is a state of doing; cure is a state of undoing, and so turns back time. (For a detailed treatment, see the online care and cure courses at www.EvolveMedicine.us.)

Strategies

Because late modern strategies are overwhelmingly influenced by industrial and algorithmic thinking, you may use strategies constantly and yet be very rusty with respect to forming one that has rational biomedical utility. Begin by becoming aware of the strategies that you are using now and of what they do and don't accomplish with respect to the future of evolved life. Be prepared for how destructive they may be and how difficult it is to think strategically. Be on the lookout for better strategies that you can adopt. These may inspire your curiosity and invention.

Skills

You have a wealth of skills already. Unfortunately, most may have to do with bureaucracy and data processing, and may be crowding out your clinical skills—which, as we all know, do not stand up in court. If you have practiced outside the country, you may have had the chance to come up to speed and to think about the values of what Dr. Philip Tumulty called the laying on of hands, and about the wastage of resources on the electronic record. In any event, you may discover that it is useful to develop skills for rescuing living systems, and that disengaging from dead ones makes for a good start.

On the following pages, you will find a description of this text's use of playwork for becoming care and cure.

Playwork for Becoming

Because the vitality of your becoming depends on your state of being, which depends on your posture, it is essential for you to observe and care for your body continuously as you would a kindling fire, so that it does not die out nor erupt into a blaze that destroys what it should protect.

If you have experience with inner work, some types of playwork may come easily while others may be entirely new. If you have no such experience, you will have the chance to be like a child again, and to learn something as basic and beneficial as movement. Be patient with the process and allow it to reveal the delight of developing new abilities that support your creation of a living future.

Expect to fully engage the whole book three times or more. The first time, form the habit of reading and doing some part of the playwork every day. Right after you get up or right before you go to sleep—or both—are generally best. The exrcise pattern ways of becoming that may take time to revive or to develop; the working questions prompt insight and perspective in daily life and depend on circumstances.

The second time you engage the book, dwell on those practices that actively enhance your present degree of self-care. The third time through, choose whatever practice may do the most for you on any given day. As you progress, allow your vision of a new and better life to develop along with your ability to read your body and to move your state of being toward deepening care and more perspicacious cure of one as all.

An alternative to using this book several times is to use it once, then take take all of the online courses at www.EvolveMedicine.us, and then return to any or all materials at will.

Note that the inner exercises are designed to catalyze the dissolution of obstacles to care as part of patterning it. Depending on your past and your state of being in the moment inner exercises may yield results easily, noticeably, and immediately, or none of the above. Occasionally, a practice may trigger unexpected emotions. Be ready to consult a counselor or bodyworker for support. And, of course, be prepared to consult a doctor other than yourself if you have new symptoms, or if any existing symptoms change.

If you are unable to use the following playwork or working questions to your advantage, pause to take all of the other online courses prior to joining DLI and resuming contemplation of your medical legacy. Note that self-care is most thoroughly addressed in the hardcopy of *The Chronic Illness Owner's Manual*.

Obversely, as your well-being increases over time, feel free to allow it to spill over into the life that surrounds you. Most of the playwork is drawn from ancient and enduring practices set in an emerging—that is, post-post-modern—framework. Specific instructions follow with each section.

A NOTE ON THE WORKING QUESTIONS

The method of the working question is adapted from the work of G. I. Gurdjieff, who trained in part as a doctor and a priest, and then became a self-styled guru. The method is intended to interrupt the inner "automatic pilot" that individuals form early in life and tend to see as inevitable. This interruption allows you to observe daily life in ways that increase insight and perspective, and thereby pattern objective self-assessment of behavior. This may be difficult at first as doctors are presently discouraged from exercising any form of self-determination. When you do 'get the hang of it,' go slowly enough to allow your experience to reveal itself. Do not shy away from painful experiences or skip over joyful ones. Hurry is counterproductive.

Working questions begin as objects of contemplation and become tools for observation in daily life that allow the experiences of your flesh to surface and inform your transition to a wisdom role such as medical historian, philosopher, or mentor. As with all resources in the books and courses, you will get as much out of the questions and exercises as you put into them. With their aid, you can learn to apply your accumulated experience to the completion of your lifework and the creation of your living legacy.

Your lifework is the medical career that you built after training, and your living legacy is your contribution to a thriving future for your profession and species—with its essential living context. A key aspect of your completion and legacy is embodiment of inspiration, joy, and loving care that add to your pleasure and fulfillment, and that you share with peers and juniors as you go.

These steps may prove useful:

- Choose a question to work with that catches your eye, or that you feel resonates in your flesh.
- As you fall asleep at night, keep the question in your mind briefly and then let it go.
- In the morning, take five minutes or more to sit or stand quietly with an anatomically neutral posture and contemplate the question. Perhaps your understanding of the question will change; perhaps not.
- Read the question aloud. Allow your body to respond to it. Reword it and rewrite it until it 'unlocks' your response.

- Hold the question in the back of your mind as you go through your day. Pause to observe and question your habitual reactions. Put your automatic responses on hold so that you have a chance to think before you act.
- Allow it to come to the fore when prompted by events.

When the working question has allowed you to see something about your behavior, go on to another or make up your own until—over the months—you have created a repertory of questions that have tractiol at present, and that you can update as needed to update your changing patterns.

As a question becomes useful, write what you have learned in your journal so that you can refer to it as you become more aware of the choices that are available to you. Over the course of the next year, use any 'juicy' working questions to instill a process by which you discover, act on, and make note of your evolving self-knowledge in a way that brings you alive and reveals your unique life purpose, and so informs your capstone and legacy.

If the working questions prove to be good tools for you, extend this natural process of investigation and discovery by expanding the journaling or the contemplation by which you gradually come to comprehend and communicate the discoveries that you make in your 'aha' moments. Record your experiences and the problems and solutions that they reveal, and those that delve deeper and deeper into the mystery of being.

You can then look back on the record every month, every season, or at the end of the year and so expand the scope of your awareness, see more deeply into habits both old and new, and contemplate and create the meaningful change that you desire. If you do not wish to record your experiences at present, you can return to these questions and to the question of journaling in the course of a second or third engagement with the new habits that you are patterning with the aid of this book.

Learning to Play with Eldering

Consider the questions below and choose the one that appeals most as your first working question for June. A promising question for you may be one that you can answer glibly but that, on reflection, you feel that you haven't answered well or at all. A question like that may be opportunity in the guise of an obstacle. Seize it.

You will know that the question has begun to work when you lose your fear of not knowing the answer, when you regain a childlike wonder about the answer, and when daily life prompts an 'aha' moment in which you apprehend something new. This something new is like a wedge or 'toe in the door' that enables you to engage in an incremental or fundamental expansion of mind.

WORKING QUESTIONS

Employed Physicians

- How can I make time for a breather every day?
- How can I make time every month to stop, look, and listen to my life experience?
- How can I make time at least once a season to think deeply about the past, present, and future of my life, including my medical life?
- How can I take a locum or sabbatical that will allow me to leave my habits behind for six months at least, and so create the opportunity to imagine a better life?

Self-determined Physicians

- What experiences refresh me with love, joy, and contentment, and how can I create the opportunity to enjoy more of such experiences?
- What prompts my zeal, and what lies behind it?
- What can I do all day long and enjoy it the whole time?
- To what living context would I wish to adapt? To restore? To integrate with?

Note: when things go well, give yourself a 'carrot' to replace the incentives that have drawn you away from your unique life purpose. In other words, take change of and choose your own rewards.

EXERCISE

- Thinking back on your past experiences for a few minutes, what are the top ten things that seem now to have defined the arc of your life story?
- Record the list of ten in your journal. Take this as the baseline spine of your personal narrative, and—without referring back to it—write another list at the end of each quarter.

(If you're using your tools well, each list will be different, and the final one will be truest to the genesis of your character, values, and deepest concerns.)

Essay

How can I best engage my profession in ensuring a living future for my grandchildren, my grand-nephews, my young friends and mentees and their descendants? If you like, write an introduction now and come back to add notes and make a project of it to organize your thoughts over the course of the month or the year. This is, for many of us, the most important question to hold as we contemplate the time that remains to us.

Field Trip

In what habitat do you spend most of your time? Obtain a map of the habitat and go out into it with a field guide in hand to get to know the other species that comprise it. If a guided nature tour is available, consider taking that. If habitat is being restored in your area, take a day to observe or join in the work.

Supplementary Reading

The following list is given in priority order with respect to the formation of this first version of the emerging paradigm. Feel free to choose those that speak to you, and to use any that you like in future months—as occasionally prompted by lists in other months.

1. Elizabeth Kolbert. *The Sixth Extinction: an Unnatural History.* New York: Henry Holt and Company, 2014.
2. Rachel Carson. *Silent Spring.* Boston: Houghton Mifflin Company, 1962.
3. Charles C. Mann. *1491: New Revelations of the Americas Before Columbus.* 2nd edition. New York: Vintage Books, 2011.

4. Charles C. Mann. *1493: Uncovering the New World Columbus Created.* 2nd edition. New York: Vintage Books, 2012.

5. Laura Dassow Walls. *Henry David Thoreau: a Life.* Chicago: The University of Chicago Press, 2017.

6. Charles Darwin. *The Autobiography of Charles Darwin.* Edited by Nora Barlow. London: Collins, 1958.

Encountering Deep Time

According to Dunne, [time] doesn't exist in itself, but is always relative to the person who has the idea of Time. [As] Maeterlinck [put it], standing in the Present, on the highest point of the curve, you can look back and see the Past, or forward and see the Future, all in the same instant. Or, if you stand off to one side...your eye wanders from one to the other without any distinction.

— M. Wylie Blanchet in *The Curve of Time*

Having seized control of the biosphere through desperate, short-sighted, and narrow self-interest, our species is devouring, destroying, and poisoning the body of life and all of the unique and essential lives that are integral to it. The task ahead for all humans, especially doctors and others versed in biomedicine and dedicated to caregiving and the save, is to now step up to care for and to cure it—or else lose it to the void of extinction. Doctors—along with clergy, field biologists, and others—still have the chance to put into perspective our late modern human ways of life, which doctors can frame as galloping consumption of the body of life. This long view makes it possible to create and model new ways of living that draw on your stout heart and that reverse the habits of neglect and abuse imperiling the future of life. With your support and leadership, your juniors and others in your bioregion can form new habits of care and cure that revive and restore life as well as ensure its future survival and thriving here on earth.

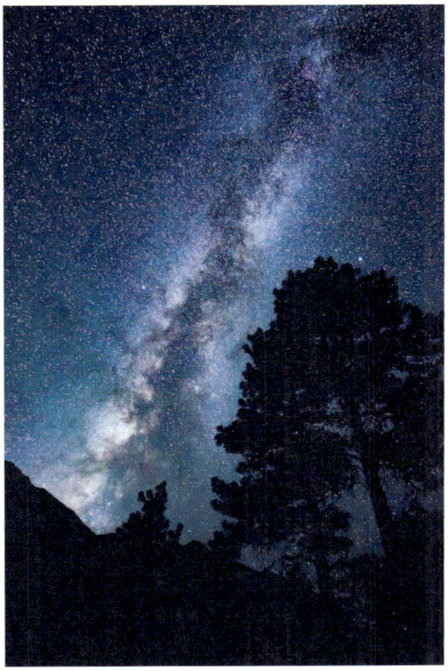

You cannot shepherd this transformation until you find your place in time. This requires you to extract the best of your embodied past and to use it as the raw material from which to craft a better future from your core, which you then share in the most strategic way possible. The work has, believe it or not, been done for you; others have gone first and shown the way. The Mayo Brothers' motto was said to be never be the first and never be the last, and

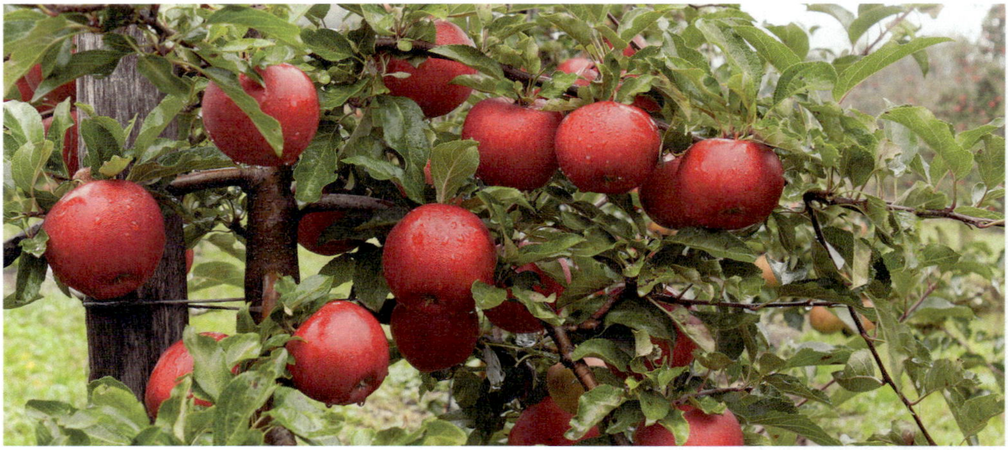

this motto can also serve you now. All you have to do is what doctors have always done at end of an era: align with the leading edge of a dynamic parent culture that is already in the midst of transformation and that is calling out a new way of life.

Organic farmers began what some now call local, living economies. Architects and designers are developing what they call the living building paradigm. These and other constructs are seeding the new paradigm now emerging in all fields. This new paradigm, which has been called post-post-modern, emerging, or living, is generating new views, frames, and constructs that doctors can interpret and adapt to serve care and cure. This book—with the corresponding courses offered by Evolve Medicine—offers a first emerging medical paradigm that builds on precepts from other fields, such as: contextualization, human scale, biomimicry, avoidance of red list chemicals and other sources of harm, appropriate technology, self-sufficiency, active rather than passive use of human tools and structures, and so on. This paradigm is inspired by the seven petal living building paradigm and references the work of Amos Tversky and Daniel Kahneman, Dr. David Sackett, Richard Levins and Richard Lewontin, Dr. William Foege, and many others. It crosses boundaries by integrating global medical traditions with evolutionary and field biology, theology, cognitive psychology, and medical history. As such, it hitches deep human and biological time to the here and now. Within this long view, you can repattern the timeline of your life as integral to those of your near and distant predecessors and descendants.

When you embody your relation to deep time, you can use the emerging perspective to harvest the fruits of your history with medicine and also your interpretation of those you discover in the recorded history of medicine. By pondering primary sources such as the writings of the transformative and integrative physicians of the past—Hippocrates, Galen, Avicenna, Maimonides, Vesalius, and the doctors of the Scottish Enlightenment—you can take the long view of the work of more recent medical thinkers such as Drs. Mervyn Susser, Oliver Sacks, and David Sackett. You can then interpret their ideas for today—as clergy might put it, to do an exigesis or drash—of postmodern medical thought. You can then take your place at the moving front of time, own a long view of medicine, and create a dynamic personal interpretation of the medicine of the species: public health. You will then be well-prepared to evaluate the role and betterment of newer tools of clinical science such as clinical epidemiology, long narrative case studies, and qualitative case series. You can also downplay data and information to create essential higher-level tools such as knowledge and wisdom.

The work of medical elders like you can free the profession from its late modern bonds, which will allow it to transform in sync with the parent society and to craft new ways of practicing that include medical detection and biologically context-sensitive care. These methods will prepare the field to become rapidly responsive, dynamic, sure-footed, and evolving, and so to respond to rising epidemics and disasters—whether natural or man-made.

In our profession, context extends inside the body—especially into its organ systems—as well as outside it. The living part of that outside context, we here conceive of poetically as the bodies of species, of habitats, and of all life on earth. These congregal bodies are like the body of Christ or the guru in large form, in that they aggregate many instances of life.

Is the stuff of transformation mind-blowing? Yes! Thank Heaven, yes. We are in desperate need of fundamental change, and others have already changed their minds and shown us how to change ours. We have every chance to make good on the science of ecology and use its methods to comprehend sequential processes and complex webs of cause and effect. We also have every chance to gather and harness ancient and modern views, frames, constructs, and narratives as we aggregate and synthesize a practical philosophy that will enable us to care for each and every life as one.

ANECDOTES FROM MEDICAL LIVES

I have a growing collection of sacred places. I find them wherever I go. Some are corners of parks, others are abandoned lots, and one is my wild garden at home. They are usually places where I can sit anonymously among old trees, grass, the earth. Sometimes I feel mournful, but then for a moment I feel free.

— Dr. James Orbinski in *An Imperfect Offering*

If you have come to terms with your own mortality, matured a religious or spiritual practice, or pushed yourself to extremes, chances are good that you have come up against deep time. For the purposes of this book, we define deep time in biological terms; for example, the lifetime of the individual, species, habitat, or life on earth. To meet with deep time in this period of respite, visualize yourself stepping outside of your routine. This will allow you to consider the time that remains to you in this life, the time that remains to your species, and the role of medicine in making both those periods as rich in experience and action as is feasible. Keep in mind as you do this that your state of ability and vitality may not continue as they are for as long as you would like, and that you will inevitably, at a time that you cannot predict or determine, leave behind this wondrous and incomprehensible gift of earthly life. We are, as Newton and others have said, standing on the shoulders of giants as we do this, and are thus continuing a venerable tradition of engaging deep time, seeing the big picture, and impacting all those lives that have, in the course of our lives, become entwined with our own.

Paul: the Example of AIDS

Paul was born into a blue-blood family with high ethics, high standards, high expectations, and a close connection to the Catholic Church. Free of motives such as gaining status or money, he had always been a little different, and chose to go into medicine in order to pursue a noble profession. Like many introduced to the Church in the 1950s, he was oppressed by it; he responded by eschewing inner structures that depended on the intangible, and by pursuing science and medicine both as a way of expressing his commitment to the material world as it was, in addition to realizing their potential to effect real transformation.

After graduating from medical school and qualifying in Infectious Disease, Paul joined a thriving practice in Southern California, bought a house with a stunning view where he became acquainted with neighbors in show business, and worked hard to build a practice. Not long after his arrival, an exceptionally gorgeous young man came to see Paul for medical care and fell in love with him. Medical ethics forbid doctors from taking advantage in such situations, but this patient's declaration of love propelled Paul into a period of questioning, conflict, and confusion, from which he emerged as a gay doctor madly in love with a patient dying of a new plague about which Paul could do little. The new and wholly unexpected love of his life died in his care.

Paul went on to treat countless cases of AIDS. With historically unprecedented speed, the medical care establishment responded with the crowning glory of modern medicine (excepting the eradication of smallpox): the rapid development of tests and drugs for the control of AIDS. A decade on, Paul had used new technology to save countless lives, and had extended his practice into the era when most of his new patients were women who couldn't imagine how they'd contracted the disease.

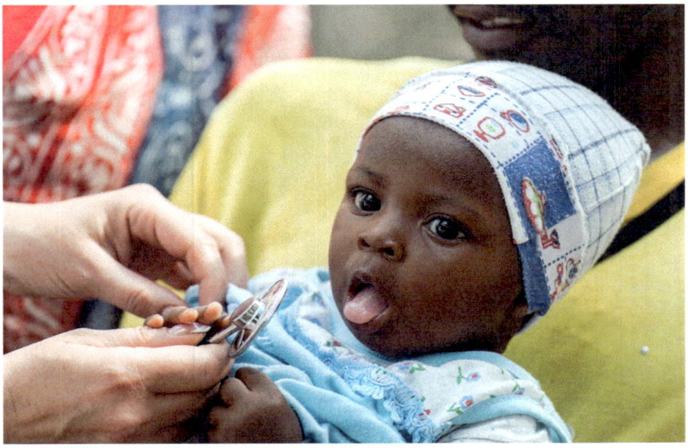

In other words, in a brief and harrowing time, Paul touched mortality on an intimate and pandemic scale by way of a disease that came out of distant, stressed habitats, ran through species including primates, and impacted humans around the globe. He had undergone a trial by fire through which he and his loved ones and community were preparing our species for the problems that we were about to encounter, problems for which we remained resolutely unprepared: human-caused non-infectious as well as infectious epidemics that imperil the body of life and all of the lives—individual and congregal—that depend on it.

Jacob

During Jacob's residency, it became obvious that while he was an excellent clinician and could choose from many career paths, his heart's desire was to become a historian. Which he did. He has since developed a multidisciplinary career that has touched on many areas of scholarship. Some years ago, when I was sick and had been reading a biography of Darwin to my daughter, I noticed that Darwin's mysterious symptoms were much like mine. They were generally constitutional and non-specific, so I wasn't surprised to discover via internet that many other people had wondered whether his life story might relate to an illness of one kind or another.

The similarities between Darwin's condition and mine haunted me. I decided to call Jacob, who had become an academic medical historian, and who was kind enough to take a telephone call to discuss my case and Darwin's. Quickly, a note of exasperation entered his voice, and I could picture him rolling his eyes. He had heard many opinions and discussions about Darwin's case, and wanted to be sure that I knew that disease was at least in part socially constructed—enough so that even if Darwin had been given a robust diagnostic label during his lifetime, it would be impossible to generalize from the last century to this one. For example, he said, the consumption of the nineteenth century was not the tuberculosis of today.

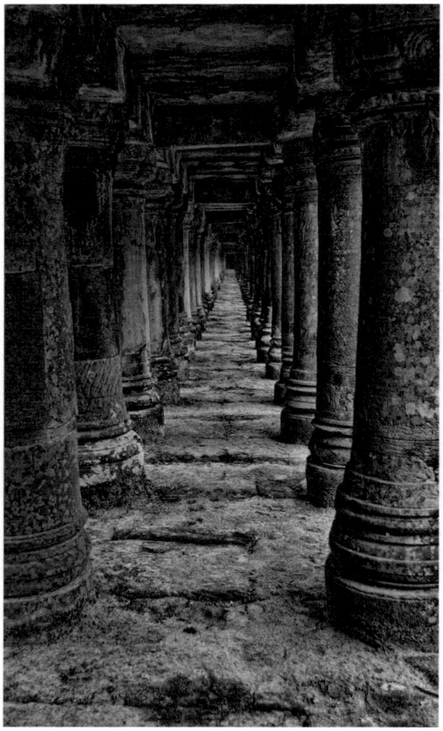

At that time, I had not looked into the lives or works of those doctors whose work marked key eras in our profession, such as Hippocrates, Maimonides, Vesalius, and Snow, the first to arrest an epidemic by tracing it back to its source—a London well contaminated with *Vibrio cholerae.* Jacob and I both remembered Howard Ricketts, who had died identifying the pathogenic agent of rickettsial diseases, and whose portrait looked out on a corridor at the University of Chicago medical school as if giving us fair warning of the cost of medical progress. This time, Darwin's disease remained a mystery, as it will likely be for all time. The past was thus mute, and I did not crack his case, nor mine. I did, though, encounter deep time as the long history of learning embedded in the profession that is now yours and mine to carry forward as best we can.

Dr. Tom Hornbein

Not long ago, my daughter and I went to see Jon Krakauer and Tom Hornbein in conversation at a Seattle Mountaineers celebration of the fiftieth anniversary of the first ascent of the West Ridge of Everest by Hornbein and his team. They were discussing Dr. Hornbein's new edition of his book *Everest: The West Ridge.* His team included Willi Unsoeld, who stood with Horbein on the roof of the world, and who—years later—took a fatal fall at age fifty-two.

I had avoided Krakauer's books, which seemed to me to disseminate—or perhaps trigger in me—secondary post-traumatic stress disorder. As he spoke, I quickly developed a deep sympathy for him. His closest childhood playmates were Willi Unsoeld's children, who had been left fatherless when their alpinist father rationalized taking voluntary risks for the sake of bagging peaks. Krakauer asked penetrating questions of Hornbein, who had survived against the odds to explain his commitment to climbing to the world's highest places. He acknowledged that the chances of coming back from the West Ridge were even, and no better, and that the next generation—including Krakauer—were traumatized by the costs of climbing glory.

It was a profound conversation that touched on the meaning of life and the choices that we face consciously and willingly or thoughtlessly and inadvertently. Perhaps because of his work as an anesthesiologist, Hornbein was much clearer than most climbers about the risks he chose to take—and the consequences to his closest friends, many of whom had died taking those risks. Other climbers with whom I've spoken look resolutely away from valleys and shadows; their world has no risk because everything that matters is known and under control, and those who lose at the Russian roulette game of climbing have only themselves to blame. In other words, they suffer from bad cases of what cognitive psychologists call the illusion of control.

Hornbein had some time ago come to terms with the risks of life and with his own mortality. He spoke of grief without regret of those whom he and Krakauer had known, and who had sacrificed their lives to a passion to reach the heights. Unlike Icarus, whose wings were made of wax, Hornbein had flown on wings that could not be seen or touched. What remains of his—and his team's—achievement is the inspiration to do the impossible, to see what is important to us, and to know and own our choices. Doing so is the only way that we will be able to face the problems we are avoiding and to solve them now, while we still have the chance.

BETH LOOKS BACK:
Your Past as the Raw Material of Your Future

On a religious quest that is both medieval and modern, [Samuel Sewell] judged himself. In doing so he became an unlikely pioneer of civil rights for powerless groups. [To] put [his] ideas into perspective, the widespread belief in the equality of races and genders in America lay more than two centuries in the future.

— Eve LaPlante in *Salem Witch Judge: The Life and Repentance of Samuel Sewall*

History is changing. I didn't realize this when I first noted that a budding crone's thoughts turn to biography and history. That was in medical school, when a close friend's mother and her peers read as if to keep New York publishers in the business of putting out non-fiction. Around that time, my mother sought consolation from the writings of Emerson and Marcus Aurelius. Then, I held to my girlish framing of historic figures coming from the same time, the past, and the same place, a bookshelf in my childhood living room.

When I got sick in midlife, I stopped reading fiction limited by inexperience, ignorance, or defeat and groused at publishers who—catering to the addictive tendencies of late moderns—profited by putting out addictive genres. I came to think of books as drugs—usually depressants. I sought out books that were inspirational, and began to write ones that aimed to be transformational. Eventually, I, too, started to read biography and history, and encountered writers who were contextualizing lives. They viewed the past through a lens formed by post-modern deconstruction and emergence. I saw then—right in front of my eyes—that history was changing, partly because of new knowledge and partly because writers were making new sense of the past.

My explorations of transformation began to take root in history as well as in the inner spiritual work that I had learned from emerging theologians who were also harvesting the past afresh. From them, I learned of the ancient Indian spiritual practice called tantra. An adept—a *tantrika*—might do inner work that can be interpreted allegorically as weaving together threads of personal and shared history to create the fabric of life. In other words, tantrikas might consciously construct the present moment or the current era by bringing forward warp threads comprised of essential and perennial human habits and by adding others that form a new pattern. This alters the future. If you run with this idea in your personal narrative, you can identify and perpetuate useful habits that stabilize your life, replace any that were dropped or cut off prematurely, restore those that are essential but failing, and add any or all through which you may enhance the future of the body of life. The value of this metaphor is that it puts the loom and shuttle in your hands. It allows you to consider the psychic and social fabrics that you are creating, and to improvise new patterns of beauty, utility, and stability as you come to terms with the past and envision and form your future.

For me, this metaphor has been integral to developing an interest in my ancestral and cultural heritage, which I can personalize as far back as the dawn of modernity. In 1550, an ancestral Alderman was born in Ipswich and gave birth to descendants who became pilgrims. At nearly the same time, a Johannson was granted land in Halland, Sweden in payment for military service. These threads of human history resonate with my evolving medical life, such as the religious dissent of medieval England that makes it possible to think independently in English, and the marauding Viking berserkers who savaged a wide swath of humanity in search of fertile soil, spun off Norman culture, and eventually produced peace-loving cultures.

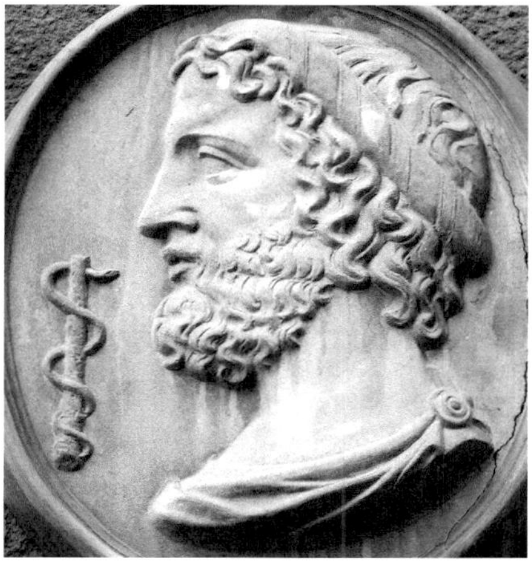

I had begun to personalize the past in medical school with an improbable—given my heritage—desire to go to Africa to look for American roots. Some years later, I went to Sweden to visit distant relatives at a family farm that my mother remembered fondly from her childhood. Her ancestors—like my pilgrim ancestors and their Congregational descendants—could be viewed as tribal, and suspected of inbreeding, though this idea owes more to the fact that I carry genes for slow metabolism than to any sober study of genealogy or genetics.

This realization informed my opinion that the late modern enchantment with genes and other molecules can be dispelled by recognizing that human genes haven't gone viral—at least not yet—and don't account for any epidemic. They enchant us because they flatter our illusion of control, because they provide products to patent and profit by, and because it is easier to deny thorny problems than to solve them. When we use cognitive psychology to hone our insight, perspective, and common sense, we can see our errors and integrate medical thought across cultures, disciplines, times, and places. We will then be prepared to devise emerging ways of practicing medicine that rescue the body of life in deep time from modern mistakes.

According to wise elders like the late Reb Zalman, who coined the term "Age-ing to Sage-ing," wisdom entails celebration of past accomplishments—which can be very difficult for doctors, who make decisions in good faith and do their level best, yet still feel the stinging tail of regret. Wisdom also entails gleaning the life lessons you gained through experience but have yet to recognize and utilize. This inner work is augmented by taking advantage of the life harvesting of others by family members, public figures, and historians—and by whole communities, as reported in *The Story of England* by Michael Wood. Both the outer and inner work prepare you to share your joy and to ease the pain and suffering you have embodied through your life experience. This is how I view my fifteen years of pain: as the raw material of my diagnosis, cure, and medical philosophy.

Comment on Encountering Deep Time

The word 'Anthropocene' is the invention of Paul Crutzen, a Dutch chemist who shared a Nobel Prize for discovering the effects of ozone-depleting compounds. The importance of this discovery is difficult to overstate; had it not been made—and had the chemicals continued to be widely used—the ozone 'hole' that opens up every spring over Antarctica would have expanded until eventually it encircled the entire earth.

— Elizabeth Kolbert in *The Sixth Extinction: An Unnatural History*

We can encounter deep time in the long view of the individual medical life, the modern era preceded by so many others, and the body of the profession that has metamorphosed again and again with the body of our species—and that is set to metamorphose once more. This time, we know that our planet is not at the center of the solar system or of the universe and that our species is not at the center of life on earth. We are become, in our modern ways of living, a case of galloping consumption, a nuisance turned lethal by its poor reckoning of time.

Ancient traditions taught young boys to visualize or meditate on their own deaths. They also taught men to die before they died—to become, as Paul of Tarsus put it, new men. These rites of passage are still passed on in medicine,

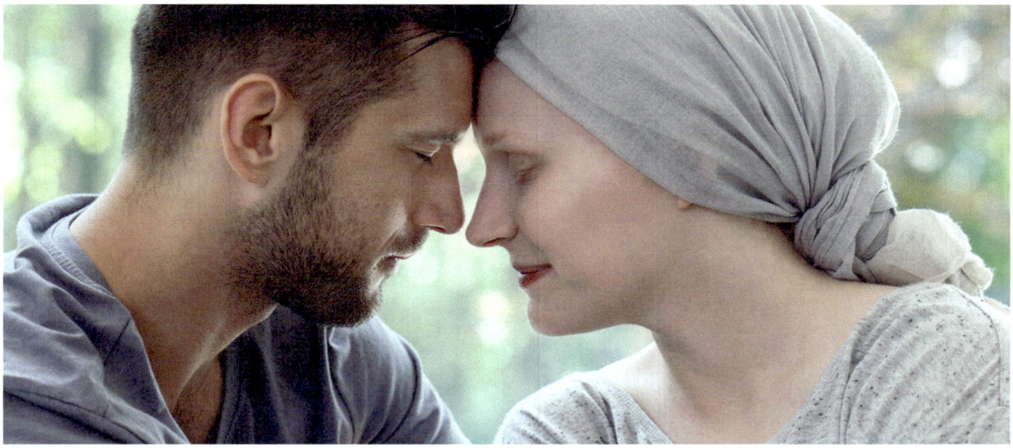

as when you take call during your third- and fourth-year clinic rotations and 'see one, do one, teach one,' and when you recite the Hippocratic Oath on taking your medical degree. When you see this, you can recognize that you are going through a rite of passage as an eldering individual, as a member of a perennial human profession, and as an instance in the aggregated lifetime of our species. You can look for a rite of passage such as a sabbatical—self-funded, if need be—or retirement. You can review the past for raw material from which to co-create the future, and so leave your mark.

When my mother was diagnosed with metastatic cancer, her surgeons urged her to accept procedures that would have caused pain and suffering and likely interrupted her life for as long as or longer than any months she might have gained from them. They were unable to accept that she had been ready for her own death for some time. She had always sustained a high degree of personal responsibility along with ethics free of the illusion of control. She had been ready for the "undiscovered country from whose borne no traveler returns"—perhaps too much so.

Through my mother's care, I came to see the greatest advance in medicine in my lifetime as the advent of home hospice care. This 'advance' offsets the institutionalization of modern medicine and allows those with common sense to leave this life gracefully with love, well-chosen last words, and blessings on those who remain. May her life—and yours and mine—be for a blessing.

ENCOUNTERING DEEP TIME

I have a sense—which is nearly impossible for me to describe—that there is a task waiting for me, that now something is expected or required of me. I feel strongly that I am destined for something, to do something.

— VIKTOR FRANKL through Haddon Klingberg, Jr.

WORKING QUESTIONS

Employed Physicians

- What era in medical history is of most interest to me: the one that followed Hippocrates? Galen? Avicenna? Maimonides? Vesalius? Boorhaeve? The Munros of Edinburgh? John Snow?
- How far back can I trace my ancestry? How far into the future may my bloodlines continue?
- How much Denisovan or Neanderthal DNA do I have?
- How can I make time to think every day? How can I make time for several days each season to think deeply about my place in time and my impact on what follows?

Self-determined Physicians

- Will what I am doing right now affect the course of the Anthropocene era in a life-negative or life-positive way in the here and now?
- What choice can I make right now to favor a living future? To avoid harm to wildlife?
- Is my present behavior a relic of ancient times? Can I drop it now?
- Do I need to consume this now?
- Do I need to purchase this poison? What consequences might it have in the distant future?
- How can I apply here what I learned from what I watched or read this month?
- How can I minimize the destruction of life by the consequences of my behavior?

EXERCISES

1. This month, do some searching in the library or online for self-education on habitat restoration, living futures, and the emerging paradigm in medicine. As part of your search, browse the following sites:
    - Society for Ecological Restoration, ser.org
    - Bullitt Center, bullittcenter.org
    - International Living Future Institute, living-future.org (Investigate the seven petal paradigm by purchasing and downloading PDFs from the website.)
    - Future Medicine, www.FutureMedicine.us
    - Evolve Medicine, www.EvolveMedicine.us
2. While you're at it, trace the beginning of the Anthropocene era and determine its present extent, and trace the evolution of the human species from the migration of the first Australians sixty-five thousand years ago; or from ancestors of humans passing through the Forest of Deane over four-hundred thousand years ago; or through Beringia from fifteen to twenty thousand years ago.
3. Recently, British law required all developments to do an archaeological assessment prior to digging. Israel has a similar requirement; Greece, Italy, Egypt, and other countries are expanding their history by incorporating new archaeological findings into their knowledge bases. Take advantage by:
    - Watching the first half of Michael Wood's *Story of England*, BBC, 2012, or
    - Browsing online or in the library recent issues of *British Archaeology*, *Archaeology*, or *Biblical Archaeology Review*, or
    - Reading *1491* by Charles Mann and *Henry David Thoreau: A Life* by Laura Dassau Walls.

Now, create an annotated timeline in which you reconstruct the deep history of the place you live now, where you grew up, or the place of origin of your ancestors. Include humans and their living context.

Essay

How can I best engage my profession in ensuring a living future for my young relatives, friends, and mentees?

(If you like, do an introduction now and come back to add notes and make a project of it to organize your thoughts over the course of the year. This is, for many of us, the most important question to hold as we contemplate the time that remains to us.)

Supplementary Reading

History

1. Moses Maimonides. *Ethical Writings of Maimonides.* Edited by Raymond L. Weiss with Charles Butterworth. New York: New York University, 1975.
2. Daniel Defoe. *A Journal of the Plague Year.* London: E. Nutt, 1722.
3. Tara Womersley and Dorothy Crawford. *Bodysnatchers to Lifesavers: Three Centuries of Medicine in Edinburgh.* Edinburgh: Luath Press, 2010.
4. William H. McNeill. *Plagues and Peoples.* New York: Anchor Press, 1976.

Tree of Life

5. David Quammen. *The Tangled Tree: A Radical New History of LIfe.* New York: Simon & Schuster, 2018.
6. Adam Rutherford. *A Brief History of Everyone Who Ever Lived: The Human Story Retold Through Our Genes.* New York: The Experiment, LLC, 2017.
7. Tom Phillips. *Humans: A Brief History of How We F****d It All Up.* Toronto: Hanover Square Press, 2019.

Living Future

8. David Suzuki. *Letters to My Grandchildren.* Vancouver: Greystone Books, 2015.
9. Jared Diamond. *Collapse: How Societies Choose to Fail or Succeed.* Revised edition. Penguin: New York, 2011.

Initiating Your Lifework and Legacy

What difference then can be seen between the purpose of him we call physician, who is an acknowledged handicraftsman, the discoverer of the mode of life and of the nourishment suitable for the sick, and his who discovered and prepared originally nourishment for all men, which we now use, instead of the old savage and brutish mode of living? My own view is that their reasoning was identical and the discovery one and the same.

—HIPPOCRATES in *Ancient Medicine* via W.H.S. Jones

WHEN YOU CONTEXTUALIZE your destiny, you prepare yourself to create a meaningful, dynamic vision of the future that is particular to you and that sustains you and draws you forward in the moment. You also form a pattern that holds your stance and in which your dynamic motive purpose propels you toward your vision; sets and attunes your direction as needed; and leads you to develop the strategies and skills that you need to effect your purpose. This process enables you to complete your lifework and leave the legacy that only you can create in response to experience.

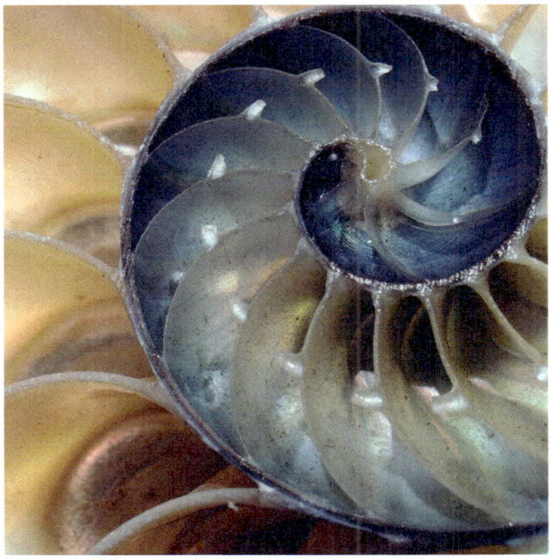

Therefore, if you do not establish a clear and evolving narrative purpose, you may lose the chance to make good on your experience—including any unresolved or painful bits. You may miss the opportunity to define an elderhood in which you delight in the time that remains and gain the peace of mind that comes with fulfillment of your unique destiny. Put differently, you may lose the chance to repattern your becoming and doing to support your eldering. The working questions and exercises in this book, as well as the online courses in care and cure, are designed for you to adapt for this purpose.

ANECDOTES FROM MEDICAL LIVES

That is the difficult thing: getting doctors who have begun feeling they are more and more knowledgeable and omnipotent to appreciate that they do not know everything.

— Dr. Thomas Chalmers in *Can Med Assoc J* Sept. 15 1996; 155 (6) p.759

The most impenetrable obstacle that any pre-modern doctor would face in the days when there was no access to information beyond medical training, personal experience, and whatever networking might chance to be available is the same one that divides late modern doctors from using their scientific training to solve new medical problems: the imposition of static paradigms on mutable biological realities. Fortunately, some doctors can respond despite these, for example infectious disease doctors trained in medical detection who respond adaptively to new pathogens like the AIDS virus.

Solving the intractable or big problems thus comes down to the few of us who are not employed, whose employers support them in responding to unplanned problems, who are paid to do the right thing, or who have devised ways to become independent of late modern systems of care. As you enter your elder years, you can choose to take on problems that you could not address in your adult career, and look for inspiration to peers who crafted their lives to suit their vision of living medicine.

David: a Life of Compassionate Action

When David was in the midst of his career as a staff doctor, teacher, and mentor at a university-affiliated veteran's hospital, he and his wife Susan became concerned about people who were living in places that lacked the advantages offered by modern medicine. Their humanitarian concern eventually came to focus on children in Southeast Asia who had lost limbs to land mines. They arranged their lives so as to be free from time to time for periods of a month or more to travel there and fit limb prostheses. So, having developed this concern and the expertise to address it, he and his wife extended their life of service to people in other parts of the world.

Over time, they spent more and more months of the year living and working in various parts of Asia and Africa, often in close concert with groups of religious who had dedicated the whole of their lives to service to their own communities or to distant ones. It was then that Susan became aware of the profound ethics of their Muslim security workers and the compassion of the

Catholic sisters who worked at great risk and with just enough material reward to sustain lives of service.

David and Susan brought this wealth of experience into their gentle mentoring of younger physicians. In their home, they kept mementos of the places they had visited and told stories of their fulfilling adventures in far-flung places. Like Dr. Paul Farmer, who cares for patients from all sides in strife-torn Haiti, David cares for casualties of war at home and abroad and thus for the body of the species within which we move into the unknown future.

Dr. Paul Zimmet

Whenever and wherever I see Paul, he is taking photographs of the obese. His growing collection includes photos from many countries, and serves as a resource for Australian journalists that are drawing public attention to the obesity epidemic and attempting to engage nationalist sentiments in weight loss, as when headlines warn Australians that they are becoming fatter than Americans. Perhaps that is the reason that, when he visits Seattle, he is delighted to take snapshots of the morbidly obese people struggling along the sidewalks.

Like a young physician on call, Paul seems to have established no firm circadian rhythms. For many years, he spent half his time in the air flying from one place to the other, using his seemingly endless energy to provide international leadership in his chosen fields of research—and in the implementation of policies consistent with biomedical realities. He is a maverick in his medical life and—as far as I can tell—has been one from the very start. When he realized that the system in which he was working would bar him from creating the career he envisioned, he sought funds from private and international sources, including the National Institutes of Health.

Having acquired data that policy makers could put to good use but also tended to ignore or to approach fatalistically, Paul entered his eldering years by stepping up and extending his leadership in research to public health policy at the national and international levels. He consulted with political leaders. He appeared on talk shows. He collaborated with organizations that had a stake in addressing the growing epidemics of diabetes and obesity. As these epidemics and their sequelae did more and more harm and caused greater and greater expense, he did more and more to stem them. Not one for idle learning—and well aware that information was insufficient to induce change—Paul spoke on national television and button-holed politicians of all stripes. Years on, he continues to complete his destiny by sharing the fruits of his lifelong labors with any and all who will listen and who may choose to act with him.

Dr. William Carlos Williams

Williams moved—as the saying goes—from blood to ink, that is, he wrote poetry that expressed his creativity and books that conveyed the essence of his professional life, most particularly in *The Doctor Stories.* Many others have captured and examined the human experience through medicine in plays, poetry, fiction, and non-fiction—including Anton Checkov, Arthur Hertzler, and Oliver Sacks, to name a few. Others, like James Orbinski, have written to formulate new narratives and to propose new solutions to pressing problems.

While doctors since John Snow and Lemuel Shattuck have used counts and statistics to analyze the roles of social factors in health and disease, and social workers since Jane Addams have done the same, artists have been freer of constraints imposed by the limits of medicine, religion, and science. We see these sent up in the plays of Moliere and in films like Akira Kurosawa's *Red Beard,* which explores medical practice and mentoring.

Some say now that narrative is the most basic element of patient care, and that the purpose of every doctor-patient encounter is the creation of a shared narrative that supports subsequent care and cure. Should that narrative fail, the doctor-patient relationship will fail. This presents tremendous obstacles to doctors and patients who are infatuated with technology and who expect expenditure of resources to lead to proportionate increases in health and well-being.

Gentle disillusionment with the past and new inspiration for the future are required to set our profession on solid ground. This ground will support the construction of narratives that match fast-changing social and biological realities and convey better ways to use resources. One task that lies ahead of our generation of medical elders is to use biography and autobiography as well as art to capture the truth of the human experience and then use that to construct post-modern medical narratives that go beyond the myth of rescue. We can therefore consider creating a legacy of writing that will inform and inspire those who come after us. To prepare for this, we review, reconcile, and integrate the lessons of a lifetime of learning and share them as narratives.

BETH LOOKS BACK: Future Love

Our Bodies, too, are Incessantly changing, and what we were, or are, is not what we will be, tomorrow: once we were seeds, the hope of our fathers, and lay concealed in the womb of our first mother; creative Nature willed otherwise: took us in hand, and out of the narrow confines of mother's expanded viscera, sent us forth into the open air, homeless!

— Ovid in *Metamorphoses* via Charles Martin

There is such a thing as a medical celebrity. I don't like to admit it because it seems to trivialize the sacred. I'm not talking now about doctors who become rich and famous by appealing to the public; I'm talking about leaders of the profession who dazzle us and turn us into wannabes.

I'm talking about that poised and gracious speaker, Dr. Sir Richard Doll, who discerned and documented the impact of smoking on lung cancer in his time, and who made it seem that medical breakthroughs came of classy, effortless grace. I'm talking about Dr. Arthur Herbst, who listened to his patients and clothed his findings in data that persuaded others that the diethylstilbestrol (DES) women took while pregnant caused vaginal adenocarcinoma in their daughters. He was an ambassador of Obstetrics and Gynecology who was eager to recruit to his specialty the gifted young women who did not accept that it had been, or should be, seen as second-rate. He was a surgeon and mentor who kept his temper at all hours and under all circumstances, though I did once see him sweat while doing an extenteration.

I'm talking about Dr. William Foege, who I saw rather than heard at a national meeting, where he was speaking in a large room that was packed to overflowing. Tired, disillusioned public health functionaries and taken-for-granted caregivers entered to figuratively touch his hem and take away some of the darshan of his involvement in the first-ever cure of our species, the eradication of smallpox. That tired audience was soon sitting at attention, then pouring out of the room smiling, eyes bright, spirits restored. He hadn't given them funding; he hadn't managed their project or shared their work; he had revived and renewed them with the mere force of his personality. It seemed that Osler lived again in a new and—to me—better guise: a doctor who could see the big picture and help to do the impossible for the body of our species, and who heralded emerging care and cure of the body of life.

It was these celebrities—and even more the everyday mentors I met in training and practice—who sustained me when my profession let me down in every possible way. When I lost my career and my credibility as a patient—not appearing to have a 'real' disease like cancer or AIDS or cirrhosis—I became very isolated. I watched films and drew on past inspiration. Fueled by that inspiration, I took my problems in hand and found a new way of looking at my body that allowed me to access every possible form of effective healing and cure, and a new way of looking at the context that enabled me to discover and remediate the causes of my pain and suffering—tangible and intangible alike. I was ready to enjoy the emerging paradigm that encompassed new-economy vocations such as organic farming and sustainable construction, and that presaged vocations such as habitat restoration and integration.

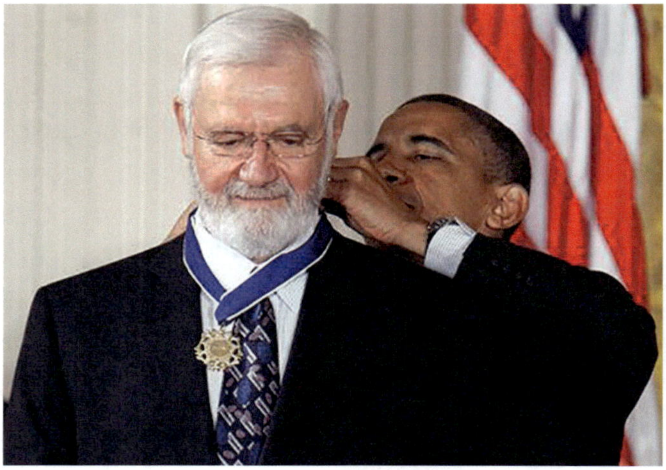

Dr. William Foege receives the Medal of Freedom

Doctors have yet to engage the new economy or to do the work of the century that could, if we moved with speed and wisdom, prevent the catastrophe that threatens every life on earth present and future. We have yet to do the hard work of accepting problems that we deny, enacting the science of engaging the unknown and creating the necessary tools for care and cure in context, and allowing the healthy disillusionment with idolatry of statistics, drugs, devices, and procedures that blind doctors and researchers to the devastating consequences of ignoring the living context on which all humans—born and unborn—rely.

It will be harder for doctors to engage than it will be for people in many other lines of work. Like farmers, we fare poorly in a monoculture. We also face the tricky task of sustaining essential services while devising better and more sustainable ways of working. You can prepare for this heroic task by taking a breather. You can stop running, take a long and broad and deep view of the profession, and do the right thing by your body and—as able—by the future of evolved life. Looking to the giants of the past who inspired us will ease the way.

CONSTRUCT 4

Care States

Deep care states prepare the body for better sleep, supplement sleep, and relieve the stress of daily life and challenging times. Abiding in them is a form of what some call energy medicine.

Preparation for Energy Work

You prepare for energy work by creating a conceptual framework. You can recall that your body is a conductor that can draw lightning on a playing field. You know that doctors measure aspects of energy through the electrocardiogram and electroencephalogram. You may know that scientists know very little about the autonomic nervous system, and that the little that is known tends to be based on pathology studies, that is, on dead rather than living flesh. This need not impede your self-care. Rather than approach your subtle energy body through your understanding, experience it directly through your awareness and focus, as adepts have done for at least two and a half millennia.

Your awareness is a marvelous inborn scanner that is dynamic, adaptable, and resilient. No one could devise a scanner better able to serve your intention to be and become care—that is, to deepen care continuously in daily life. To teach your awareness to detect and interact with your energy, you do playwork like that which follows, which draws on ancient living traditions.

You also prepare by purposing to become able to align your posture to enhance the flow, balance, and integration of the circulationof energies and the sustenance of care states and actions. To ensure your safety, you also learn to ground the energy body as if it were an electric circuit. In this paradigm, actively ground every aspect of the body as detailed below.

Grounding Awareness

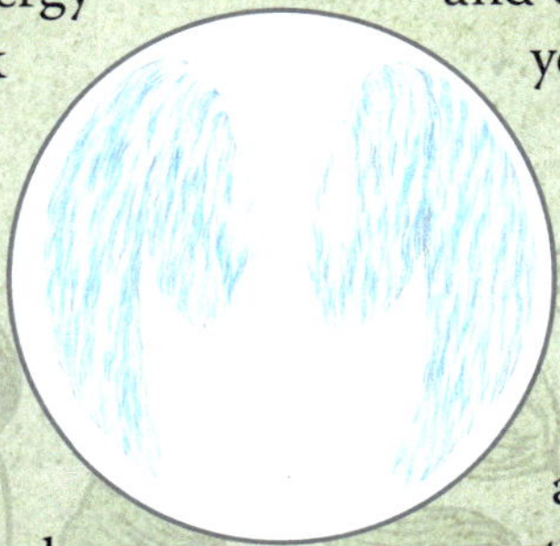

On the level of awareness, grounding lowers your center of energy so that you can fully relax into alertness and safely sustain intense degrees of attention and concentration sufficient to calm the agitation of the intangible body and to anneal the fragmentation of flesh and interbeing. Without grounding, you may lose your focus and disregard care and cure. Without grounding, you cannot set intentions to guide your care, sustain or deepen care states, focus intently on subjects or objects, or increase the scope of depth of your awarenss in life, location, or time.

Grounding Understanding

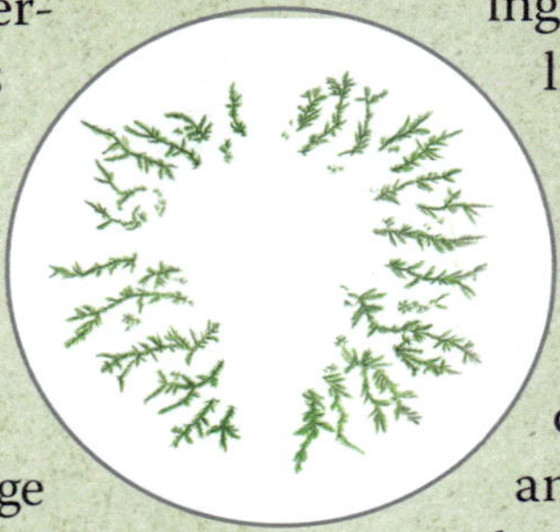

On the level of understanding, grounding is the objective reality that enables you to distinguish fantasy from comprehension and to know harm from healing. Without grounding, you cannot gauge the effects of ideas on actions or of actions on care. Without grounding, you cannot recognize the limitations of ideas and may waste your awareness on fruitless notions and on useless or harmful fantasies. With grounding, you can gauge and hone your analyses and syntheses, and so learn to guide yourself toward care and cure.

Grounding Perceptions

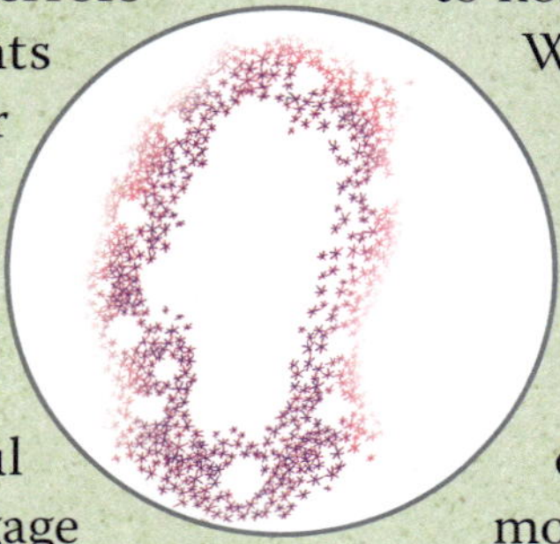

On the level of perceptions, grounding alerts you to errors in your reading of events and to harm done by your habitual responses to them. Without grounding, you may respond to misperceptions that trigger useless or harmful reactions rather than engage reality and miss the chance to use moment-to-moment experiences to hone your habits as needed. Without grounding, you may undermine your understanding by basing it on wrong assumptions or systematic errors. With grounding, you can discern what matters in the moment, where you are, and where you are going.

Grounding Sensations

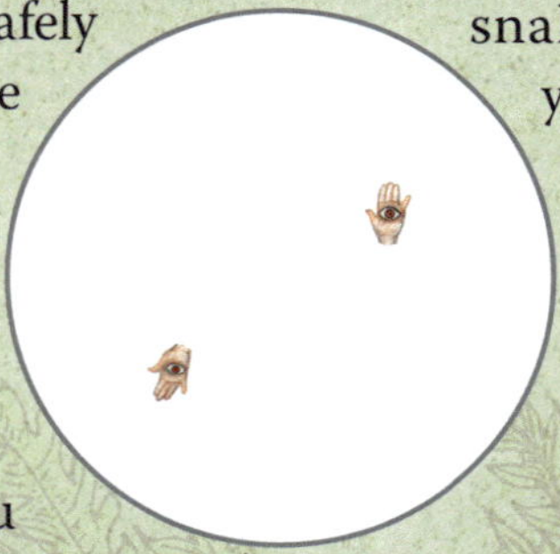

On the level of sensations, grounding enables your senses to safely join your awareness with the tangible world. Without grounding, your senses and sense awareness may become dissociated from matter and interrupt your interbeing, as when you mistake a coiled rope for a poisonous snake. You may undermine your perceptions by dividing them from sensory experience. With grounding, you can sense the intangible and tangible, and inform and align them.

Grounding Energy

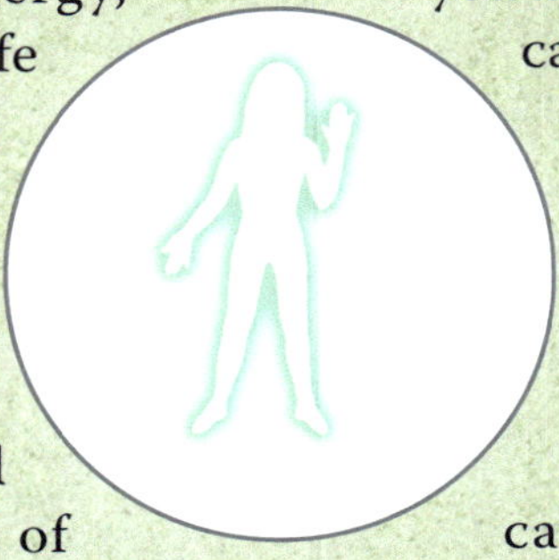

On the level of energy, grounding holds you safe and steady as you receive, conduct, transmit, enhance, and transform the ineffable dynamism that interpenetrates all levels of being and animates all processes of becoming. Without grounding, you may undermine all of your care states and processes. With grounding, you can align and harmonize all aspects of the sevenfold body and sustain the energy-intensive focus that mediates and catalyzes your purposes, care states, skills, and transformations.

Grounding Flesh

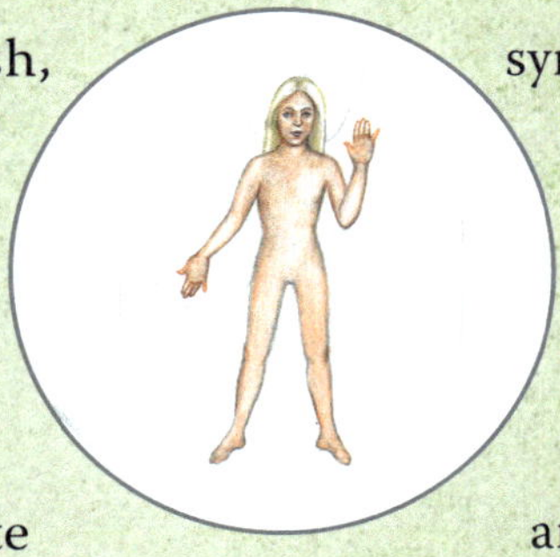

On the level of flesh, grounding orients the exquisitely orchestrated electromagnetic processes of cells, tissues, organs, and systems. With grounding, your flesh can join with energy to create synchronous, dynamic resilience. Without grounding, you waste precious energy and obstruct the connections between your intangible body and the body of life in time and eternity.

Grounding Interbeing

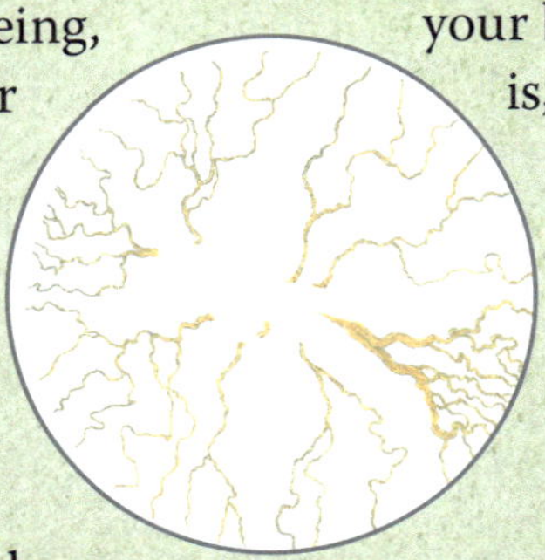

On the level of interbeing, grounding orients your body in life, space, and time. Without grounding, you may participate in sustaining shared illusions and delusions that obstruct your ability to align your action with your being and becoming—that is, wth the dynamic unfolding of life in space, time, and eternity. Without grounding, you cannot be wise. With grounding, you can make good on your being and becoming.

Discovering Care States

Though moderns do not yet comprehend or objectify the subtle body, you can apprehend it directly as the ancients did and use it to advance your care states. Discovery of a care state of compassion, lovingkindness, joy, and resilience begins with enhancing your relaxed, alert, clear awareness; sustaining and eventually intensifying your focus; deepening and broadening your serenity; strengthening and balancing your care skills; and dissolving obstacles that interfere with your self-patterning.

While doing energy work of any kind, remove your body and being as much as possible from poisons such as artificial energy fields. Turn off all the electrical and electronic technology that you can, preferably at the breaker box, or better yet do all your playwork while sitting or walking outdoors in a healthy forest far from communications towers and the power grid.

In addition to grounding your whole body, become more aware of your orientation with respect to your lifetime and to the body of life evolving in time and eternity. If you sense that your energy is straining forward or pulling back, refresh your serenity and invite your energy to rest at the moving front of time in eternity. You may find it helpful to allow your eyes to remain somewhat open and unfocused so that your sense of sight can help to ground you in your milieu.

Now, bring your breath and awareness to your alert relaxation, a skill that supports care states that embody compassion, joy, serenity, wisdom, and altruism. If you settle for harmful states created by caffeine, alcohol, anger, or adrenal arousal, you may be caught in a cycle of stimulation and depression that is difficult to break.

In general, your outer life begins in the morning and your inner life on which it depends may begin late in the evening or not at all. Because the outer life may be more complex and stimulating, your body may become imbalanced. Activity may dominate over contemplation; the sympathetic nervous system may dominate the parasympathetic nervous system; and wakefulness may dominate sleep. All of this may lead to chronic adrenal stress. All of this may compromise your self-care to an unpleasant and unhealthy degree, to which you become hardened and come to take for granted.

Eventually, when you are able to remain in a state of alert relaxation at all times, your awareness will not contract, and you will be able to sustain mindfulness of states and take a step toward continuous self-care.

Continue bringing your inhalations and awareness to your state of alert relaxation. If you discover a care state, abide in it for ten minutes or more, as able. If you do not, or you wish to deepen your state, try one of the maneuvers below.

Enhancing Alertness. If you feel lethargic, stand or sit in a favorable posture and allow your head to tip back. As you breathe in slowly, deeply, and silently, lift your chin and breastbone toward the ceiling or sky. Taking care not to overdo, continue the slow deep breathing, allowing the breastbone to rise higher with each inhalation.

If you like, you can add arm movements. Stretch your arms straight out to the side, palms up; then breathe in, tip the head back, and sweep your arms upward to bring your palms together above your breastbone. Pause briefly on the in-breath and then allow your head and arms to return to their starting positions, and exhale slowly, fully, and silently. Do not pause on the out-breath, which is called the death breath. You can repeat the cycle three times and then, if you like, repeat it again a few minutes later.

Alternatively, you can use acupressure. Stand or sit in a favorable posture, breathe in deeply, gently, and slowly, and press a fingertip gently on the point at the center of the forehead, midway between the eyebrows and between the brow and hairline. Massage the point lightly for ten slow counts or longer. You can wait several minutes and repeat or shift the fingertip up to the midpoint of the hairline and massage that point.

You can also do gentle scalp massage, spreading the fingertips and massaging with just enough pressure to stimulate the circulation without causing discomfort. If you like, do this as you wash your hair, and allow the flow of water to enhance the self-massage.

Caution: if your spinal mobility is limited or you feel lightheadedor uncomfortable when you tip your head back, substitute acupressure or massage for spinal extensions.

Easing Agitation. If you are too restless or jittery to focus, or if you are having trouble going to sleep, do forward spinal bends to relax. Standing or sitting in a an anatomically neutral posture, allow your head to tip all the way forward and then hold this position as long as you like. If you still feel tense or distracted, sit on a chair and fold your body forward at the hips until the chest is resting lightly on your thighs. If your belly is pregnant or large, spread your thighs to avoid cutting off your circulation. If you are comfortable resting thus, allow your head and arms to dangle and hold the position as long as you like.

Options

Yoga: Many people, especially men, lack sufficiently-honed proprioception to do yoga safely. If you are not experienced, consult an expert teacher or attend a class. If you have experience with yoga, you can enhance alertness with a sun salutation. This salutation is a series of sacred yoga poses or asanas rich in spinal extensions and well-suited for morning use. Sun salutations may be particularly helpful for those who live in the far north and seek to counter the depressing effects of short days and limited sunlight. To learn this practice, take a gentle class in hatha yoga; consult a book like Donna Farhi's *Yoga Mind, Body and Spirit: a Return to Wholeness;* view Jane Fonda's *Yoga Workout;* or search online or in the library for Rodney Yee's *Yoga for Beginners.* You can likewise relax with asanas like child's pose that feature forward bends. To learn these asanas, you can take a hatha yoga class or access Rodney Yee's *Yoga Practice for Energy.*

Returning to Care: Whenever you lose your relaxation or equanimity, take time to deepen your care state. Before advancing to the playwork below, satisfy yourself that your care state is relaxed, alert, grounded, and free of force, clutter, stress, or tension. If you cannot do this easily, pause and take time to do the Care course first—either online at EvolveMedicine.us, or through the more detailed material in *The Chronic Illness Owner's Manual.* Note that every time you lose your care state, you have an opportunity to practice discovering it.

Initiating Your Lifework and Legacy

People like you and I, though mortal of course like everyone else, do not grow old no matter how long we live; [we] never cease to stand like curious children before the great mystery into which we were born.

— Albert Einstein via *Wikiquote*

EXERCISE 1

Introduction

In this exercise, you pattern yourself to become a source of compassion and sympathetic joy by offering well-wishes to your sevenfold body, including your interbeing. If you are not yet accustomed to thinking of interbeing, you can visualize your body as touching a Huon pine tree, which has a single root system that supports acres and acres of trees. While each tree appears on the surface to be separate, all are connected underground. You body relates in this way to one trunk, and through it to all trunks. Likewise, through your local area of the body of life, your body belongs to your dynamic ecosystem and to the whole web of life in time and eternity.

Purpose

You do this exercise for relief and wellbeing and to develop your compassion and sympathetic joy.

Instructions

In this exercise, become a source of compassion and sympathetic joy for your own body by repeating well-wishes. The first three express your wish to free your body of suffering and the last three invite your body to experience wellbeing. Offer the phrases from the heart as able, inviting rather than compelling your body to experience joy.

May I be free from disaster
May I be free from disablement
May I be free from defilement
May I thrive in form
May I thrive in essence
May I adapt easily and well

As you say the phrases, focus on their meaning as follows.

When you say *May I be free from disaster,* think of events that create discontinuity and wish your body free of them. These are events that disrupt the web of life, as when tsunamis destroy farmlands and cities. They may disrupt the social peace, as when force displaces people. They may disrupt your peace, as when betrayal causes a break with the past. As you think of misfortune, you can put your suffering in a larger context and remember your good fortune in having escaped many kinds of disasters.

When you say, *May I be free from disablement,* think of events that reduce your tangible abilities and oblige you to develop new ones. These are events that lead to loss of function of one or more parts of the body.

When you say, *May I be free from defilement,* think of intangible habits that divide you from care. These habits may be linked to highly charged memories of trauma, to behaviors such as overeating, or to thought patterns that depress your immune response.

When you say, *May I thrive in form,* think of caring for the flesh and its functions—that is, of creating supreme wellbeing through the tangible aspects of your body, including your anatomy and cellular structure and function. You can envision specific types of care, such as the union of a fracture, the elimination of a cancer, or the recovery of your immune function.

When you say, *May I thrive in essence,* think of healing the intangible aspects of yourself, such as your awareness, understanding, perceptions, and energy. You may envision specific transformation of suffering to wellbeing, restoring vitality, or enhancing relief and wellbeing through blessing.

When you say, *May I adapt easily and well,* think of behaviors you can change to enhance your relief, wellbeing, and recovery, such as eating better, freeing your thinking of harmful habits so as to lift your mood, and changing your perceptions to relieve your body of hatred or craving.

Repeat the phrases until your time is up and then dedicate your time and effort to deepening your care state. Then note anything that you may wish to remember.

Options

Advancing the Practice. You can adapt and extend the practice by devising and adding new phrases that suit you on the day, such as, *May I dwell in peace.* You can also use these phrases to enter into care states as they evoke in you a warm glow of love of life to which you can return and in which you can abide. You can then use the phrases to become care by allowing them to move your baseline and extreme states of being in the direction of care.

When you are strong enough, advance to sharing the phrases with others. For example, silently offer them to a pet as you feed him, to a child as you put her to bed, to a stranger as you ask for coffee or directions, or to a tree or flower as you pass it. When your awareness is spacious, you will be able to share your phrases easily and gladly with all aspects of the web of life that you contact.

To work more with well-wishing, you can consult books that feature the path of blessing such as *God is a Verb* by Rabbi David Cooper, *To Bless the Space Between Us* by John O'Donohue, or *The Force of Kindness: Change Your Life with Love and Compassion* by Sharon Salzberg.

EXERCISE 2

Go on a treasure hunt for simple pleasures in nature and record the day's top ten in your journal. Take special note of things that delight you and record any such moments in your journal.

EXERCISE 3: *Season Finale: The Autobiography*

Read *Making Stories: Law, Literature, Life* by Jerome Bruner (2002). Without referring to anything you wrote before, and ignoring Bruner's idée fixe that art is meant to articulate problems but not solutions, write a 1000-word bio of your life as a set-up for your capstone and living legacy. Feature your living treasures and gifts, however harrowing, and make it biocentric.

EXERCISE 4: Contemplation

Once a day, spend twenty minutes or more holding the following questions in sequence as you remain aware of all levels of your body. If you can make time, do this two or three times a day, or for extended periods of time on free days.

Is my mind relaxed and alert?

The purpose of this question is to become aware of your habitual state, in particular whether you tend to be tense or relaxed and sluggish or alert.

Where is my attention at this moment?

The purpose of this question is to increase awareness of your usual habits of attention. As you observe your habits, you will find out whether your attention is usually fragmented or unified, stable or flighty, and responsive to your purpose or to your external circumstances and internal reactions. As you become familiar with your habits, you do not yet attempt to alter them. You 'take a baseline reading' that will enable you to wisely guide your personal evolution.

How deeply am I able to concentrate right now?

When you are familiar with your habits of relaxation and attention, you can become familiar with your concentration and it's fluctuations.

You can do this by noting your ability to become absorbed in the subject of your attention, such as a conversation or a piece of music; a trip across town; a map or jigsaw puzzle; the taste of a sauce or juice; the texture of a fabric, tile, or carving; or a memory of a care event. If you find it difficult to observe your concentration on the fly, you can challenge your focus by doing a task such as finishing a crossword puzzle, painting memorizing a poem, drawing an image from memory, or pursuing a hobby.

WORKING QUESTIONS

This month, you will prepare to contemplate the big questions by withdrawing from multitasking and developing your ability to focus on a topic. This will support and deepen your contemplation of a living future and your place in its creation. Take time each morning to come to know aspects of mind and being on which wisdom depends.

As you look ahead to elderhood, you may find that the meaning and purpose that shaped your earlier career are still alive in you—that is, your passion for medicine has grown or remains the same, and you are ready now to envision a lifework and legacy and to fulfill that vision. Or, you may find that you have lost the passion that once drove your career or your life or allowed you to take action to bring about a better future for yourself.

If you find that you have lost your passion or your ability to harness it, you may have to create and hold working questions about your specific meaning and purpose for the rest of this year of transition—or for however long it takes to discern the future that your body is set to create. However you discover the highest level of your most intimate personal dreams, you can use what you discover to formulate working ideas of meaning and purpose, such as making the world a better place through medicine. Those can be used as guideposts when considering your future and its big-picture context, used until you break through to become aware of your deepest meaning and purpose. Then you will be able to keep an eye out for choices that open to you, and be prepared to take advantage of them.

Employed Physicians

- Is the task I am doing likely to make life better for my children and grandchildren?
- Is what I intend to do immediately after this urgent, important to a living future, both, or neither?
- If my actions contribute little to the future of life, what could I be doing instead?
- What can I be doing for my body now, today and every day?
- What can I be doing for fun and delight?
- How can I live sustainably so as to model a joyful elderhood?

Self-determined Physicians

- What past resources of problems, pain, suffering and unprocessed memories can I access and take as raw materials for the priming of my lifework and the formation of my legacy? What experience is gathered in my flesh and ready to make good on?
- Where can I find books, films, or conversationalists who will challenge me to delve into my body, expand my awareness, explore the full scope of my life purpose, or extract meaning from the phenomena that life imprinted in me?
- What else do I want to accomplish before I die? What would I like to be able to have done for my juniors when I'm lying on my deathbed?
- What gifts of the past, what past and present wisdom and mores, belong to my body through my kindred, my culture, my species, my habitats, and life on earth? What lights live on brightly in my soul to support me in becoming part of the change that contributes to the continuation of life on earth?
- Where can I find inspiration now?

Supplementary Reading

1. Yvon Chouinard. *Let My People Go Surfing: the Education of a Reluctant Businessman.* New York: Penguin Books, 2005, 2006.
2. David Suzuki. *David Suzuki: the Autobiography.* Vancouver: Greystone Books, 2006.
3. Anything on previous lists that you have not already read.

Contextualizing Your Destiny

A lot of the dinner-table conversation was inevitably about medicine, but the talk was never just about "cases." A patient might present as a case of this or that, but in my parents' conversation, cases became biographies, stories of people's lives as they responded to illness or injury, stress or misfortune. Perhaps it was inevitable that I myself became both a physician and a storyteller.

— Oliver Sacks in *The Mind's Eye*

When you view your body as one instance in the body of life as we know it—that is, as one in countless billions of entities that survived the fifth extinction or came into being after it—you can see that your personal destiny is part of something that is far greater than any individual. When you view your destiny as also belonging to larger bodies such as species, ecosystems, and the body of life at locales in time, you see that you and you alone can care for your body—that is, the sum of your material and ethereal existence—in accord with the bodies in which yours nests and on which it relies for life.

When you see that the miraculous body of life is comprised of systems of a complexity and timespan that human brains cannot encompass, you may feel overwhelmed by the task of caring for it. It helps to recognize that reductionist thinking that fails to account for biology or that focuses on molecules vastly increases complexity, confuses and befuddles, and undermines common sense and experiential learning. This thinking is the reason that doctors have been slow to see and respond to the emerging epidemics of chronic exposure and related ailments. The trick to seeing life in all its complexity is to see it through a new simplicity. One element of this is a change in scale. In the emerging paradigm in habitat

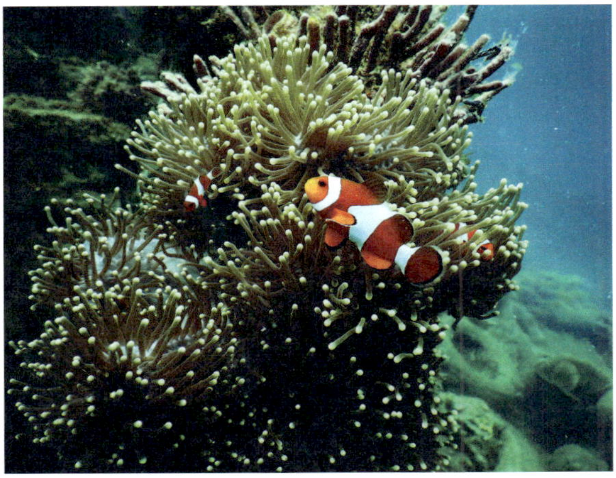

care, you focus on the next five centuries; in organic farming on preserving and enhancing living soils, watersheds, and seed diversity; in architecture, you focus on all of these and on local living economies; in medicine, on organ systems and patients, their habitats, and the next twenty generations at least. Data overload and reductionism are likely to be of little use in creating a destiny that rescues the body of life and averts the sixth extinction, and so sustains your professional and personal descendants as well as their care and cure.

EXTINCTION EVENTS

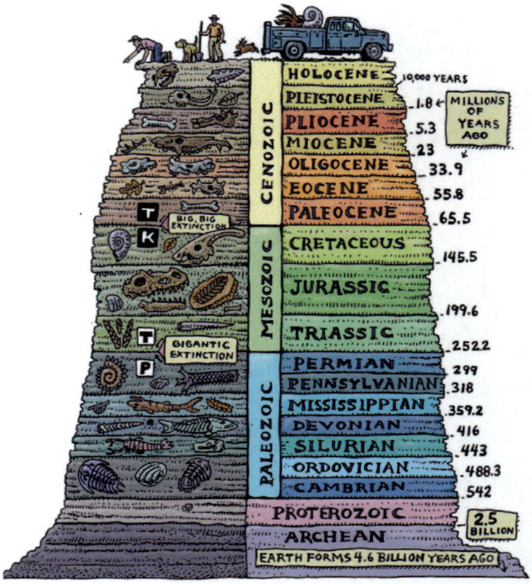

This book therefore defines your personal destiny as the future that you—and only you—can effect in the time that remains to you. This destiny is sensitive to your context in space, time, and life as a whole as it is now, and now, and now, and so on with every breath from now until your last. To choose and create your personal destiny, you can approach life and the profession as sacred; take your embodied experience as the precursor for your completion; take a stance that joins and aligns your being and doing with the bodies in which you nest and on which you rely like a baby in the womb; and act from your conscience as directed by your developing vision of—and faith in—the future of life.

ANECDOTES FROM MEDICAL LIVES

When one of our friends pointed out that more than a third of American men in my age group were retired, and that we could expect to live until we were eighty years old, I had one disturbing reaction: What was I going to do with the next twenty-five years?

—President Jimmy Carter in *The Virtues of Aging*

In the course of your medical life, you will have contextualized your career to fit your locale in life and time. You will in turn have impacted your locale—most often unawares. Now, as you contemplate your elderhood, you have the chance to rethink your context and your relation to it, and so to alter your impact on your locale. If you join with a group of like-minded peers, you may be able to exert a large enough impact to sustain the heart of the profession through a period of deep change that is unprecedented in the history of life on earth. This change will test all of your inborn and acquired talents because it will call you to support modern standards of patient and community care as you devise ways to care for the bodies of species, habitats, and life on earth—or at least ensure that you are not contributing to their demise.

Dr. Buchanan: a Keeper of the Flame

In the 1970s, a faculty member of the University of Chicago School of Medicine named Dr. Buchanan sustained the tradition of the medical narrative by passing on to medical students beautifully-crafted case histories that perfectly illustrated various diseases. He was said to have trained in the Edinburgh school, a mysterious and wonderful thread of the medical tradition that was praised by Thomas Jefferson and closely connected with the Scottish Enlightenment. Buchanan's stories and other mentors' use of Hippocratic aphorisms kept the ancient roots of the profession alive in day-to-day practice and helped to form our common sense, which was, as the saying went, uncommon.

Times had changed since horse and buggy days, when medical students might throw shoes at a dull professor, but we were still a tough crowd. Dr. Buchanan was one of the few professors who—even as his hands trembled with age—could hold a theater full of glassy-eyed, grumpy students rapt and breathless with the narratives for which we had waited our whole lives and that he passed on with pithy, earthy simplicity. His case histories revealed the miraculous and hidden order of the body, and so made sense of the art of medicine—the art that has existed for longer than any single life or era.

A hundred years earlier, when the majority of Harvard-educated physicians were illiterate and could not take a written exam, the oral and practical traditions—especially the medical narrative—were essential to the practice and continuation of the profession. Buchanan's art thus reminds us that while indoctrination by information and infatuation with technology are understandable in view of the discovery of antibiotics, the advent of hygiene, and the eradication of smallpox, technology bears little relation to the human body and may fail to impact its changing ailments—apart from contributing to human-created ones such as nosocomial infections and those that form the focal points of new specialties like occupational and aerospace medicine.

Thus, as we move forward into elderhood, we can resume the tradition sustained by professors like Dr. Buchanan and writers like Oliver Sacks, and so leave behind distracting and extraneous information. We can also respond to modern devolution by bringing forward perennial narratives that are still useful and by creating new ones that make sense of the seeming chaos that characterizes biological and social metamorphoses.

Dr. Fernando Vega: a Pioneer in Integrative Medicine

Dr. Vega had an unusual upbringing. His father was a marine biologist whose work took his family to far-flung places like the rain forest of the Philippines and Kodiak Island, where young Fernando bore witness to the Alaskan earthquake of 1964. After graduating from the University of Washington medical school and qualifying in Family Medicine, he opened an office and waited for patients to seek care. Business was slow at first, so a friend suggested that he team up with a woman who was practicing Chinese acupuncture.

Their joint practice succeeded beautifully, attracting far more patients than did their individual practices combined. Over time, the practice grew by gathering practitioners of all sorts, many of whom offered new and promising modalities that sank or swam depending on the currents of the marketplace. It became a center of complementary and then of integrative medicine. It suited its time of over-systematization—which did so much for trauma care and so little for primary care—as well as its location in a Pacific Rim city enriched by a highly-educated, well-traveled population with a history of independence, self-sufficiency, and active participation in self-care and cure.

Thirty years on, as the practice—now called Seattle Healing Arts—continues to invent and innovate new treatment modalities, Dr. Vega looked ahead to elderhood. Having long faced mysteries that lie beyond the cutting edge of care, he considered retirement. We here suggest that those who have successfully practiced invention and innovation, as he did, enter into a phase that offers respite and also the potential for contemplation of and contribution to contextual care, which we include here as an aspect of medical eldering.

Harui: Family Care in Retirement

Harui was born in Hawaii into a Japanese-American community that sustains many Asian traditions, including that of filial piety. After attending the University of Washington for his medical education, he remained to undertake medical training that led, eventually, to his becoming a Professor in the School of Medicine. During that time, he and his wife raised their children in

Seattle, and those children went on to pursue their educations and to develop work lives and families in the lower forty-eight states.

Aware that diabetes was increasing in many groups, including descendants of Japanese immigrants to North America, Harui developed and led a series of studies of the causes and consequences of diabetes in members of the Issei, Nissei, and Sansei generations, and also began to look into the health habits of the multiracial Yonsei. Through these studies, which he performed with government funding and in cooperation with Japanese-Americans and, increasingly, Japanese colleagues, he found that small increases in retroabdominal fat deposits could sharply increase risk of diabetes in people of Japanese descent.

As Harui approached the age that many Japanese consider to be the age of retirement, he considered how best to sustain his responsibilities as the eldest son of a Japanese-American mother, as a doctor, and as a mentor of many colleagues both in his own city and overseas. It seemed to us—who watched from the outside—that he was, like his home state of Hawaii, enmeshed in a tangle of historical threads, each defined by a distinct way of reckoning time and place. We wondered if he would find a way to sustain all of his responsibilities, each on its own terms.

After thinking things through carefully, Harui and his wife returned to their home state, where they built a new house near his family home on ground that had been cleared and covered by a relatively recent lava flow. From there, he traveled to Japan several times a year to serve as a consulting academic. He also kept up collegial working relations with former mentees who worked to fulfill the aims of the projects that he had begun in the States. And so, like more and more doctors whose responsibilities encompass many locales divided by time and space, he devised a way to sustain the disparate threads of a complex life even as he drew his old career to a close.

BETH LOOKS BACK: Physician as Priest

Just as the Church of the Holy Sepulchre covered up the very ground of history it was there to honor, so too, all our institutions tend to hide that which they were created to celebrate.

— Rabbi Ted Falcon in *Getting to the Heart of Interfaith*, with Pastor Don MacKenzie and Sheikh Jamal Rahman

The first thing they do is lie. I've seen it time and again. It breaks my heart. Here's an example: I'm at a religious retreat deep in the heart of the Catholic

Church, in a place where priests live and where nuns and other religious and serious lay people come to stay for silent retreats and profound encounters with scripture. It doesn't occur to them to ask if I'm Catholic, or if I've been baptized, or if I belong. I don't. I'm unaffiliated. I explore and value all faiths.

In that way I'm a bit like Elie Weizel when he stopped on the steps outside the door of the synagogue, deeply desiring to enter but unable to do so. I can't enter a door built by Rome, or say I believe when I belove—as Marcus Borg translates the word in scripture. I can't be honest and claim a creed other than my own because I am an intellectual, an investigator, a seeker. It wasn't a choice. It was my answer to the questions which—as Dr. Viktor Frankl put it—life was posing. In the way of Dag Hammarsjöld, I saw such questions as arising from common ground. Though my deep roots go back to cultures born of Christianity and dissent, I was blessed to evade indoctrination and am free to encounter the sacred and the infinite without fear or antipathy or set expectations.

When those at the retreat find out that I am not Catholic, they feel consternation and yet they accept me, for now. They like that I am there. They know that I am not lying and they are secretly pleased to be reminded that they do not control God. They don't want to. They like to see the Gospel do its work, and to meet the stranger who is, for an inexplicable reason, able to bear witness to the truth of their faith from a perspective of conscientious inquiry and open expectations that they in turn can witness.

After weeks of periodic silent, cloistered retreats and home prayer, we have met for the weekend, concluded the retreat, and exited to the parking lot outside the chapel door. I am walking with a pleasant woman who is wearing a black wig and who has been circumspect in her remarks while I myself have blurted—politely I hope—whatever was in my mind or on my heart. She and I have been talking all weekend about faith, life, spirit, love, and the teachings of the human Jesus and his fallible followers. We have talked about life and death and—from my side at least—have opened to God, the Divine, the Truth, the Other, the Way. We did what we could to go deep.

As she puts a box of her things into the trunk, she confesses that she has cancer and expects to die in the next few weeks. She came for consolation and to reconcile with her Church, but found that she couldn't trust it. She couldn't be truthful or open; she feared that they would invade her, dominate her, spoil her last hours. Even now, when her need was dire and she ached for union, she couldn't trust them. Like children of my generation who attended Catholic

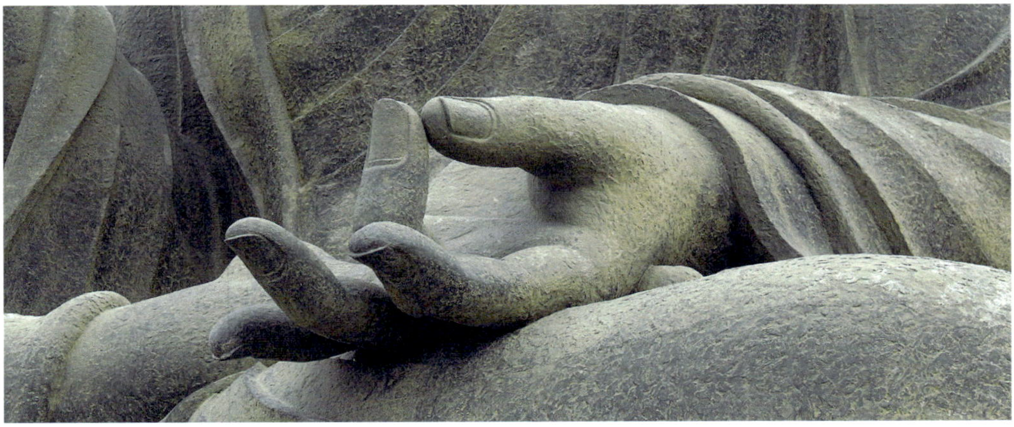

schools, she made things up to say in the confessional so that she could keep her faith in her heart and shield it from the trivialization of rote judgments and irrelevant, degrading punishments. I didn't know what to say. She didn't want me to say anything. She wanted me to bear witness, as doctors do, to the faith that finds no expression in the realm of the religious.

How does anyone become free to place their heart or, as Buddhist meditation teacher Sharon Salzberg puts it, to form the faith that comes of trusting their own deepest experience? How do we encounter the infinite unknown without falling into the role of the child who never grows up, or into the forms of comprehension that bar apprehension and recognition, and supplant naked reality with a human projection? How do we know what it is to be a "child of Man," or to rest in God, or to fill with Spirit, or to reach the limits of our being and becoming, to rest with ease in the place where we know nothing and where we may experience the vertiginous freedom in which we penetrate all of our notions without losing our minds? I don't know.

I do know that if you are well-grounded and open, you will encounter the unseen and unknown and find your present ways of comprehending the finite and infinite insufficient. The task ahead of you then is to engage other fields through methods that you may see as historically spiritual or scientific. As you seek a way to integrate human tools that will encompass the unheard-of in ways that enable you to comprehend the care of one as all, you may follow the Way, wrestle with God, do the Work, comprehend Newton and Einstein, surrender to the nothing that is the all, or form a spirit body that will endure. These will prepare you to fully embody and contextualize your medical life, and so to enter into the secret heart of the profession where you encounter and engage the eternal.

Your Destiny

We are often asked, 'if dolphins are so intelligent, why aren't they ruling the world?' My very considered answer is—they may be too wise to try… it is a very insecure position to want to rule all of the other species and the vast resources of our planet… One's fears and one's angers are being projected on others outside of oneself.

— John C. Lilly in "Toward a Cetacean Nation" in *Between Species*

WORKING QUESTIONS

Employed Physicians

- Is what I am doing right now necessary or desirable?
- What is my experience telling me now?
- Why am I behaving this way right now? Is this right for me? What would serve my purpose better?
- Is what I am expected to do right now the right thing to do?
- What is this meme supposed to mean and what does it reveal about truth and lies? If it's misguiding me, how can I filter it out?

Self-determined Physicians

- What is the ultimate purpose of the life that I have been creating? What do I want my life purpose to be from now on?
- What meaning can I draw from my personal past? From the pasts of my kindred, of my community, of my profession, of my species, of my habitats, and of life on earth?
- What purpose can I glean from the history of my profession, my species, and the body of life? From the evolving human response to its context?
- What do I want my purpose to become as my life reaches its fulfillment?
- If I were looking in J. K. Rowling's *Mirror of Erised* (which would show my deepest desire), what would I see right now? Would I see something that I want because others want it, or would I see something that comes from my truest self?

- When you are lying on your deathbed, what will you look back on with relief? With satisfaction? With regret? With gladness?

EXERCISE: Biography

Look for an autobiography of a doctor or several doctors whom you might wish to emulate in your elder years, and see if you can pinpoint what it is that inspires you in terms of priming, stance, states, strategies, skills, and vision. In other words, discern the life processes and visualize them as potential life processes for yourself.

In your journal, note down aspects of the life narratives that inspire you as well as pitfalls that you would wish to avoid.

FIELD TRIP: Organize a Medical Pilgrimage

Doctors tend to be great travelers to places of significance in medical history. Depending on your interests and resources, consider going to Kos to see the tree and temple of Hippocrates; the birthplace of Maimonides in Spain; the medical museums in Edinburgh; or another location closer to home. Read up on contemporaneous medical history before you go, and go as soon as convenient.

Or, do some local eco-travel and read more about habitats and practical ecology or living buildings in anticipation of living forward.

Supplementary Reading

1. James Orbinski, M.D. *An Imperfect Offering: Humanitarian Action for the Twenty-First Century.* New York: Walker & Company, 2008.
2. Tracey Kidder. *Mountains Beyond Mountains.* New York: Random House, 2003.
3. Oliver Sacks. *On the Move: A Life.* New York: Alfred A. Knopf, 2015.
4. *Bodysnatchers to Lifesavers* (see June list). A ready source of brief bios that may suggest a subject.

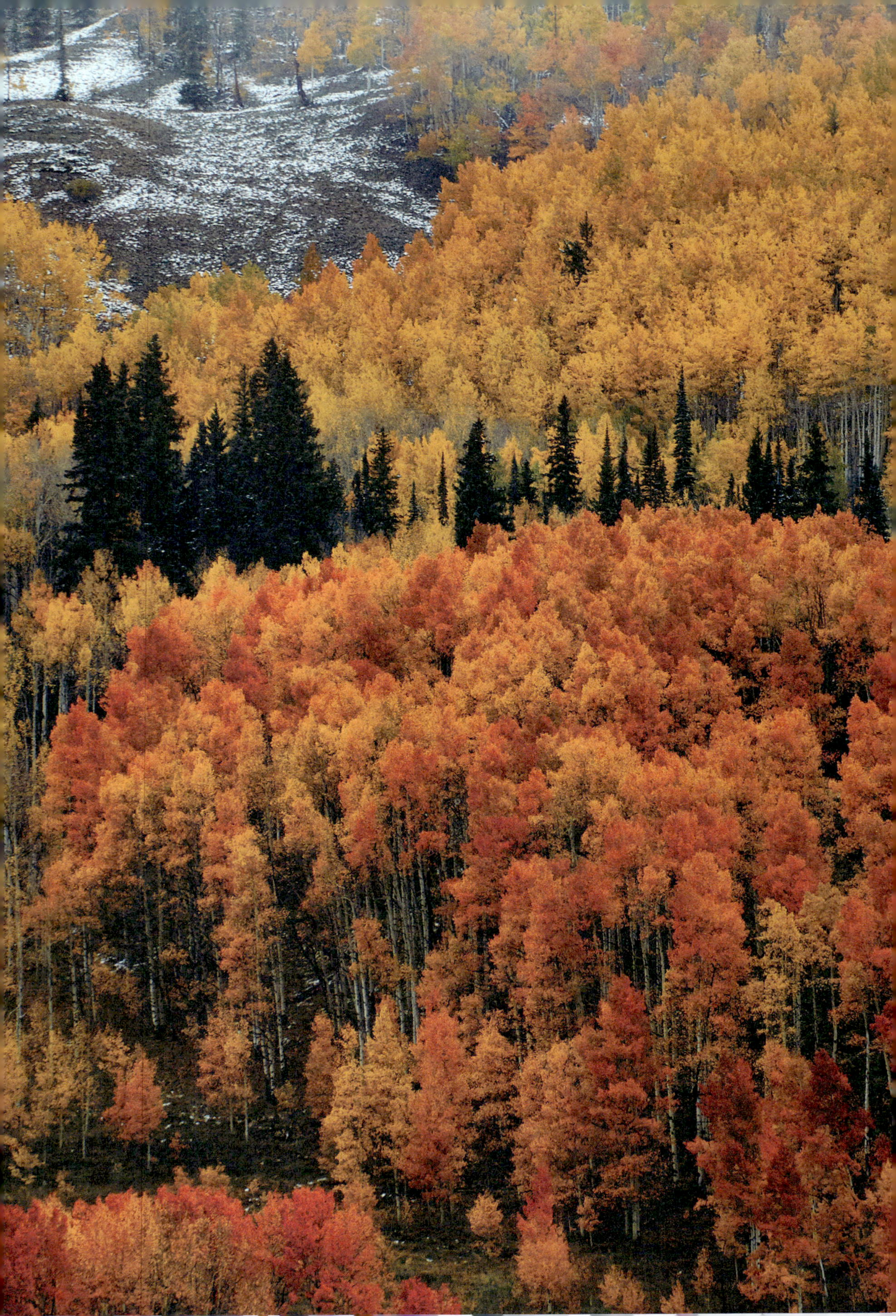

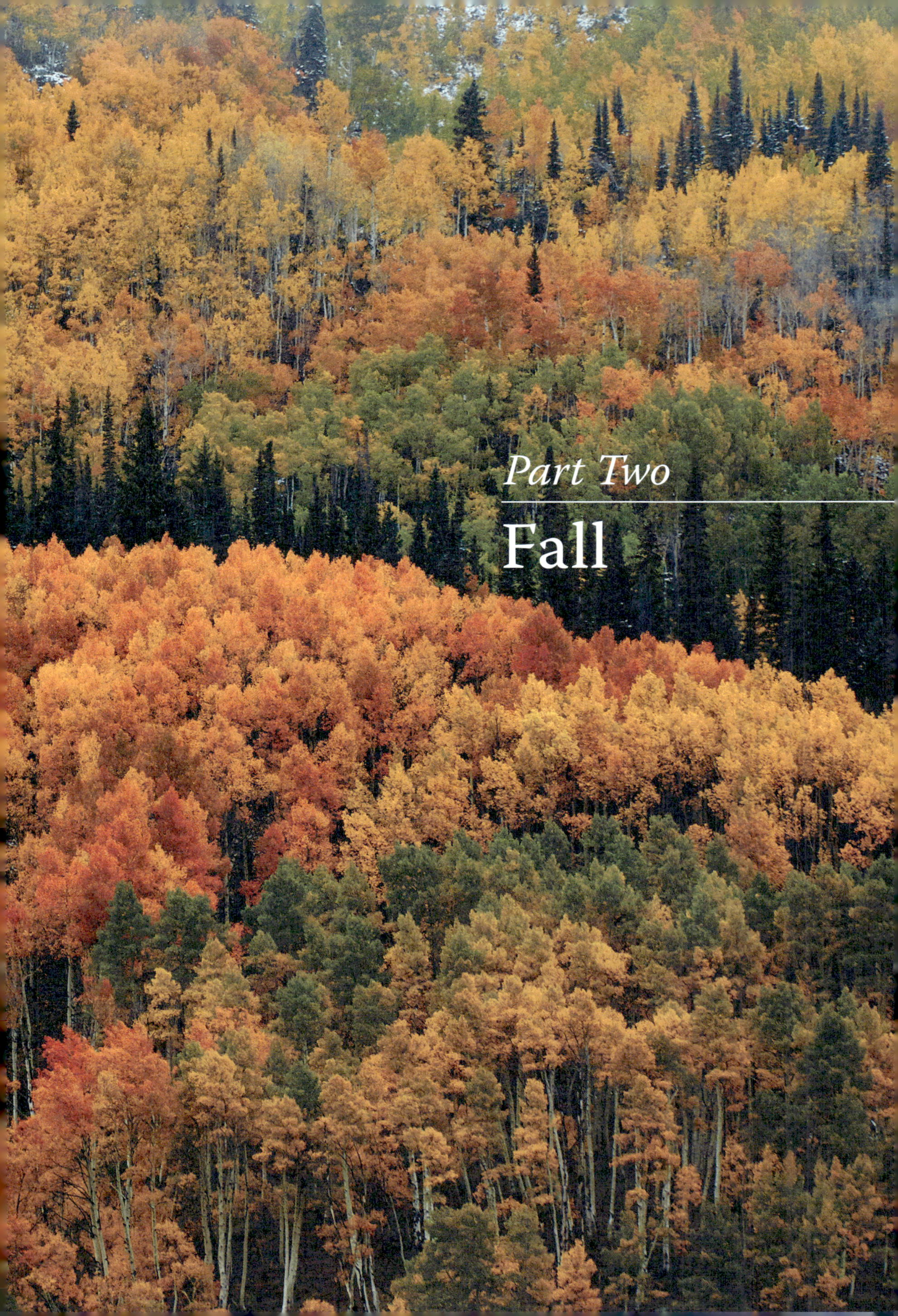

Part Two

Fall

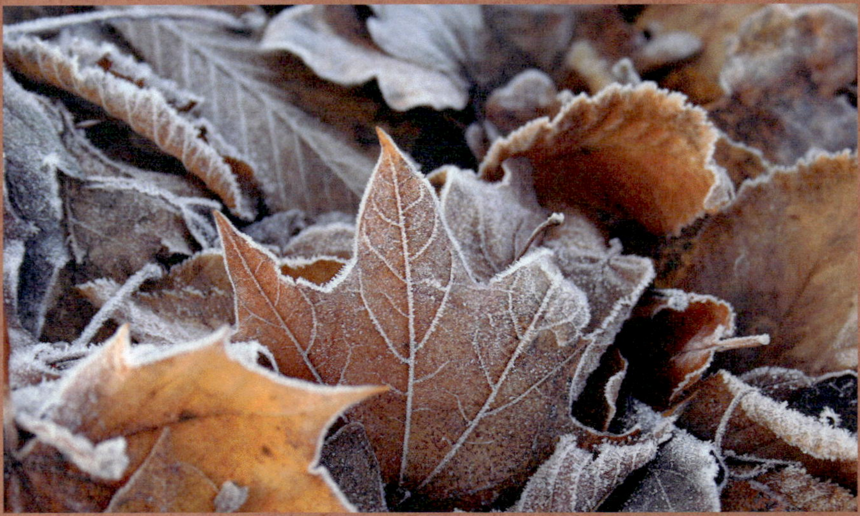

THINK ABOUT ROUSING YOUR CURIOSITY AS TO HOW THE SPECIES AS A WHOLE IS DEFINING THE FUTURE OF LIFE. THINK OF MAKING YOUR WAY TO THE MOVING FRONT OF TIME AND ABIDING THERE AS YOU MAKE THE FINAL CHOICES THAT WILL DEFINE YOUR LIFEWORK AND LEGACY FOR THOSE WHO ARE TOUCHED OR CHANGED BY YOU.

Opening to Wisdom

Fool: Yes, indeed. Thou wouldst make a good fool.

Lear: To take't again perforce—Monster ingratitude!

Fool: If thou wert my fool, nuncle, I'd have thee beaten for being old before thy time.

Lear: How's that?

Fool: Thou shouldst not have been old till thou hadst been wise.

— William Shakespeare in *King Lear* through Alfred Harbage

FALL

In fall, the colors of turning leaves, the migrations of animals, the beginning of a new academic year for youth may fill you with anticipation even as the waning light and the holidays remind you of the inherent transience of a life. Fall is thus the ideal time to prepare for the wisdom years by gathering the fruits of your lifetime of labor and ease. Reflecting on your life as a whole and on its context leads naturally to your reorientation to biological time and to life on earth, and to the revision of your life narrative as part of the story of life on earth.

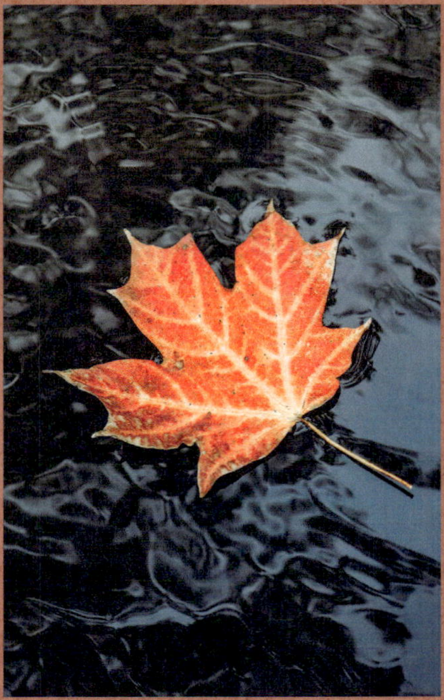

In fall, holidays like Halloween, Day of the Dead, and Thanksgiving may remind you of your fears, your connection to the past, and your reliance on the bounty of life since it began. They transcend your frailty by their recurrence across generations, cultures, and habitats. They endure through human cultivation and care of the sources of life.

This fall, in order to put your past to rest and prepare to focus on your future, I invite you to delve more deeply into your present context in time and life while continuing to tend to your body. You can play with this process of reorientation in your journal by using the reporters' five W's to observe events: who, what, when, where, and why—leaving the modern favorite, how, for the spring.

As you catch the smell of fallen leaves, see lights go on as dusk comes earlier, or put on dark clothing against the new chill in the air, take time to identify fall-blooming flowers like dahlias or asters. Observe birds preparing for winter, and enjoy the cozy feel of a warm hat or coat. Ponder the moving front of time where a plethora of possibilities is reduced to a moment of countless choices that becomes one shared past. Think about rousing your curiosity as to how the species as a whole is defining the future of life. Think of making your way to the moving front of time and abiding there as you make the final choices that will define your lifework and legacy for those who are touched or changed by you. This work—the last expression of your living fertility—will take time and thought and love of life, especially of the remainder of your lifetime, the final chapter of the personal narrative you have been forming and reforming in response to events in time.

Because your life makes no sense out of context, use your growing wisdom to envision a way to bring forward the best of your personal and shared past, to transform past problems into present solutions, and to leave a legacy for your posterity that enriches the living future. Notice that the species is becoming more aware of biology through sustainability, and recognize that the big picture is supporting your reorientation to your lifetime as integral to biological time. Ease this process by taking a page from the work of Dr. Viktor Frankl, founder of the third Viennese school of psychotherapy: revisit your life as you consider your personal narrative; frame it as a continuous source of profound questions to which you are responding by constructing your unique character arcs, plots, pauses, and themes.

This fall, a season of transition in your year of transition, is associated with the harvest and with turning inward. Let it be a time of winnowing, when you contemplate modernity, life on earth, and your own deeply felt experience. Discover old tasks and concerns that you are ready to leave behind. Set in front of you unfinished business that will cease impeding your thought and creativity when you finally finish or let go of it. If you are haunted by something that hijacks your attention, as traumatic memories or disproportionate regret may do, consider supplementing your transition with targeted counseling, a do-it-yourself adaptation of a twelve-step program, or a self-made ritual of writing and burning confessions and atoning as needed to reconcile your conscience.

Orienting Your Being and Doing in Time

The paradox that now emerges is that only a system with short memory can follow the environment. But the optimum parameters of the tracking system depend on the mean, variance and autocorrelation of the environment, [and] these can only be estimated accurately by a system with a long enough memory."

— Richard Levins in *Evolution in Changing Environments*

To guide your moment-to-moment existence as a post-employment doctor, and comprehend the present challenges of the profession you vowed to keep, you must orient yourself with respect to person, habitat, and time now and continuously into the future. You cannot rely on media or books for this; you must examine your life experience and then contextualize it by using your knowledge base, adding to it as needed. As you try on this version of the emerging paradigm, avail yourself of current work in other fields such as history that will give you a new perspective from which to view your past.

We are at the end of the modern era. Modernism arguably began with the pandemics of bubonic plague that formed deep-seated habits of possessive individualism—that is, the beginnings of privacy and personal hoarding. These deep changes in turn catalyzed the Protestantism that subsequently nurtured freedom of thought and experimentation, including the medical work of Boerhaave and the doctors of the Scottish Enlightenment. This freedom came at the cost of a power struggle between states and then between doctors and clergy that all but divided doctors from their religious and spiritual context and led to a schism between clergy and the living, evolving systems of the natural world.

In Shakespeare's Hamlet, late moderns can revisit the genesis of new habits of conscience and personal responsibility that primed humans to undertake essential global change from the periphery, culminating in the hygiene movement and the grassroots rights movements of the past century—including independence from colonialism.

This extraordinary and well-recorded process of human social evolution informs our use of the wisdom that developed with modernity, such as the realization that fatalism is a choice. The Enlightenment idea of optimization and the desire for active, effective patient care—that is, heroic medicine—spurred doctors to face the unknown with sanguine optimism and determination, to hold open questions, and to try to save lives. Unfortunately, the old illusion of control combined with the old fear of the wild unleashed unprecedented disregard for living systems. At the same time, the virtual reality of industrial and information systems relegated doctors to the role of employees. The old way by which doctors used shaming to punish unusual or dangerous doctor behavior—the morbidity and mortality conference—has given way to management by metrics administered from afar. There is, in short, a weakened group dynamic that could make way for freer learning but is negated by excessive obedience, money, and management that precludes thinking and common sense. Moreover, to play it safe from lawsuits, we had to be 'DDDs'—that is, dumb dedicated doctors. And so we are. And so the modern idolatry of data and technology is minding the store—with its hand in the till.

To place modernity in the context of the evolution of Hippocratic medicine, we recall that Hippocrates was practicing a form of indigenous medicine grounded in ancient elemental thinking. He transformed this thinking with his theory of the four humors, which linked the signs and symptoms of disease with the fluids of the body. His naturalistic view, which informed what we might anachronistically call his guild, gave way over time to the medieval model of globalist medical doctors like Maimonides, whose comprehensive integrative thinking encompassed the material and ethereal. His unitive view of the body was far more sophisticated than the elemental view or the naturalistic view, and was sustained by rabbis. It has been forgotten by doctors, scientists, and seminal analytic thinkers in theology, medicine, and the natural sciences. Thus the modern era deconstructed body-centered wisdom much as Freud, Babinsky and Charcot later deconstructed clinical neurology.

To consider what best to do next, recall the advantages of globalism. The Silk Road that once carried wisdom to Maimonides and that was interrupted by the flow of human history has opened again in an era of dynamic communication in real time. We are coming into contact with modalities of care and cure that developed in many habitats and across a wide swathe of the living cultures on earth. We therefore have an unprecedented opportunity to take the long view, the broad view, and the deep view of human evolution and existence. In doing so, we can orient our views of medicine to deep time as well as to the immediate moment.

This connectivity comes at a critical moment in your career and in the history of the body of life, including our species. As presented in popular books such as Charles Mann's 1491, Elizabeth Kolbert's *The Sixth Extinction*, and James Lovelock's *Healing Gaia*, as well as the body of work by geneticist and communicator David Suzuki, we can no longer afford to ignore the consequences to life on earth of the reckless, unintentional, and—unfortunately—complete experiment of modernity. As mentioned earlier, it is useful to liken the consequences of our recent ways of living to a case of galloping consumption of the body of life. To ignore this disease is to relapse into passivism and to risk the future of the living world that we late moderns now control.

To bring this point home, we can become more familiar with our global and historical contexts through archaeologists, who have been obliged to coin the term Anthropocene to take account of the fact that humans have altered the face of the globe. In North America, modern humans have erased 95% of habitats. Worldwide, we have developed, dug up, or deforested 80% of the earth's landmass.

In other words, we have no choice but to care for and cure the body of life—with no more data, information, knowledge or wisdom than we have now. As doctors, we are among the few mainstream groups—like farmers—who gather extensive knowledge of life and who are accustomed to taking direct action and responsibility. Like common sense, this union of knowledge of and responsibility for life is extremely—even hazardously—uncommon in this era of urbanization. Lest our species go the way of the habitat-integrated peoples who are now gone because moderns 'triumphed'—that is, lest we all disappear from the earth—we late moderns must step up and amend our deadly habits, which are now entangled with medicine as well as with conventional agriculture and architecture. To do this, we doctors must work in concert with wisdom keepers who have been divided from us by modern ways—e.g. clergy, field biologists, and veterinarians—and with emerging stewards of life such as habitat restorers, communicators, and habitat integrators.

ANECDOTES FROM MEDICAL LIVES

I kept trying to remind [my fellow] geneticists of the disastrous consequences that had resulted from claims made by equally eminent geneticists only two generations before. It has been a lonely role for a geneticist to raise issues of concern when there was and is so much enthusiasm and so much apparent potential for revolutionary applications.

— DAVID SUZUKI in *The Autobiography*

At the turn of the last century, innovators moved beyond anatomical primacy and began to recover and to advance knowledge of the intangible body. This knowledge was known to Hippocrates and Maimonides, lost in the mechanical thinking of the industrial age, and rediscovered by pioneers such as Drs. William James, Carl Jung, and Sigmund Freud, and later also by Adler, Frankl, and many others. Their experiences remind us of the hazards of discovery that we see in Dr. Sir Arthur Conan Doyle's profile in the book *Lifesavers to Bodysnatchers* and in the film *A Dangerous Method*, which recounts the difficulties that Drs. Jung and Freud experienced on attempting talking cures of doctor-patients Otto Gross and Sabina Spielrein. In Doyle's case, he and his fellow student physicians risked their lives to find the right doses of anesthesia; in the case of Jung and Freud, giving up their gounding in the flesh left them without a gold standard to guide their work.

As you look back on your life and seek to comprehend the route and result of your experiences to date, you can explore the works of poets and preachers who perceive a life's journey in terms of paths taken—or, as with Robert Frost, in terms of roads not taken. Emerson, from his Concord-based perspective on westward expansion, advised students to go "where there is no path and leave a trail." As you move forward into the unknown future and perhaps forge a new path, take time to look back at the paths you took and did not take, where they led or could have led you, and where you might like to go next.

As you consider your unique sequence of forays into the modern world, contextualize them by comparing them to those taken by your contemporaries or near contemporaries, especially any who took it upon themselves to solve fundamental medical problems. These include doctors who participated in the eradication of smallpox, e.g. Larry Brilliant and William Foege; who provide medical relief, e.g. Paul Farmer and James Orbinski; who study or criticize the profession from the inside, e.g. the mavericks like Alvan Feinstein,

David Sackett, and doctors of integrative medicine; and explorers at the frontier of patient self-care, e.g. Andrew Weil, Dean Ornish, Mehmet Oz, and Deepak Chopra.

Julie

Julie has always been independent-minded, and devised her career accordingly. Formed by a childhood in the self-reliant, independent-minded culture of Alaska, and inspired by a close female relative who was an executive at a major network when women in such positions were rare, Julie believed that she could do anything she chose to do, and set out to push back the frontier of modern medicine. She was the first to administer AZT in a human being; participated in the development of effective delivery systems for cholera vaccines in Bangladesh; and, at an age when others might retire, joined a start-up developing an effective treatment for Menière's disease.

In other words, Julie has managed—despite living in the late modern context in which employment defines most doctors—to own her own life and define a cutting-edge career. If you choose to forge a career path in your wisdom years, you will come to hone your judgment as to what is most important to do in the moment. You will create the independence that is integral to eldering and essential to those who follow. You may go where no one has gone before and prepare the way for the species to move forward at a critical juncture in its history by finding ways to care for one as all. Then you will own a concrete and essential task rather than a social and virtual one.

If you have been defined by the expectations of others through incentives set by an institution or system, you may lack habits of thought and action that catalyze invention and innovation. You will find, however, as you look at your past, that there was a time when you were curious; when you developed the ability to observe patients as a naturalist would observe the living world; the ability to view biological entities objectively in context; the chutzpah to act when others could or would not; and the ability to think critically about claims from both the mainstream and the fringes. You will find seeds of perspicacity, personal agency, interpersonal agency, and the ability to act wisely in response to important problems. As you transition to elderhood, you have the chance to look back and gather all of the adaptive responses that you developed over the course of your lifetime, and to apply those to care of the profession that is integral to ensuring the future of evolved life.

Dr. Thomas Chalmers

The problem with cutting-edge developments in new methods and concepts—especially statistical and technological ones—is that they are often taken at face value and then taken for granted. When others follow suit and come to depend economically on a particular method, it becomes socially fixed, its development stops, and scientific learning ceases. For example, investigators rush to win funding from their peers by looking into 'hot' molecules. Well-paid researchers do not look to life but to the dream of finding a key drug that will prove profitable and do some good. Examples include the floods of studies on the effects of prostaglandins, leukotrienes, statins, and the dazzler that crosses decades—DNA.

For the well-regarded investigator who devises new ideas and methods—and has the integrity to learn from experience—a momentary glimpse of order in a pile of absorbing details may be taken for a breakthrough and used to establish a new social consensus. Fundability and publishability are conflated with knowledge and wisdom. The social approach to biological phenomena is thus limited by habits of thought that arrest innovation and dampen—or preclude—new biomedical learning in response to disease as it unfolds.

In the United States, the social process of medical research has been mediated in large part by the National Institutes of Health, which considers proposals for studies on topics of interest to the research community. Peer committees evaluate proposals on a periodic basis, rate their merit, and disburse available funds to those rated most highly. Oftentimes, funded studies are inconclusive in whole or in part, and others are done to attempt to resolve the issue. Eventually, a whole string of studies on the same topic yields conflicting and seemingly irreconcilable results, with years upon years of work and millions upon millions of dollars of investment for naught. Conscientious investigators develop the creeping suspicion that they have been wasting their lives. Others may declare conclusive results. Confidence in centralized management of the unknown slips. Morale wavers.

Into this breach stepped the eminent, well-intentioned, and kind investigator Dr. Thomas Chalmers, who devised a solution that allowed investigators to pool the results of myriads of studies. He called this solution meta-analysis. With this approach, his peers and juniors pooled data across studies. Investigators sighed with relief. Their methods must be working! A flood of analyses was reported. Those who devoted their lives to this system—which

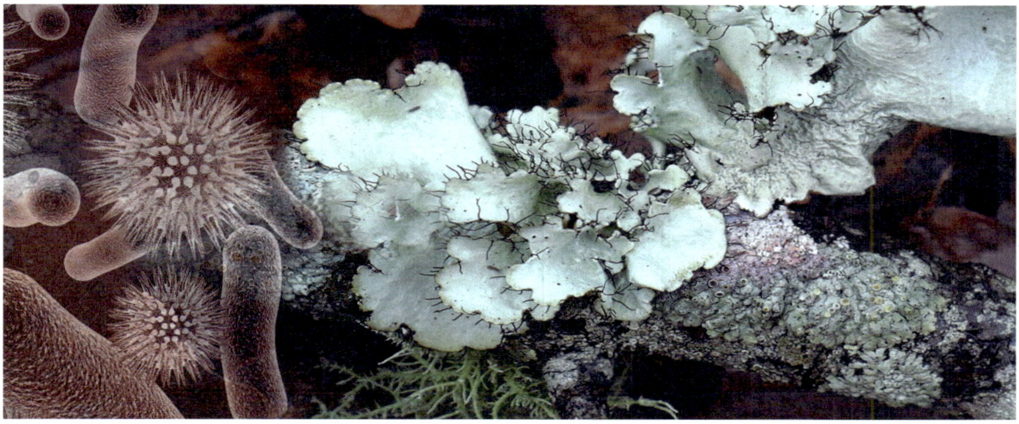

was, unfortunately, as good as it got—continue to believe that they will be able to make the status quo work. The country—the world—continues to rely on this system years after the acceptance of meta-analysis. Dr. Chalmers did not.

I had the opportunity to see Dr. Chalmers give a talk. He was in his wisdom years and was well-loved as a leader in his field. He was speaking to a room full of well-dressed, successful researchers and other colleagues who had used meta-analysis to advance their careers. After speaking for a number of minutes on the topic that he had been asked to address—namely, meta-analysis—he began to share an anecdote about a patient whom he had been seeing. He was taking a new approach, the N-of-1 randomized trial, which had enabled his chronically-ill patient to discover which of the available symptomatic treatments gave her the best result. In her case, as in any individual case of chronic illness, he pointed out, the results of studies in groups of patients did not matter; what did matter was her personal experience.

The room kept an impassive silence like the one that greeted Dr. Carlos Finlay back when he reported that yellow fever was transmitted by a mosquito vector, a fact that was only believed when Dr. Walter Reed verified it with an experiment that involved loss of human life. It was as if the perceptual filters of Dr. Chalmer's audience made them impervious to a particularist view—particularism now being a footnote to generalism in college philosophy courses—as well as to the possibility that clinical evidence might trump the social consensus in 'evidence-based' medicine. In other words, they seemed to be patiently indulging the musings of an old man who they hoped might return to his former way of thinking.

I appreciated Dr. Chalmer's kind humility and honest integrity, and wonder to this day if anyone else noticed and appreciated that he had continued to learn when others would have wished him to stop. I wondered if they, too, had noticed that the production chain of research that gives us end-to-end control has become disconnected at both ends from ecological realities, and so is failing to keep up with clinical realities. Wise elders are free to take the long view, to gently lead others to examine the well-oiled machine of modern virtual medicine, and to experiment anew—at least at the periphery—so as to learn in real time.

Dr. Alvan Feinstein

It is easy to love leaders who show us the way to an inspiring vision; it is less easy to love self-appointed critics who prod us on, or to love conscientious thinkers who burst the bubbles that seem to be carrying us toward a victory lap but that are in fact taking us toward an unforeseen fall. These critics poke us and thus awaken us from a false and perilous feeling of comfort; for so doing, they deserve our gratitude and praise. This will be easier to see and to accept in the elder years, when you are more inclined to think of what you can give to posterity than of what you can take from it.

One figure on whom I look back with gratitude is Dr. Alvan Feinstein. I recall reading one of his articles in which he pointed out that studies of the hazards of everyday life were subject to hazards of their own. I had read many and more critical articles that gave formulae for knowing which studies were sound, or that quibbled with specific points that had escaped the social consensus, or that urged new studies to fill in the gaps in the medical database or to correct its errors. I had also read a few—those by Kenneth Rothman, Jamie Robbins, and their close peers—that pointed out fundamental errors in our methodology, and others—those by Tversky and Kahneman and members of the Society for Medical Decision Making—that pointed out fundamental errors of human perception and comprehension that were, once you got them, all too easy to see. I had yet to see any of this reach or influence doctors or researchers, or to hear anyone say publicly that institutionalizing clinical research also divided it from life.

Around that time, I had the opportunity to see Dr. Feinstein address a group of researchers at the annual meeting of the Society for Medical Decision Making. The hall was packed, and the energy in the room was high. Dr. Feinstein moved freely on the stage as he spoke, stopping once to mime doffing his cranial vault like a hat. "Please," he said, "fill my empty cranium." He was mocking the tendency of doctors to adopt the dogma of other fields in hopes of improving clinical care. These included law, which worsened the glut of lawsuits clogging the legal system and that led doctors to validate the obvious with expenditures intended to 'treat the chart.' They also included business and economics, which were intended to fuel competition but in fact—predictably so, given studies on willingness to pay in times of medical crisis—fueled the proliferation of unsustainable 'products' such as tertiary-care hospitals and precise imaging modalities of marginal diagnostic utility.

Feinstin was sardonic, sharp, quick-witted, irreverent, and a rascal. He was a devil's advocate. Unfortunately, he represented the epitome of post-modern analysis—that is, the criticism that comes from a view that offers just enough perspective to tear a system down but not enough to put it together again. When a member of the audience—which was filled with his juniors—asked him what they should do to correct errors and right wrongs, he shrugged his shoulders. He was mute. I saw then, as never before or since, that we were too like lemmings for comfort. Though disillusioned with the status quo, we were still waiting for answers to descend from above. I also saw, with some discomfort, that wasn't up to him to provide an answer: it was up to each and every one of us.

BETH LOOKS BACK

We need planetary medicine. Its approach may be empirical, even at times unscientific, but it is all that we have...The mere employment of a hundred new and brightly polished doctors of philosophy...is most unlikely to achieve anything other than provide them with secure and comfortable employment.

—James Lovelock in *Healing Gaia: Practical Medicine for the Planet*

Some time after the beginning of my post-employment years, while I was searching for a more constructive way to frame, model, and engage health and disease, I began to see the flaws of methods used by modern epidemiologists. These methods had functioned well in the early years of quantification and estimation of risks related to overwhelming causes of disease, such as smoking and alcohol. As noted by critic Dr. Alvan Feinstein, these methods didn't function as well in studies of the ordinary hazards of everyday life. They may have been the best we had, and yet they led to confusing and inconclusive results that better reflected the nature of our tools than the biological realities we purported to reveal. The persistence of dependence on these methods had more to do with sustaining the social consensus and the illusion of control than with any realistic search for truth or comprehension.

Effective leaders of the past overcame inertia and friction well enough to sustain morale and to keep modern and pre-modern social systems going in spite of their inadequate premises and pointless frictions. Such leaders were—like Churchill—Godsends in a pinch, but they could not lift the status quo. In academia—as in all institutional systems—the status quo is generally taken as sacrosanct and is rarely subject to questioning from 'below' or to revision through experiential learning. The greater the inertia of a system, the more it behaves like a spinal reflex in which the afferent part of the loop has been cut. This is the reason that we continued using methods that might or might not be better than lore or reaction to lore, and that substitutes scientism for science, which involves risky encounters with the unknown. It is safer in the short run to meet, exceed, and reinforce social expectations.

If that was not the safe road, we would not prefer our models to reality. We would not lump when we should split just because it makes our statistical methods work; or externalize from our models the interdependent aspects of life—which includes almost all biological processes that matter; or continue to use methods that we have exhausted; or continue to reason from the general to the particular as if the inverse were not the other half of a dynamic equilibrium essential to personal and congregal learning. When there is no solid clinical science, and a case study has the chance to solve at least one case, particularism is the best choice: the N-of-1 study is the only way to remove the noise due to confounding and effect modificaton by uncountable interconnected processes that obscure signals pointing to etiopathogenesis.

And so, I began to read and to appreciate the value of anecdotes and long medical narratives, particularly those of William James, A.R. Luria, and Oliver Sacks. I also began to see the value in investigating pressing biological realities with the best available rather than the expected methods; honoring experiential learning; recognizing that moderns have already destroyed or damaged much of life on earth; and responding to presnet realities by constructing new forms of comprehension of the body and its ills.

And now, as I look forward to medical eldering, I have written an N-of-1 case study that I hope may inspire those who keep faith with the profession: *Medical Detective - Chronic Ambient Poisoning*, which links the dying planet with emerging epidemics of chronic disease.

Comment on Orienting to Medical Time

If anyone actually visits the Amazon or the Arctic expecting to see what they saw in a film, they will be very disappointed, because the one thing nature needs is the one thing television cannot tolerate: time.

—David Suzuki in *The Autobiography*

As we move beyond the now-facile methods that are passing away with the modern paradigm and in their places draw on the wisdom of habitat-integrated peoples, we face the daunting but exciting task of forming a paradigm that promotes long-term survival. The lead time introduced by late modern management can be cut by an emerging paradigm for discovery that is interactive, iterative, and efficient with respect to the emerging epidemics of chronic exposure. We thus have a crucial chance to free medical innovation of the ill-fitting, high-inertia, costly, top-down, and complex systems that disregard devolving biological realities.

Those of us who step up to guide the profession though a time of fundamental change face the task of forming provisional views and constructs to support the rapid evolution of coordinated but diverse and dispersed experiments in the care and cure of each as all. That is, we have the chance to envision and—perhaps—to practice big-picture medicine that does not put our species at the center of the universe, or impose early or false consensus, or value time or money above life. This approach, which is like networking but is alive and therefore is more than a tool, may enable us to solve our most pressing self-created problems in time to rescue the patient that includes all patients: the body of life.

If we do our work well, our juniors will be able to stand on our shoulders and look ahead, perhaps to a vision of how our species can act as the immune and nervous systems of the body of life, or as an adjunct of all systems, and so catalyze and coordinate care and cure across species. They may then grasp in ways that we cannot foresee the ancient visions of prophets like Isaiah, who foresaw a time when the lion would lay down with the lamb and peace would prosper—and with it, our profession and our species.

Our first task is to mind the store. We have not been doing our work as allopaths; we have been effecting centralized policies that might or might not hold up to common sense. We can begin by welcoming those visionary polymaths who have stepped up in our place and formed the emerging paradigm that crosses the mountains of data and chasms of ignorance that divide medicine from fields such as religion, field biology, veterinary medicine, and the simpler so-called hard sciences. To draw on the historical views and constructs created by our species, we must put our heads together now, for no single mind can hold all of the strategies and skills required to solve any one of our pressing global problems.

We must therefore welcome the good intentions of scientists like James Lovelock, who work outside the mainstream and who make the mistakes that we are all bound to make. When he conflated animal, vegetable, and mineral, we pushed him beyond the pale. Let's hope that those who step up to guide other fields are more charitable to us when we prove unable to solve linear equations in our heads, or to distinguish one type of sea gull from another, or to provide an exegesis for a scriptural passage, or to interpret a passage of ancient epic poetry.

As we step up to elderhood, one of the tasks of integration that we face is to make sense of the overly detailed—not to say shattered—late modern view of the body. This excessively detailed view has lulled us into the false belief that we can care for life one molecule—or one class of molecules—at a time. We cannot. We cannot even care for one species or one habitat at a time. We can only care for each as all and for all as one. As we seek to create new simplicity from overwhelming complexity, we can be aware that while we may be able to envision unity, we will not be able to analyze it—at least not yet. Our brains can hold only three to seven variables at once; a group mind may, if all goes well, be able to comprehend many more between its members.

Constant change—in past times most often incremental or marginal—is integral to keeping up with biological realities, which we are now impacting—mostly annihilating—as a species. The creation of new problems cannot be avoided, but it can be slowed so that our ability to create living solutions is able to at least keep up. To create change that is continuous and that responds to consequences in real time, we will have to accept that we cannot foresee our errors and must always be looking out for them—both where we might expect them to occur and where we might not. We therefore save ourselves headaches when we anticipate that no new solution will be good enough to endure without adaptation, and that even it if were, the context would change and necessitate continuing transformation.

Orienting Being and Doing in Time

There is a kind of contagion that affects the imagination unconsciously much more than we realize. It emanates from things like advertisements and from all the spurious fantasies that are thrown at us [and become] a form of tyranny.

— Thomas Merton in *Christian Mystics* by Matthew Fox

WORKING QUESTIONS

Employed Physicians

- What would it feel like to take a black bag on an airplane and travel to a place off the grid where doctors are needed?
- If I had no technology at hand and had to rely on my clinical skills and the medications I brought along, could I be of use to patients?
- If I had to treat people who live in the wild, would I have any idea what health risks they might face? If I went to an unfamiliar healthy habitat, would I be able to make use of local flora for patient care?
- If I had no MRI, would it change my outcomes?
- Does imaging that is more detailed seem more informative? Is it detecting preclinical findings that may resolve spontaneously? What diagnostic tests do I use that the patient could not do without?

Self-determined Physicians

- What were my usual stance and state of being during my early years? What were they during the peak of my career? What are they now? What would I like them to be in the final phases of my personal life and my medical life?
- What events or circumstances in my early life primed me to go into medicine? What primed me to transition to eldering? How will I refresh my priming in the future?
- If I had a time machine, what period in medical history would I visit, and who would I seek out to share conversation or action? What aspects of the living future capture my interest? What enduring impact would I wish to have on the future of life?

EXERCISE: Representing Your Temporal Context

Now that you have had a chance to ponder deep time, revisit it and connect it with your priming and your evolving stance. Begin by creating a visual representation of your lifetime from the year of your birth to the actuarial expectation of your year of death. Draw this representation on a wide sheet of paper, or a number of pieces of letter paper joined in landscape aspect. Use 1 cm or 1 inch per year.

Then, using your memories as they are now, draw in your major life events, the ones that are easy to recall. Once these are in place, think of the things that you have done, and draw those in. You may find your timeline broadening to accommodate everything that has been meaningful to you, such as gatherings of extended family or participation in public or professional events. Do not feel obliged to include things that had little significance to you. Now, see if you can depict events that changed your baseline state of being or marked you emotionally in one way or another. When you finish, go back and record any periods of darkness or happiness or peaks of distress or celebration.

When your personal timeline is finished, make several others that encompass longer and longer periods of time:

1. A timeline of the past 100 years showing historical events that impacted your lifetime and your parents' and grandparents' generations. Include any biological events that you know of.
2. A timeline of your legal ancestry back to your eight great-grandparents, or farther if you know your more distant ancestry. Include any medical information that you recall.
3. A timeline that highlights the past "Big Five" extinctions and known periods of glaciation. Include the locations of continents at those times.

Now, compare and reconcile the timelines. Which carry emotional weight in your being? Does any reveal what you are "spring-loaded" to accomplish in your lifetime? If so, does it reveal something of your present stance?

Next, do a timeline of the history of medicine. Record on it events that move or motivate you. Does this reveal any other priming or inform your present stance?

If these questions reveal little, return to them again and observe your feelings carefully as you look through what you have created. Pay special heed to any tension, joy, heartache, or pleasure that is prompted in you by past events. Then reflect on your priming and stance. Repeat until you develop a connection to your embodied experience. Record your findings carefully in your journal. Each time, continue to elaborate on your exploration as long as you are in 'the zone'—that is, able to make it productive.

Supplementary Reading

Lifetimes

1. Jerome Bruner. *Acts of Meaning.* Revised edition. Cambridge: Harvard University Press, 1990.
2. Don Richard Riso and Russ Hudson. *The Wisdom of the Enneagram: The Complete Guide to Psychological and Spiritual Growth for the Nine Personality Types.* New York: Bantam, 1999.
3. Terry Tempest Williams. *The Hour of Land: A Personal Topography of America's National Parks.* New York: Sarah Crichton Books/Farrar, Straus and Giroux, 2016.
4. Apricot Irving. *The Gospel of Trees.* New York: Simon & Schuster, 2018.

Generations

5. Thomas Berry. *The Dream of the Earth.* New York: Random House, 1988.
6. Wendell Berry. *What are People For?* New York: North Point Press, 1990.
7. Matthew Fox. *The Reinvention of Work: A New Vision of Livelihood for Our Time.* San Francisco: HarperSanFrancisco, 1994.
8. Aldous Huxley. *The Perennial Philosophy.* New York: Harper & Brothers, 1944, 1945.

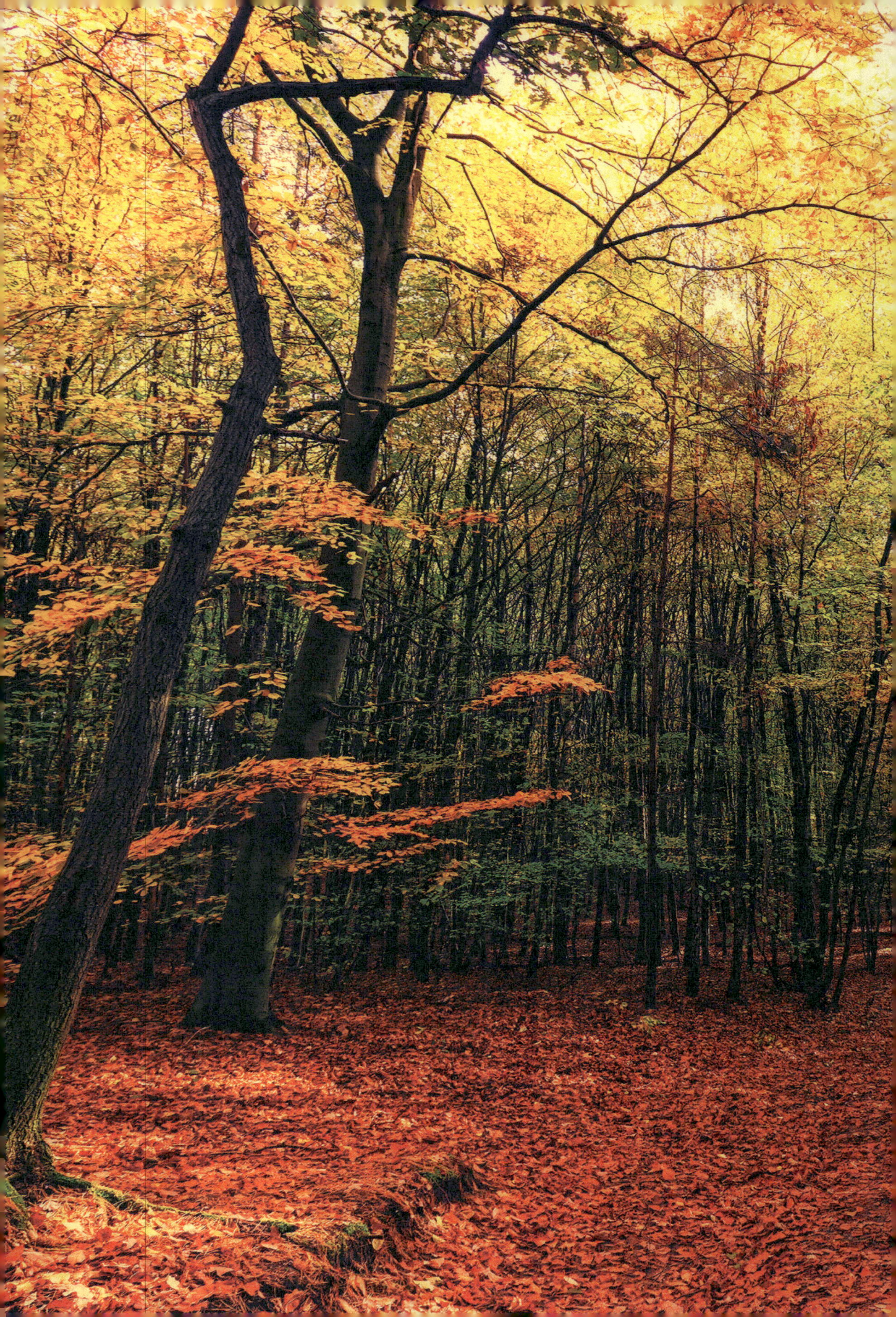

Orienting to the Body of Life

After the Hippocratic era, fundamental advances in the concepts of disease were few and long in gestation...In the ecological model, the interrelationships are appropriately described by terms like "web," "network," or "configuration." Nearly all the interactions between factors in the particular system we have examined are reciprocal and multiple.

— Mervyn Susser in *Causal Thinking in the Health Sciences*

Both inside and outside your skin, your body—which includes the highest integrative functions passed on through your vocation—is in a perpetual dynamic equilibrium with the living world of which you are an integral part, and with the substrates that support it. For example, your body is at every moment engaged in an exchange of material resources with other generators of the living world. You are exhaling carbon dioxide that plants turn into oxygen. Your resident bacteria are making essential nutrients like vitamin B12, and you are gathering and ingesting nutrients to support them in turn. Activity in gravity and calcium exchange in your gut are remodeling your bones. All the while, your highly-adapted liver and kidneys are cleansing the milieu of your being and sustaining your ephemeral, miraculous life.

In this book, I borrow the term 'interbeing' from Buddhist monk Thich Nhat Hanh, who likens the sum of all being to an ocean and each being within it—that is, each instance of generative life—to a wave on that ocean's surface. Herein, your body generates your interbeing, which joins you—material and ethereal—with the body of life and its substrates. The most proximal reach of your interbeing is the body of the species into which you were born and on which you rely for the ability to define your purpose. As a generative and social species, humans form a species body that shares processes like: sexual union with partners, family bonding with formative teaching of strategies and skills, transmission of genetic material across generations, social aggregation for invention, innovation and evolution of shared arts such as communication through language, creation of meaning through narratives, and sustenance of states of being that have the potential to nourish shared survival and thriving.

As you orient to aggregated living entities beyond the body of the species, the next body is that of the habitat. This may correspond closely to inanimate features of the earth that support life, e.g. river basins, climate zones, soil, clean water, and essential minerals. Hippocrates described habitats favorable to humans, as did others after him right down to the late modern era that is proving to be unsustainable and therefore ripe for thoughtful transformation with the recovery of useful but lapsed wisdom.

If you practice in a tertiary care institution surrounded by a vast urban area, you may strain in the fall for a glimpse of red leaves that signal the change of the seasons. If you live and practice in New York City, for example, you may take a bus to a city park, or drive north to Bear Mountain or travel to Quebec City to see the indigenous crimson maples. Even when your connection to your habitat is tenuous or invisible, and you struggle with strained social norms that further isolate you—or even overwhelm you with anomie or nihilism—you can become aware of your habitat and value it.

If you do not, you may lose your grounding in the body of life. When you are the doctor, and you wall off realities with which the profession has dealt poorly—such as social and habitat deprivation disorders—you may have to exert yourself to reestablish your grounding in your habitat and the body of life in order to help arrest or reverse the life agnosia that comes of social and biological isolation. Then, your patients and mentees can learn to care for our species in situ—in the intricately interconnected body of life on which we depend as completely as a fetus does on the womb.

If you are modern, you may try to create an artificial womb, and so reach heights of absurdity. If you are post-post-modern, and desirous of becoming one of the wise elders who guide our juniors in giving birth to the emerging, living paradigm that can rescue and—eventually—enhance life on earth, you comb human history for ready solutions such as ways the ancestors modified habitats, as described in Charles Mann's *1491*, or sustained agricultural land for millennia, as described in Michael Wood's BBC series, *The Story of England*.

ANECDOTES FROM MEDICAL LIVES

[This human-dominated] Anthropocene [epoch in geology] will be...a product of the current extinction event on the one hand and of the human propensity for redistributing life on the other...Future evolution will take place from the

surviving (and frequently anthropogenically relocated) stocks. Or, as Zaliseiwicz would have it, rats.

— Elizabeth Kolbert in *The Sixth Extinction: An Unnatural History*

If you are like many late modern doctors, your professional life may be expressed through your function in a hospital or other large institution, while your personal life may be embedded in an urban enclave. If so, your association with nature may be limited to dumpster-diving rats, a child's pet gerbil, or a struggling potted plant. Alternatively, you may live in a town where you cultivate a kitchen garden, care for a farm or woodland, and walk in nature on the weekend. Or, you may practice wilderness medicine in a place where your whole life can be immersed in nature.

In other words, your career may have placed your relationship with the natural world in any frame from out of sight and out of mind to palpable and integral to your daily happiness. Put differently, your relation to your body—and its relation to the bodies in which you nest—may fall anywhere on a spectrum from habitat-starved to habitat-integrated.

Wherever you sit on that spectrum, you will have interfaced with life in a way unknown outside the profession. You will have cared for the ills of the body of humanity while viewing it in in various lights, such as cultural and psychosocial. You need only extend your care to the patients' nested bodies, and the relation of individual ills to those of the smaller aggregated bodies—such as the microbiome—and of the larger ones—such as the biome. That is, you can begin to think and act as a doctor of life in a setting that supports you to do so, such as an emerging paradigm clinic or practice. The need has always been present; being ignored, it has reached the point of crisis and begs your fast response.

Noah: Questioning Technology

Noah trained in family medicine and then did an academic fellowship that would enable him to both research and teach. Exceptionally well-trained and accomplished, he was hired by a major university right out of training. He was to head and build an academic department devoted to primary care. Shortly after being hired, however, the administration of his university did an about-face: they decided that it would be better for their finances, prestige, and community relations were they to withdraw from primary care and rely strictly on referrals.

The residents would learn about primary care from community doctors and then go on to prestigious sub-specialties offered only by referral hospitals.

Noah's salary was safe, but his career had lost its meaning and purpose. Because his present employer also employed his new wife, he sought another post nearby. He soon joined the faculty of another highly-regarded medical school in the same metropolitan area. Now among a faculty motivated by compassion and by the desire to care for those families most in need, he regained his original purpose. He used his training to move the profession beyond the hand-holding that characterized the fee-for-service era and also beyond the reliance on lore in which decisions about patient care were based on statements that began, "Where I trained under the renowned doctor so-and-so, we always did thus-and-such."

In other words, Noah became free to help others to the best of his ability using all that he had learned. Being energetic, he was able to give his all in good faith despite living in an era wherein attention and energy was increasingly diverted to self-involved institutions dissociated from their locales. His good faith continued through all of the bureaucratic overhead imposed on him and his colleagues, until he became somewhat discouraged by the imposition of an 'updated' medical record that gave him no place to record his thoughts. The potential of placing modern medicine within a rational, scientific framework was giving way to managerial overload and excessive automation. The system was engineering delivery of data instead of supporting physicians in their ephemeral bids to offer rational, responsive, customized, humane, and fully human care.

Leah: Interspecies Joy

Like many physicians with a busy practice, Leah trained and worked at a series of referral hospitals in major urban centers. Her chosen specialty of Maternal and Fetal Medicine, which she now practices in a large city on the eastern seaboard, requires long working hours, frequent call nights, and a hobby that is engaging enough to relieve her mind of the potentially crushing responsibilities posed by her livelihood. She found that hobby in partnership with her beloved Doberman dogs: she and the youngest of those dogs compete in agility.

In the sport of dog agility, the human and her dog partner learn to navigate an obstacle course together, the dog in the role of course-running competitor

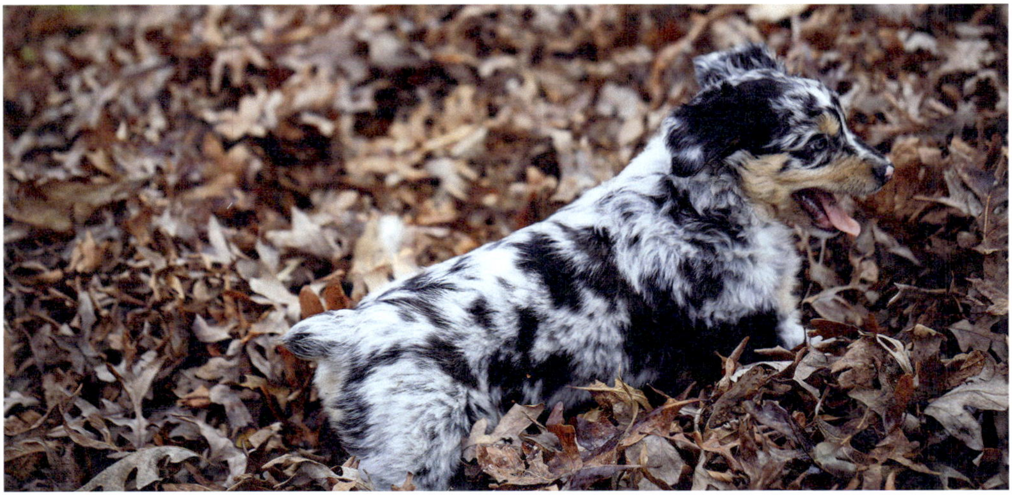

and the human in the role of trainer and coach. The sport may involve enjoying each other's company, attending sporting events, belonging to a kennel club, and socializing with other members. Like many other sports, it has spilled onto social media, which allows the human member of the team to share it at a distance with friends, family, and colleagues. Like many sports, it involves exercise and time in nature, and so allows for a whole-body experience that is shared by humans and their familiars.

In her sport, Leah has formed an interspecies bond with a dog. Many of us may have cared for an animal as children, perhaps as members of an organization like 4-H or Future Farmers of America, and others of us may have been active in farming or ranching and through that formed animal partnerships or practiced animal husbandry. For some of our emerging partners in care, bonds remain strong, such as those who sustain sacred indigenous traditions such as calling whales, singing to seals, or making music or rituals with wild birds. Some biologists in the field are learning to communicate, as with naturalist Joe Hutto, who learned many turkey vocalizations while 'mothering' a brood of turkeys, or zoo keeper Francine Patterson, who speaks gorilla sign language. As the body of our species recovers the ability to relate more fully to the bodies of other naturally-evolved species, we doctors have the chance to become more aware of evolved relations with other members of the body of life.

Sydney: Wilderness Medicine

Shortly after the middle of the last century, Sydney moved to Alaska to work for the Indian Health service. There, she lived in a city surrounded by an

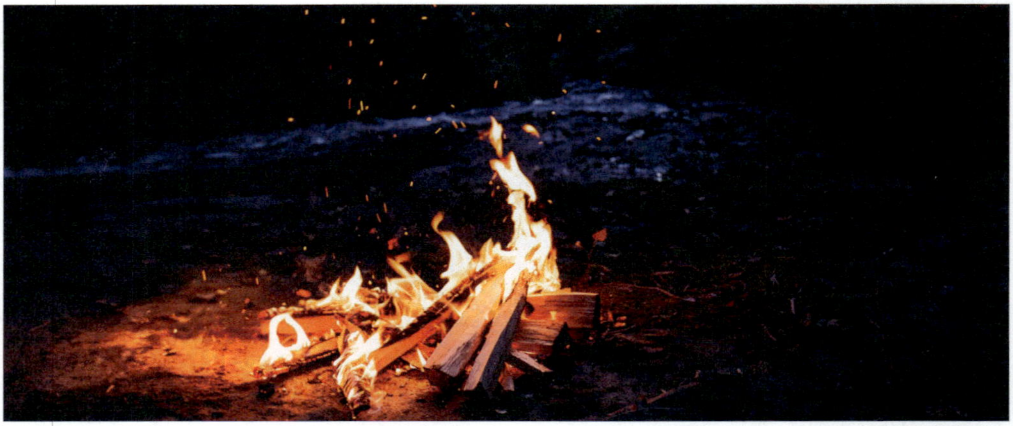

unfamiliar culture and immersed in a vast wilderness in which the indigenous people had long played integral roles through hunting, fishing, and gathering. Adjusting to this environment meant learning strategies to cope with hazards; these strategies included avoiding rutting moose grazing in the yard, carrying a shotgun on nearby hikes where she and her children might encounter grizzly bears, and carrying an ice axe that she could use to arrest a fall.

Her life in Alaska entailed new pleasures such as skijoring, which is cross-country skiing behind a dog—or team of dogs—as they run across the snow. It also entailed new sorrows, such as caring for habitat-integrated peoples who were giving up their traditional ways of life—and in the process developing tastes for junk food, alcohol, and other forms of undernutrition combined with overnutrition correlated with fast-increasing rates of diabetes, birth defects, and other modern ailments. Sydney's new life thus positioned her to appreciate and respect the vanishing ways of life through which humans had long interfaced directly with the body of life and shared in its health and its ailments.

Because she was living in a city, her knowledge and use of wilderness survival skills tended to center on weekend outings with the family. In one instance, Sydney was hiking with her son when slopeside ice gave way beneath their feet. They began to glissade—slowly at first—down an open slope toward a precipice. As they gained speed, she realized that she did not have access to the ice axe that was, like her firearm, attached to her backpack. Determined to save her son's life, she grabbed him and forced his head into the snow—in other words, she did a head plant and hung on for dear life. Once stabilized, she dug her son out with her hands as quickly as possible, terrified that she had injured him. He laughed with delight, saying, "Let's do it again, Mom! Let's do it again."

BETH LOOKS BACK: Habitat Integration via a Pilgrimage to the Temperate Rain Forest

Behind each cause is still another cause; the end of the beginning of all causes has yet to be found.

— Albert Einstein via Wikiquote

As ongoing ingestion of neurotoxins in food continued to damage my nervous system, I lost the ability to do many things. No longer able to use my mind as an accessory for processing large data sets, I practiced various forms of contemplation, sought out a wide range of healers, and tried various kinds of practices. In meditation and prayer, I explored awareness, experimented with inner silence, shared expansive states of being, and got to know my body from the inside out. I had done this as a girl through dance and music, but had turned away when I began medical school, adopted the point of view of anatomical primacy, and relied on visual and molecular constructs of health and disease.

I had questioned that point of view in the course of my academic life, when I struggled with the knowledge that risk factors and causes were only loosely related to the final common pathway diseases defined by modern gold standards. I also struggled with the recognition that physicians and patients believe—in the face of contradictory evidence—that the more precise an image, the greater its diagnostic utility. Now faced with the task of helping myself, I was ready to take on a new perspective; I relied on experiential learning and empirical evidence as I sought to know my body and all that it generates as well as possible from the inside out, to assess the effects of all kinds of treatment modalities, and to probe the limits of mind over matter.

As I became more aware of life energy, I became less and less able to ignore or deny the flow of energies that immerse our bodies and influence our beings at all times—energies that stymie moderns. I needed ways to detect and quantify my experience, something missing from modern materialism, so I began to hone my vestigial sensory abilities to detect these energies. Those who develop these abilities in early life or with great effort in later life are subject to suggestion, abuse, and exploitation—and, of course, emulation by charlatans or adoration from their fanciful or devotional peers. When your life and health depend on your developing such skills, however, it is remarkable how quickly you can come to disregard caution and trust yourself to move beyond the pale of medical group dynamics such as scapegoating of unrepentant outliers.

One of the new pleasures that I discovered early on while accompanying my daughter to her ballet class was 'bathing' in the life energy of young children. Like the much-older grandmothers seated at one side of the room, I was visibly lifted and revived, and soon came to a new appreciation of the positive exchange of energies that many of us experience as children when visiting loving grandparents. Through this and other experiences, I learned to detect, invite, and circulate healing vitality and chi in daily life and—slowly and incompletely—to use them to support my health and well-being. One advantage of possessing—or being possessed by—a vulnerable nervous system is learning more easily how to share vitality and life energy with the body of the species and the body of life.

While some in prayer groups can hold strong healing or ecstatic states, no group of humans can compare in restorative qualities with a healthy forest habitat. Because I was fortunate to live near protected temperate rain forest—where one's individual body can immerse in the body of a lush habitat—I have had the chance to take pilgrimages to sources of life. These untouched or enhanced habitats, which were here in North America before the arrivals of the white and gray tides, might still recover if cared for rather than consumed, destroyed, or poisoned. In them, I—and others like me who have been poisoned by modernity—can feel well, and find abundant life in spite of scriptures written in desert climes that disregarded the body of life, and that led my pioneer ancestors to deforest soil for cultivation. In forests, I can receive good tidings, as John Muir put it, and then return to the lifeless—or nearly so—world refreshed and renewed, as I hope my children and their children may be able to do after me.

Comment on Orienting Your Body in its Nested Bodies

The mnemonist [has] a memory that is peculiarly lacking in one important feature: the capacity to convert encounters with the particular into instances of the general, enabling one to form general concepts even though the particulars are lost.

— Jerome Bruner, Foreword to the First Edition of Luria's *The Mind of a Mnemonist*

As biologists say, we are the first species that has the choice not to go extinct, but we haven't made that choice. As in the *Twilight* series, by Stephanie Meyer, we threaten to kill our mother from inside her womb. As we damage

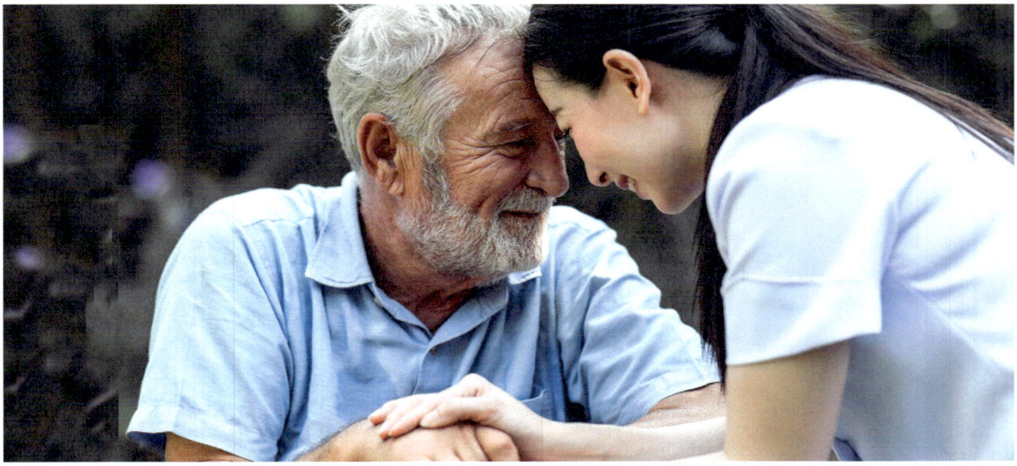

her more and more, we imagine that she is attacking us, and that our best course—other than catastrophizing—would be to run away to another planet, to seed other galaxies with our habits of self-destruction. And yet, a greater and greater part of the body of humanity is setting aside denial and disregard and facing the fact that our careless consumption, destruction, and poisoning of the body of life are not good for anyone—including doctors, patients, and the public as a whole.

To limit our thoughts to the inner workings of artificial complex systems is to fail to recognize our species' homicide-suicide plan and thus to fail our patients and our profession—to say nothing of ourselves. It is to respond insanely to the internal stimuli of socially-constructed realities that lack biological validity. It is to disregard the lessons of history, especially those pertaining to civilization—that is, to urbanization. Cities have always, it seems, divided their residents from biological realities and depleted the habitats that surround them, and so ended their own lives. Such appears to be the case with Eridu, which may have inspired Eden; with Chaco Canyon; and with the Indus Valley civilization that seeded the daughter civilizations of Mother India. All cities, it seems, turn their surrounding habitats into deserts and in so doing cause their own demise.

Even now, those of us who take pride in the cultures that immigrated to America can begin to see the shadow side of immigration in the form of the white and gray tides that inundated the natural world, and recognize that we should not emulate our forebears too closely. We may admire forebears who fled tyrannies abroad and feel compassion for their descendants and for the forests of the new world that they feared, failing to realize that wilderness was

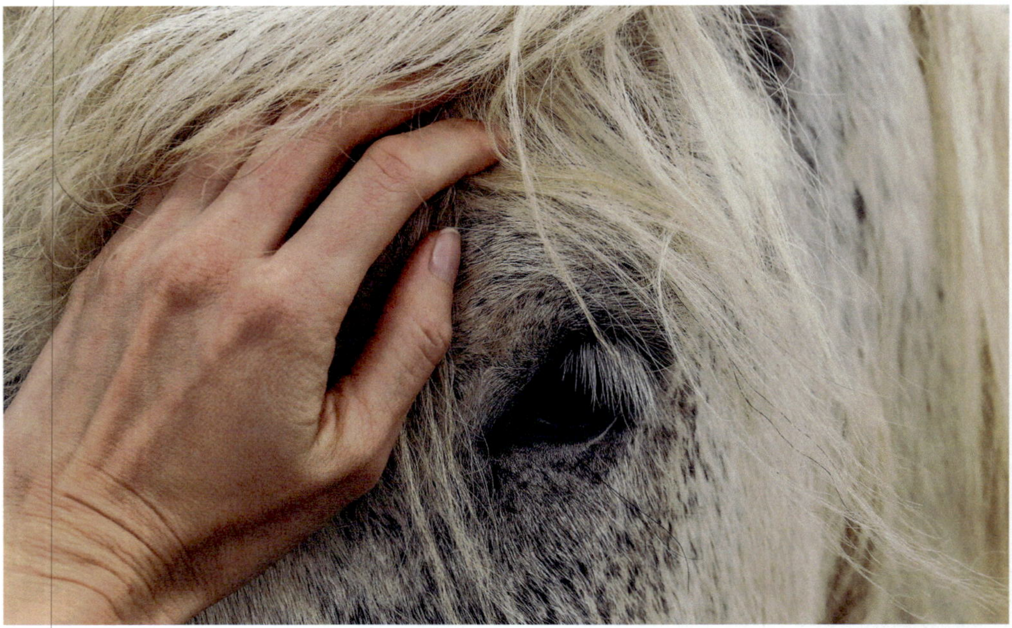

the source of pure air and water on which peoples had relied for millennia. We may value the soil enriched by family farmers who came west in pioneer wagons with their animals, and also see that many of their descendants poisoned it, and that it is up to us to stand on their shoulders and look farther and do better. This will entail restoring as many as possible of the habitats they failed to value.

To learn from the experience of your species will require extending gratitude for the efforts of our forebears to do better, along with forgiveness for their errors, which are becoming more hazardous as we magnify them. To begin doing so, take a new view of your body that looks at life from the human scale and that contextualizes all individuals and species in the body of life, which you can visualize as a protean primordial soup in oceans of air and water. Once you have recognized your place in the body of life, you can prepare to care for it as for your own body. You can put the terrors of modern warfare and their ongoing repercussions behind you and note with gratitude the fact that a new way of life is already emerging. You can see this emergence in the organic farmers who are caring for the soil, the architects who are developing living building paradigms, and the medical ancestors who—perhaps beginning with Dr. John Snow and his interruption of a cholera epidemic in London—developed population medicine and prevention.

Finding Your Place in the Body of Life

Weakness of attitude becomes weakness of character; it becomes lack of power to act with courage proportionate to danger.

— Albert Einstein

WORKING QUESTIONS

Employed Physicians

- Here and now, how is my body? The body of my species? Of my habitat? Of my bioregion?
- What ailments are my institution causing right now? My profession? (For example, you may work in an ever-expanding children's clinic in which expansion releases diesel fumes that catalyze asthma in neighborhood children and their families.)
- Has medical waste been found in local bodies of water?
- How many managers per doctor are paid for by my institution?
- What can I do today to care for those who have no care?
- Am I making a positive difference overall to life right now?

Self-determined Physicians

(Note that the first three questions may require initial research and contemplation. When you have considered them carefully, convert them to working questions.)

- What is the name of the habitat(s) in which I was born? In which I have lived most of my life? In which I live now? In which habitats do my food, clothing, and other necessities originate?
- What habitats do I most enjoy and like to—or wish to—visit? What habitats that I enjoyed in the past have become degraded or ceased to exist? Which habitat would I restore if I could take the chance to do so?
- How can I live so as to impact in a positive way the bodies of the species, habitats, and life on earth? How can I do this through my sourcing of goods and services?

- Where did this come from? Why do I have it? Must I keep it?
- Is this the right tool to use right now?
- Am I using this tool, or is it using me?
- Where is the closest stand of trees? The nearest source of surface water? The nearest toxic exposure?
- How many toxins am I taking in right now through inhalation? Ingestion? Absorption? Penetration?
- Where can I go to bathe in life energy free of artificial energy?

ORIENTING TO PLACE: Part One, Researching and Recording Your Abiotic (Non-Living) Context

You are more than likely aware of your human-made contexts—that is, of constructed manifestations of modern society like towns and highways. These represent your material social context and may seem to replace the natural one. They cannot do this; humans evolved on the abiotic, natural world—the soil and geology and non-living features of the world—as well as in the biotic one. It is therefore important to orient yourself to your pre-Anthropocene as well as your Anthropocene abiotic context.

Begin by researching the topography, waterways, and other features of the abiotic context of your primary residence. Then acquire tracing paper and draw topo maps of each layer of the surrounding abiotic surface in your journal. Fill in the waterways and mark your home. Make it as simple or detailed or artistic as you like. Make a note of any surprises. Now, on a sheet of regular or drawing paper, sketch a cross-section at the east-west or north-south midpoint and add the strata beneath the surface, including the water table and its flow. Make a note of any additional surprises. Now make a topo map on tracing paper of each under-the-surface layer to the same scale as the surface layer, and stack them beneath the surface layers so that you have a visual record of the layers of your abiotic context from bottom to top.

ORIENTING TO PLACE: Part Two, Researching and Recording Your Biotic (Living) Context

Now research your local biome and draw each wild or artificial habitat on a separate layer of tracing paper. Note separately any patches of rewilding you see as per *Rewilding Europe* by Staffan Widstrom (https://rewildingeurope.com); see also *Wild Wonders of Europe* (https://www.wild-wonders.com) and *Wild Wonders of China* (https://www.wildwondersofchina.com). For an example of such a map, see the McClosky Cascadia Map (http://www.marshamccloskey.com/cascadiamap.html). Make a note of any surprises.

Now roll up the abiotic and biotic layers, share them with some friends, and store them in a tube.

EXERCISE

Do one or both of the following:

1. Join a geo-caching or orienteering group and go on an outing that helps you get to know your area. Do excursions in other areas as well. Do you find that your awareness of your surround has changed? Get Bureau of Land Management and USGS maps for your location and put them up where you can pause and study them in the course of your day.
2. Taking the book *The Hour of Land* by Terry Tempest Williams as a template, describe all aspects of your home area in your journal. See what your body, being, and knowledge base reveal to you and record the narrative meaning that you are able to derive from them in your journal. Allow this to rapidly evolve your awareness of the Anthropocene era. Revisit the Walls biography of Thoreau and its initial orientation to the deep time of Walden Pond. See if you are able to construct a like narrative for a local natural feature with biotic and abiotic elements.

Rewilding

Even quite small areas can be rewilded... You just have to start things off... But you have to use the native species, the ones that live there naturally. That's where human management is useful, replacing the non-native with the native species.

— Staffan Widstrom

Make a plan for rewilding in your yard, a local park, or a protected but neglected area. Now make a to-do list and carry out your plan. It can be as small as a frog pond or a potted pollinator garden, or as large as a clear-cut timber farm.

Supplementary Reading

Other Species

1. Peter Wohlleben. *The Hidden Life of Trees: What They Feel, How They Communicate—Discoveries from a Secret World.* Translated by Jane Billinghurst. Vancouver: Greystone Books, 2016, 2017.
2. Peter Wohlleben. *The Inner Life of Animals: Love, Grief, and Compassion—Surprising Observations of a Hidden World.* Translated by Jane Billinghurst. Vancouver: Greystone Books, 2016, 2017.
3. Toni Frohoff and Brenda Peterson, ed. *Between Species: Celebrating the Dolphin-Human Bond.* San Francisco: Sierra Club Books, 2003.

Wild Habitats

4. Richard Preston. *The Wild Trees.* New York: Random House, 2007.
5. Oliver Sacks. *Oaxaca Journal.* New York: Vintage Books, 2002.
6. Gary Snyder, Jim Harrison, and *The Practice of the Wild. The Etiquette of Freedom.* Edited by Paul Ebenkamp. Berkeley: Counterpoint, 2010.

Modified Habitats

7. Wendell Berry. *The Unsettling of America: Culture and Agriculture.* San Francisco: Sierra Club Books, 1977.
8. Ken Druse. *Planthropology: The Myths, Mysteries, and Miracles of My Garden Favorites.* New York: Clarkson Potter/Publishers, 2008.

Orienting to Your Lifetime

It makes me think back to the radioactive clock dials my Uncle Abe used to make, and how I would press these against my closed eyelids as a child...Was I carrying an ocular melanoma gene at forty, or twenty? Or was it a mutation, one of the many, ever increasing on our polluted, carcinogenic planet?

— Oliver Sacks in *The Mind's Eye*

A popular meme is [r]evolution. This hybrid word recognizes the tension between late modern expectations of forced, cataclysmic social change and growing awareness that essential change is urgent but is only useful when it is continuous and dynamic and disseminated. Such change is evolutionary rather than revolutionary; and yet the radical experiment of modernity continues to damage life at such a speed that we have no choice but to implement prudent change posthaste. In other words, it is your destiny to use your elder years to cure yourself as you cure the body of life.

To effect wise cure on all scales, you—like all doctor elders—must effect deep inner changes that enable you and everyone you know to invent wise adaptations and transformations that will permit our species and its remnant context to survive. You begin this fateful process by owning your life experience and gleaning from it all the experiential learning that is yours and yours alone to use to effect care and cure. As an elder, you may already be free—or may make yourself free—to disengage from systems that are perpetuating and creating problems and to engage systems that are solving them. The employed are not free to undertake this task; they sustain existing systems, rather than develop and implement evolving ones designed to respect and sustain the body of life.

Chances are good that you were trained to put conformity ahead of experiential learning, and so to remain concordant with your group or system. In times past, this prevented errors. A short time of reflection will reveal that there is no need for you to be a computer or for a computer to simulate or replace you; there is a need for you to mine your treasure trove of experiential learning that has not yet been lost. In learning to own your past, present, and future, you create the chance to put failed modern forms of organization and management behind you and to invent new and better ones. Like your peers in organic farming and emerging paradigm architecture who are withdrawing from the modern paradigm, you can use your past in the context of emergence to create and embrace freedom, independence, and joie de vivre, and then to make the best of the present, and the most of your future.

ANECDOTES FROM MEDICAL LIVES

"What was distinctive in [Luria's] approach [was] his belief that human faculties could not be studied or understood in isolation, but always had to be understood in relation to living and formative influences."

—Oliver Sacks via A. R. Luria's *The Man with a Shattered World*

As you put behind you your preparation for and practice of an adult career—or careers—you have the chance to look ahead to your lifework and legacy and to figure out how to bring to bear on it the whole of your embodied experience, including parts that seem useless or harmful. For the purposes of this method, value all of it. You can use the worst parts of your past to prime change, and the best parts to enliven and guide you.

In other words, you harness the best of your life and also the errors and ills that reside in your body like imprints of unpleasant or traumatic events. These sap your energy, pull you away from the moving front of time, prevent you from comprehending or responding wisely to the now, and bar your formation of a viable future. When used to prepare you, these can push you toward change. You may at first find it more intuitive to harness the best times of your life; that is, those that connect your vitality with the vitality of your context, sync you with time and life, and support you in staying dynamic, responsive, and true. These pull you toward a better day.

But when you frame the ills and errors of the past as burdens that we herein call time debts, you can reconcile them and leave them behind. In other words, in turning your problems into solutions, you free your body to move toward joy. Your time debts reveal the drive behind your evolution, creativity, and change. When you do not overpay them—that is, do not feed them and overuse them—they can remain valid and true in changing times. At the same time, you use any time credits you have to get moving toward creating the future that you envision, and use your enduring, renewing assets—such as love of new life—to form and reform your vision. This process of purposeful change prepares you to turn obstacles into opportunities, and to turn given opportunities into more meaningful ones, as described in the anecdotes below—which are, as they say in the movies, inspired by true events.

Ruth: Patients, Class, and Justice

Ruth seemed to have been born a social activist. She had never been one to sit idly by while social dysfunction made life difficult for those who had less or who fell on hard times. She brought into medicine a socially-constructed view of the underclass as victims of neglect and abuse and as products of evil or unjust circumstances. In her career as medical director at a department of public health, she provided care to the homeless, drug addicts, and commercial sex workers.

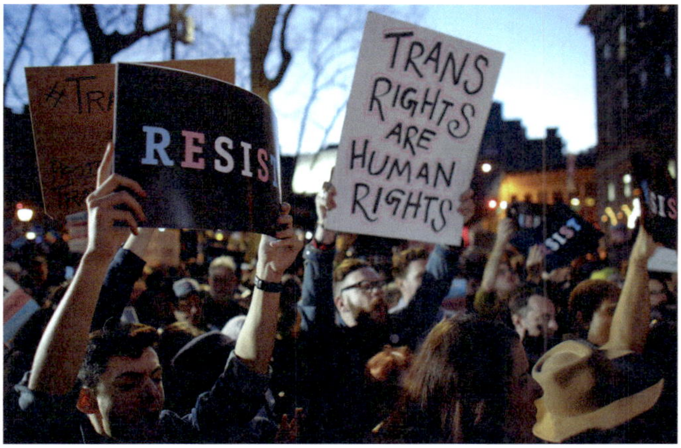

In some of them, she recognized bisexuality like hers that in their cases had led to scapegoating and a fall from social grace. Many had suffered cruelties that she had avoided by virtue of strength, privilege, determination, and ability. When she retired from public service, the stories of all her patients haunted her, as did the history of the public laws and regulations that authorities periodically invoked to punish and push down those who were targets of social frustration and who were ripe for exploitation by politicians willing to rise through hatred and persecution. She was particularly distressed by abortion laws that failed to address the realities of women at risk and that made life more difficult for her former patients.

Noting a persecutory turn in the public dialogue, and motivated by sympathy as well as empathy and maternal feelings, she decided to make their stories known. She began to write historical novels about continuing problems that offer the perspective of time. This perspective could throw into relief the forces of shame, guilt, and blame that could still be exploited, and that would—if the community failed to learn from its own history—push the weak and unfortunate into oblivion. As you reach your post-employment years, you too may face a unique mountain—low or high—of delayed gratification and unprocessed memories. As you face this mountain, you, too, may choose to talk—or write—through your time debts and credits and so develop them into the motivation that drives your life—and the lives of others like you—as you become a medical elder.

Penelope

From the time Penny was a child all through her time as a mother, she cared for family members who were struggling or ailing. When her physician husband became ill, they were obliged to leave their rural practice to live and work in a city where they had easy access to specialized emergency care. There she took a job at a health cooperative, where she took care of more patients than her peers and, perhaps paradoxically, gave each patient more attention. She was one of the final holdouts who insisted on dictating notes rather than filling out the electronic medical record while talking to the patient.

After some years of this demanding pace of work, she needed a break. Stories of her childhood in a public housing project in a major city and of her husband's harrowing treatments flooded in on her. For the purposes of the method used for this book, we would say that she accumulated time debts that she used as impetus for helping to create a more compassionate society. She was grateful to her parents for keeping the family together in tough times, and sympathetic to her doctor-patient-husband's chronic illness. She bore witness to these experiences.

Penelope chose to bear witness through artistic expression, specifically the medium of film. A typical doctor, she sought out a conventional path that was available to her and followed all the rules. She took a course; she wrote scripts; she raised funds; she gathered a following; she joined groups that supported her art. She developed a second career that she was able to pursue part-time during a leave of absence, and became an active contributor to the city's cultural life. Informed by a lifetime of experiential learning and enriched by a lifetime of service, she developed a deep well of insight and shared a broad and long perspective with affinity groups in need of both.

Dr. Addington

His friends and family thought him peculiar. According to the expectations of his time and place in life, Dr. Addington should have been a man of leisure who gave time to a family foundation and money to one of the great cultural institutions in his home city. He felt compelled to do more. By some process of quirk and fate, he felt called to practice medicine. Historically, medicine was the purview of gentlemen, and he could have taken care of the upper crust. Instead, he took a post at in an inner city teaching hospital frequented by the least among us, where he served all of his patients directly and compassionately and mentored less fortunate juniors in need of a fine—and classy—example.

Dr. Addington is not alone in turning his time credits to good use. Many physicians born into privilege choose a medical career to prove their skills, or earn a place in society, or use circumstances long on possibility and short on purpose to create a meaningful and productive life. They use position, education, freedom, and industry to make the most of their time on earth. If you are fortunate enough to enjoy a phase in life that is post-employment and post-management, you, too, can become a doctor of leisure and use the time credits—including those that you have earned through service—to fulfill an even more challenging quest as a medical elder. Then you will go to your final rest knowing that you did more than your share to rescue and restore evolved life.

BETH LOOKS BACK: Psychosocial Patterning for a Living Future

[F]luctuations are typical of any neural system that has sustained damage, irrespective of the cause...There is less reserve, less redundancy, when a system is damaged, and it is more easily thrown off by adventitious factors such as fatigue, stress, medications, or infections [or by] spontaneous fluctuations.

— Oliver Sacks in *The Mind's Eye*

One of the advantages of sustaining chronic neural damage that 'blows out' your CPU is that you have no choice but to focus on practical matters on the human scale and to test out abstract constructs of medical phenomena. Put differently, you look from the trees to the forest and become aware of life in the aggregate. You realize that you can use concepts such as the body politic or the corps de ballet to reframe life on earth as the body of life. You discover principles filled with pith and moment that supersede raw data and that form patterns far more powerful than isolated facts or reductionist analyses.

You can easily see, then, that while you have been number crunching and keeping track of details, no one has been minding the store. When I wanted advice on the progress of my medical detection, I soon found to my dismay—though not shock—that amongst all my academic connections I could turn up no allopath with a fundamental interest in allopathy, nor any epidemiologist interested in the mysteries of emerging epidemics. They were busy meeting expectations by serving social processes. They were employees habituated to caring for virtual reality, tracking and implementing medical updates automatically, and repeating safe-sounding metrics and statistics. They were too preoccupied to develop the judgment or awareness needed to pay attention to life, values, or meaning, and were afraid to be imaginative or creative and so risk violating standards of uniformity and conformity—or, God forbid, losing their peer-approved funding or plum administrative positions. I longed for the days when I had the privilege of learning from mentors who had known a time before over-management, and nimbly juggled urgency and importance. I missed the WWII vets who weren't afraid to use their wits or thwart amoral or bull-headed authorities.

When the noise of data recedes, signals appear. You form narratives that become mythic enough to suit a big-picture view of your experience or your time; this view develops like a high-resolution film print in a water bath developer. You learn to ground yourself in the particular as well as the general, and to move beyond the anatomical primacy that defines the modern era of Hippocratic medicine. You become able to integrate across fields and traditions. You begin to appreciate science; that is, the ability to encounter the unknown and develop the tools required to comprehend it so as to solve problems in their living context. You become able to imagine a kind of medicine that is like obstetrics or pediatrics in which you and the patient are the worried parents and life on earth is the treasured object of your care and cure.

From this comprehensive perspective on the human scale, you develop the ability to look inward and see the early influences that formed the patterns of thought which prepared you to become a diagnostician and clinician. For me, these included the ballet lessons and gymnastics that my parents hoped would turn me into a fine young lady but inadvertently instilled my interest in the body and patterned my kinesthetic learning. In other words, instead of becoming a lady, I became a doctor. They didn't mind—at first. But when I turned to causal studies and medical detection rather than to a well-regarded, well-paying field, they were less than thrilled. In retrospect, however, the unfolding experience they chanced to provide had perfectly prepared me to cope with the unforeseen future by using circumstances to turn obstacles into opportunities.

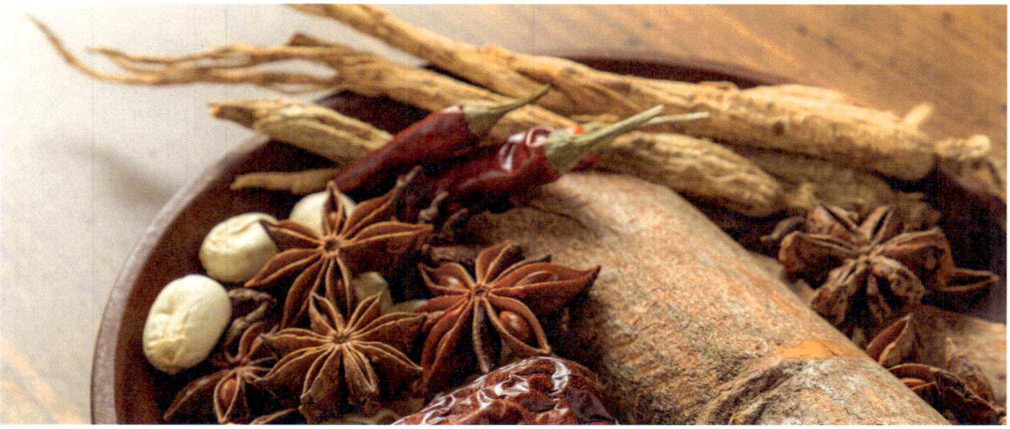

Faced by illness and surrounded by practitioners who had gathered spiritual and medical ideas and methods from around the globe, I was fortunate—and open-minded enough—to undertake an unbounded search for care and cure. I learned of treatment modalities from the East that seemed to suit endemic viral infections; of millennia of self-healing techniques belonging to spiritual and religious contexts; and of the healing benefits of nature (beyond those I encountered when working in Colorado, where many consumptives had gone for high-altitude cures).

By integrating global esoteric and exoteric—inner and outer—spiritual practices with exoteric concepts from cognitive psychology, population genetics, and interventionist medicine, I learned to pattern the joining of being and doing for the discovery of causes of illness in individual and aggregate instances of life. You may be able to use my method—which was described in Construct 3 and is reiterated here at the risk of unwelcome repetition—to prepare your body to solve problems that scientists have been passively documenting. This adaptive response hinges on transforming medicine to suit present realities. Many scientists—medical and otherwise—fail to see a way forward. They lapse into fatalism. With self-patterning, you can pass quickly through disillusionment with modernity and engage modalities that care for and cure each as all.

In brief, the problem-solving pattern begins with formation of a vision that draws you on; that is, one that gives you something to run toward rather than away from. You can speed this by adopting the emerging vision that is forming the basis of the local, living new economies with safe, organic food; bio-compatible architecture; and safe and sustainable disposal of human remains. Drawn by this vision, you form a stance that directs you to move toward that vision and prime yourself for action—most likely by taking any doubts and

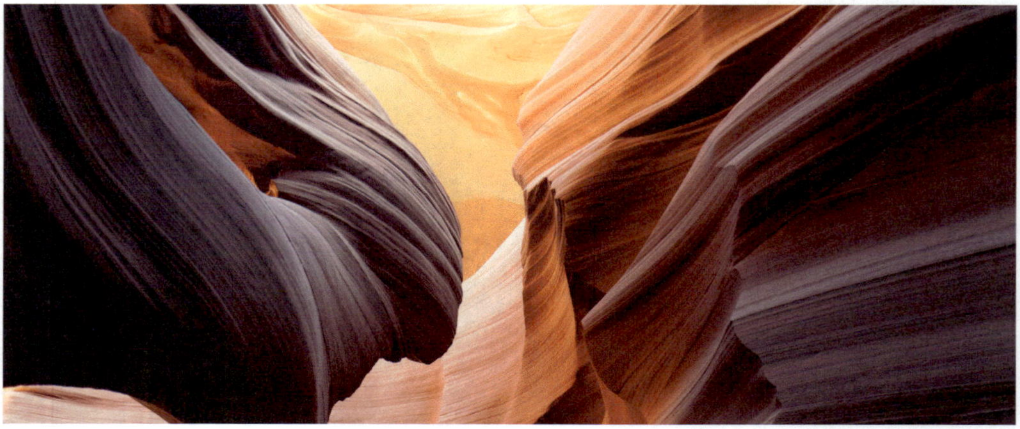

worries and living traumas that alerted you to the limits of modern ways as your impetus for change. Thus drawn and driven, you can learn to recognize states of care and cure that enable you to bear witness to and ease pain and suffering, and to cure ailments on the human scale and above.

These states of care resemble those that Buddhists call heavenly abodes, that Jewish mystics may associate with paradise, that Christian mystics may see as consolation or union, and that Muslims experience as surrender. These states draw on sources of inspiration that you may relate to self-power, other-power, or spontaneous generation—whatever frames and constructs suit your locale and allow you to abide in a state of being that is joyous and rich in wonder as well as grounded in the tangible and intangible aspects of your context. (For more, go to the online courses at EvolveMedicine.us.)

The states of cure will be familiar to you as a modern who does analysis and problem-solving—except that your field of awareness must be relaxed and your energy body grounded and balanced. The best way to ensure this is to develop care states that are strong enough to hold cure states. The gateway to these states is contemplation or meditation, which is known in all faith traditions. Early modern scientists used Christian-derived states of contemplation—like Newton's Arianism—while late moderns may draw on Himalayan or Judaic traditions.

Having developed the ability to enter into states of care and cure, you can use them to develop suitable strategies and skills for your emerging work. These may lead to different outcomes than the strategies and skills developed by late modern scientists abiding in warlike or competitive states, as with those who developed nuclear weapons and other technologies designed to destroy rather than to support the sustenance and thriving of generative life.

In sum, to set a pattern for solving the real-world problems of present-day medicine, you develop a vision that draws you forward, a stance that you prime to direct you toward your vision, states that support care and cure, and purpose-specific strategies and skills that join your states of being to the realization of your vision. As noted above, this requires broad experience: familiarity with spiritual practices, cognitive psychology, population genetics, and interventionist medicine. It also requires inner work that you will encounter in the working questions at the end of each chapter.

Comment on Orienting to Your Lifetime

A patient who is well managed is capable of helping himself to recovery, for he has been provided with insight and knowledge, hope and security, and the motivation to do whatever may be required.

—Philip A. Tumulty in *The Effective Clinician*

As you set your direction and motivate your continuation, you will find that your most precious fuel is the whole of your experience. The reason for this is that your unfinished business (time debts) can push you, while your evolving vision pulls you. When you embody them and align them with the course of your life, you form a strong predisposition for creating life-fulfilling, life-restoring actions. When you engage sequential aspects of being and doing, and they tend toward the moving front of time, you can engage one or another sequence of the strategies and skills you developed in the course of your career. With experience, you will be able to map and navigate the winding path to your completion and legacy. The challenging obstacles that you meet on your way will awaken your sleeping gifts and thereby evolve your ability to set, pursue, and revise your course in response to learning.

Your progress may hinge on how well you are able to ground yourself in life on earth and in the history of medicine. This grounding can keep you on course as you leave modernity behind, adopt new frames and constructs, and reveal hidden patterns of cause and consequence. You can then look back on the limits of late modern methods and view them with compassion that eases the confusion and frustration of transition. Put differently, you can sync with life in time and join in the processes of change that rectify past errors. This will entail iterative experiential learning that goes from the particular to the general and back again, and that you test through trial and error so that the processes you adapt can grow and develop with you. This will be—if you make it so—a grand adventure well worth the rest of your life.

Orienting to Your Lifetime

WORKING QUESTIONS

Employed Physicians

- What do I regret right now? How can I reconcile it by using it as a time debt to pay? By making amends?
- Is this regret reasonable? Will it help me do a better job? Or do I just dislike the wrong (rare) outcome of the right (best) choice?
- How did I know what to do just now? Is there a time credit—e.g. training, experience, or talent—behind it?
- Was that a win-win strategy? If not, why not?
- Is that skill what it should be?
- Do I know how I got to this point in life, and where I'm going?
- What do I want most for my species now? Is what I'm doing now promoting that?

Self-determined Physicians

- Which stances and states come naturally, and which do I have to cultivate?
- What kinds of experiences do I like, and what kinds do I dislike or avoid? What events draw me, or repel me?
- Which life experiences drive me to cultivate better states, or to develop new strategies and skills?
- When I think of fulfilling my Hippocratic oath, what comes to mind? What puts me at ease in that regard? What unsettles me?

EXERCISE 1: Drawing up a Balance Sheet

Romantics in science want neither to split living reality into its elementary components nor to represent the wealth of life's concrete events in abstract models that lose the properties of the phenomena themselves.

— A.R. Luria via Jerome Bruner in A.R. Luria's *The Mind of a Mnemonist*

To begin reckoning your time credits and debts, draw a table with three columns like the one below in your journal. Referring to any resources you choose, fill in events that are time-neutral and that will prompt your memory (e.g. family births, deaths, marriages, centennials, historical events, or the like.) Then fill in time credits, that is, time-connecting events that continue to draw you closer to the moving front of time. These may include emotionally significant events that brought out positive intentions or sacred love that rewarded you for staying in sync with time, or did more good than harm. Then fill in your time debts; that is, events that linger in you and that sap energy, distract you from life, or pull you into the dead past. These may include events that did more harm than good, that seeded regrets you have yet to reconcile, or that disconnected you from the river of life. Add as many pages as you wish until you are satisfied that you have hit upon and captured the most important debits and credits that continue to come alive in your body.

Time-Neutral	Time-Connecting	Time-Disconnecting

EXERCISE 2

Write or draw a brief bio of your life as the sequence of biotic natural environments in which you have lived, and of your relation to each in each location.

EXERCISE 3

Draw a vector diagram of one process of your life in which you harnessed your priming (e.g. your problem-based drive) to your vision (e.g. your expectation of a solution). Include all six steps shown in Construct 3, Self-Patterning, and any relation to the biotic or abiotic natural environment. Feel free to diagram any or all emerging processes that are forming or reforming in your body.

EXERCISE 4

Write a fresh 1000-word bio or memoir reframed and reconstructed based on the work and play that you have been doing. This time, feature key takes—that is, lessons 'harvested' from your embodied experiences that you might use for priming or vision. See if you can incorporate formative experiences that are pushing or pulling you toward emergence.

EXERCISE 5: Celebrating Mid-year

[Life] Harvesting shows us that we have made a difference in the world. We sense that our lives have meaning; that we have contributed to others; and that we are worthwhile human beings.

— Zalman Schachter-Shalomi and Ronald S. Miller
in *From Age-ing to Sage-ing*

Before you go on to the challenges of the extra month and the next season, winter, celebrate what you have put into your year of transition and what you have gotten from it to date. Make it a pattern: before undertaking something dark or difficult, fill your body with light and strength. This will set a pattern of self- rather than other-reward, which will support you in your conscientious independent-mindedness.

Don't worry; celebration need not be an enemy to your dedication or to your grounding in reality. Rather, it can deepen and sustain your roots in what you value most. Also, regret is pointless if you do not look back and make things right and look forward with keen anticipation when you transition to a new phase of life. More to the point, you cannot own your lifework or legacy until you are able to refresh the humanity of your calling and to show compassion for yourself as for others.

Devise a celebration that rewards the deepest parts of your body for the things that mean most to you. If you take your time and think this through, you may encounter sources of purpose, meaning, and vision that you may have missed until now. These sources are your human capital, the fertile roots of your budding wisdom. When you encounter them, you will be ready to design a celebration that is integral to a rite of passage through which your old life will cohere and end and metamorphose into a new one of pith and moment.

If you are not sure what to celebrate, list the most memorable accomplishments that you let pass without acknowledgement. When you have finished, devise a joyous celebration of one or all of them and allow everyone who cares for you to participate.

Putting Demons Behind You

The first guy through the gate gets bloody.

— *Moneyball,* the film, by Steven Zaillian and Aaron Sorkin

WHEN YOU HOLD EMOTIONALLY-CHARGED MEMORIES, they may haunt you and hold you back, in which case you can engage them to push you forward. You take them as an impetus to action in the world. You turn them from demons into angels. You may find it straightforward to resolve to do something to rectify the wrongs that bother you, and to pay your pain forward as blessing. You may also be ready to engage emotionally-charged memories of love and joy that draw you forward in anticipation of new and wonderful adventures.

Some memories are not one thing or the other. They're complicated, tangled, a mix of the tortured soul who drives herself mercilessly for the sake of others and never comes into balance with the perpetual victim who is always taking and yet always innocent. Or, they may be a mixture of other complex polarities, like those who make war to protect the sweet and vulnerable baby Jesus. These are chimeras, demons that persist to drive you in circles from one extreme to the other, often moving so rapidly that you never glimpse either extreme. When you do come to see one, it may resemble a raft of plastic refuse floating in an eddy of ocean currents. It may appear random and chaotic and pathetic and annoying. It may seem to have nothing to do with you. And in a way, that is true: it is excess baggage that you can turn into something of use such as the motivation to push you forward toward the moving front of time, and a vision to draw you toward a better future. It is not you, but your use of it is yours, and is up to you.

For the purpose of emergence, you take everything that comes to you or abides in you as a resource for loving life and mending it; as an element of care and cure useful in doctoring evolved life from the perspective of the human scale. This month, tend to a demon that is plaguing you, which you may discover as a rejected source of blame, guilt, or shame—or delight.

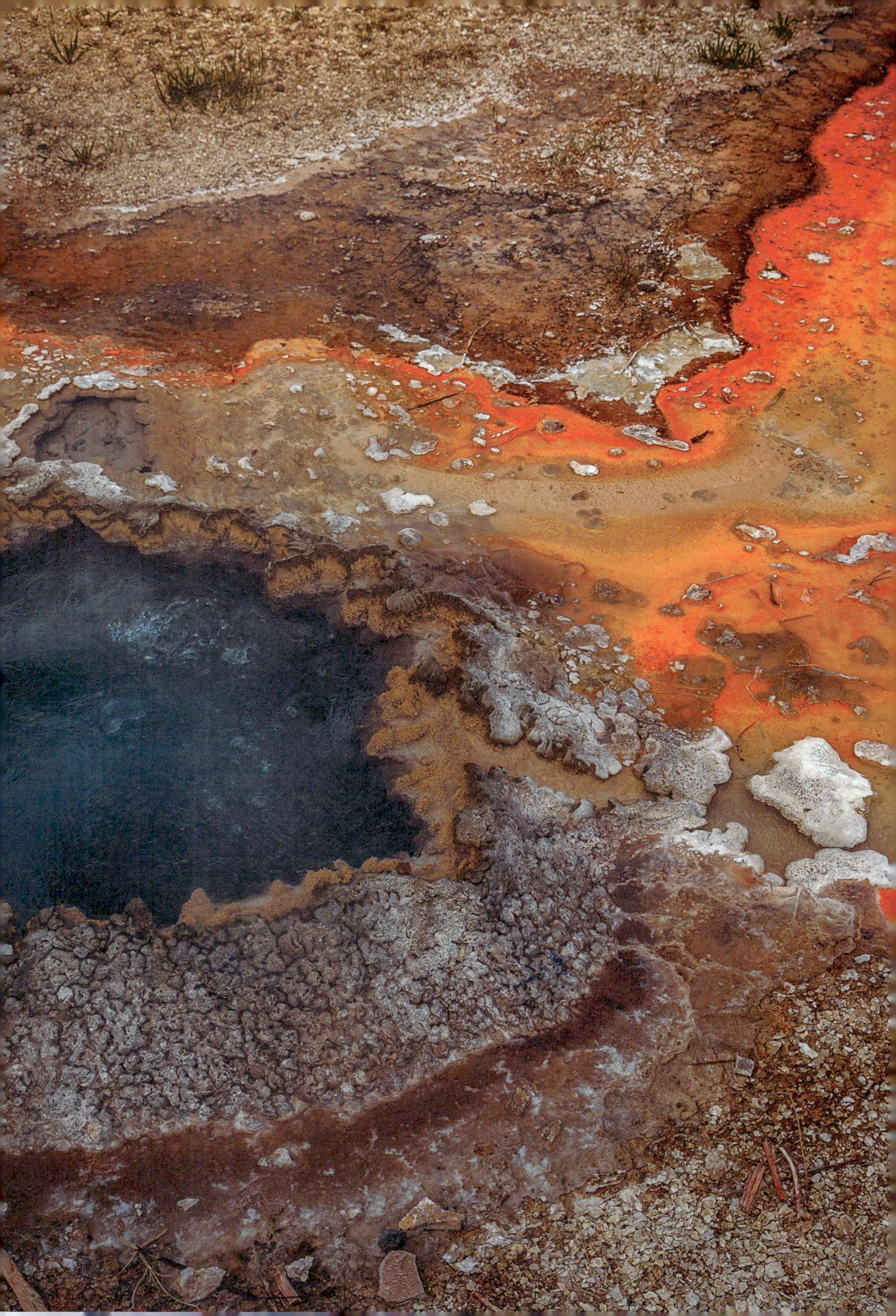

ANECDOTES FROM MEDICAL LIVES

Law looks to the past for its legitimacy, literary fiction to the possible, bound only by verisimilitude, but what shall we make of the endless forms of narrative through which we construct (and maintain) a self?

— Jerome Bruner in *Making Stories: Law, Literature, Life*

If you had to rely on information science to choose demons to use in forming your vision and priming your stance, you might scan the whole of your bodily memory, define it as a complex sequence of interdependent events, and run the data through a series of iterative analyses and still miss those that matter most. Fortunately, your embodied memory is linked to supra- and infra-rational bodily processes that can pinpoint the demons that can feed your purpose and fill your next stage of life with vital meaning. If you allow your mind to grow quiet, as in prayer or meditation, your body will reveal the demons that live in you like minotaurs in a labyrinth. They may talk to you obliquely through recurring unwelcome thoughts, feelings, or images. If you allow your body and its phenomena to signal you and also to work for you, it will then harness the demons that can best propel you toward your vision of a better future. Put differently, your body will—when respected and guided lovingly with a light hand—work to put your most potent demons behind you, and thereby prime your stances and states. It will likewise form and reform the vision that inspires you.

Anthony

When Tony was a rebellious teenager, the popular life story that he had been spinning was shattered by an unexpected diagnosis: insulin-dependent diabetes mellitus. He soon learned through hard experience that rebellion was futile. He had a new and unwelcome companion for life, and he had no choice but to own it and to turn it to advantage. Over the course of the next year, he led a brittle new life that transformed his vision of his future. He foresaw a life narrative in which he would turn from victim to hero by becoming a doctor. He would take charge of his own illness and help others as others were helping him. Perhaps he would even discover a cure. He embraced the new meaning and purpose of his life and became the author of its success.

Like many who set out to become doctors, Tony earned the future he envisioned. In college, he succeeded beyond all expectations. Afterwards, he won a place in a prestigious medical school and went on to a top-flight residency and fellowship. He earned board certification in Internal Medicine and Hematology and Oncology and joined a group practice that served a large region of his home state. His demons behind him, he envisioned and conjured a previously unforeseen medical life.

Rafaela

Like many who choose medicine, Rafaela was born into a healing process that some call *tikkun olam*, or world healing. She and her family were holding one of the fiercest of demons: the Shoah. Sent at a very young age to concentration camps, her parents survived and came to America to begin new lives. They had relatives in the new country who had not encountered the ravages of genocidal war, and who met them with something like horror. Emotionally isolated, they lived alone with the ghosts of murdered relatives until they met each other, married, and had two beloved children. They moved to a place that they later called the old neighborhood, which was home to others who bore the imprint of past hate crimes that they could neither escape nor put to rest.

Their children excelled in school, entered accelerated programs, and went on to earn advanced degrees—Rafaela in medicine, and her brother in business. Encouraged by professors of Obstetrics and Gynecology, who aimed to recruit the best of the women students who were reentering the profession in large numbers for the first time since the Flexner report, Rafaela specialized in OBGYN. She qualified at a large urban hospital in a diverse neighborhood and treated patients who spoke one or more of over sixty languages. After training, she took a position at a large urban hospital.

In Rafaela's new practice, she treated both the upper crust and those who were most in need. Many of the latter had AIDS; most were immigrants; few had health insurance; and none had doctors who knew what to do for pregnant women with AIDS or for their unborn children. Putting the grit and tears of her parents and their demons behind her, Rafaela stepped up and took care of this new wave of pregnant patients who, like her parents, had escaped horrors and come to her teeming city with the strong and yet fragile hope of raising their children in peace and safety. And so Rafaela healed her own intergenerational trauma—in part—by healing others.

The first Dr. Meacham in Wisconsin

It is sometimes difficult to remember the demons that have always driven doctors to do whatever they could to save lives. It is especially difficult now,

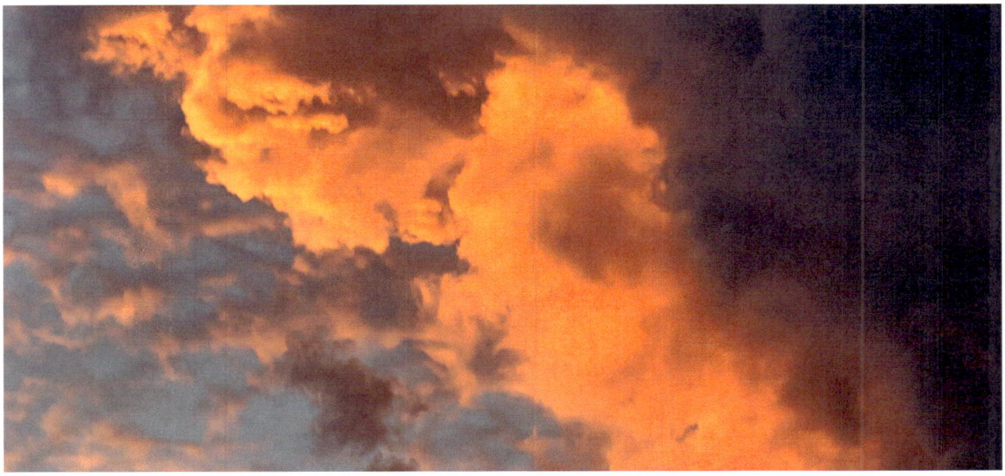

when we identify medicine with technology, to put ourselves in the shoes of doctors from frontier or horse-and-buggy days, when patients bit a piece of wood or a bullet for anesthesia. Then, as Mark Twain recalls it in his autobiography, every grandmother was an herbalist, doctors prescribed mustard plasters, and the sick would consult Native American practitioners who lived and consulted in the woods outside town.

It is easier for my friend—I'll call him Kent Meacham—to remember this. Born into a medical family, he faced a difficult choice as a young man: if he chose a field other than medicine, he would break a family tradition reminiscent of the historic Munro family of the Edinburgh School of Medicine. He would end a medical dynasty. He chose to become a 'hard' scientist, and so stopped a lineage of which he nonetheless continues to be a memory keeper.

That lineage began when his great-granduncle, a pioneer farmer living near Portage, Wisconsin, lost his newborn baby to illness. As he mourned, he became more and more convinced that if their growing community had had a doctor, the baby would have lived. Hearing of a new medical school nearby, he left his wife in charge of the family farm and walked nearly two hundred miles to matriculate at Rush Medical College. He finished his training and returned to Portage to practice medicine, as did his son and grandson.

Since time immemorial, in every culture, our species has lived in ways that have caused premature death, and the survivors have done their utmost to put loss behind them and to do something about it. Now, as our ways of living threaten to erase life itself, we can put the losses of human—and non-human—life behind us as we remove our blinkers, look around, and see what best to do.

BETH LOOKS BACK

It is man's participation in culture and the realization of his mental powers through culture that make it impossible to construct a human psychology on the basis of the individual alone.

— Jerome Bruner in *Acts of Meaning*

Demons drove me into medicine, into public health and preventive medicine, and then into medical detection and medical philosophy. They were few but potent, aligning to form an awareness of bodily harm and a desire to avert it. The demons were never entirely personal; they generally related to family, neighborhood, or peers. They included: my parents' scapegoating for situations beyond their control, namely post-traumatic stress disorder and illegitimate conception; a sexual incident at age three for which I was blamed and assigned the role of damaged goods; and an illness that marked me as a 'head case' and so ended my professional life as I had known it. All contributed to a stance of victimization, a state of isolation, and an inability to call on well-cultivated strategies and skills. Life presented the null hypothesis that I would be a fool to have faith in my species; I rejected it and embraced holy foolery.

I had already put my demons behind me, but they were no longer driving me anywhere useful. I had no goal to achieve. In the past, I had sought goals that the profession had set for me. It became literally painful to continue, and then painfully obvious that I had been locked in a direction that no one should go. The only right way to go lay in a place that was hard to get to and that lay out of sight. But what might that place be?

Once a fan of science fiction, I lost interest in fantasies of war and technology and developed new interests in theology and spiritual practice. Clergy saw me as following a well-worn path from the fallen to the raised, from disillusionment to conversion. I didn't see it quite that way; I had heard and experienced too many cautionary tales. But I did revisit my Puritan roots, which offered tales of serenity on the one hand and dissent on the other. I recognized that I should continue to choose dissent and medicine, and turned for aid to the compassionate individuals who form the beating heart of all living religions, and who offer helping hands to those thrown from the nest too early—or too far.

As I searched for solutions, I began to discover people who had landed on their feet on the other side of the failure of late modernity. They had become as uneasy about the future as their peers but had decided to step up and cure their dis-ease instead of blaming others. Blame, as anyone can see, leads to choosing up sides, building defensive walls, and shouting across them—which deepens our species' problems and leaves them to others—but to whom?—to solve. And so humans treat science as the opposite of religion, practicality as adverse to theory, and being as incompatible with doing. For me, the only guide through this valley of shadows was faith in life.

Faith isn't easy. What's worse: it isn't enough. Vision is essential. You must see where you are going in order to put your demons behind you, to let your vision draw you, and to join your being and doing to create a constructive course of action. Our push is worth nothing without the pull of faith in life. When these align to move you in a better direction, you can form and engage a sequence of steps that carries you toward your well-grounded dreams, and along the way helps you over whatever obstacles you encounter.

Comment on Putting Your Demons Behind You

I had imagined my injury...to be straightforward and routine, and I was astonished at the...abyss of bizarre and even terrifying, effects [it had. I] have since had a deeper sense of the horror and wonder which lurk behind life and which are concealed, as it were, behind the usual surface of health.

— Oliver Sacks in *A Leg to Stand On*

Doctors learn to seek the center of the herd. The select few, protected by high status, lead and the rest follow. This feels safe for the individual but magnifies any group errors; at the end of the modern era, those errors are now many and weighty. Doctors have never led such changes; we have always changed at the tipping point. Now, with excessive centralization and automation, we aim to conform, to please. We meet expectations. Now, as you reach the elder years and leave the role of employee enmeshed in an unwieldy complex of systems, you will be free to discover what is best for you to do and how to do it. You will be free to seize the day and lead the way—whether alone or with others who are heading the same way. You may blaze a new trail and live to tell the tale. With wit and will, that tale can become a part of the shared narrative that is forming to take humanity to the kind of everlasting life that consists of caring for the body of life well enough that it will continue when you leave this glorious earth.

When you put your necessary demons behind you and allow them to motivate you to do better than you and others have done before, you engage a process

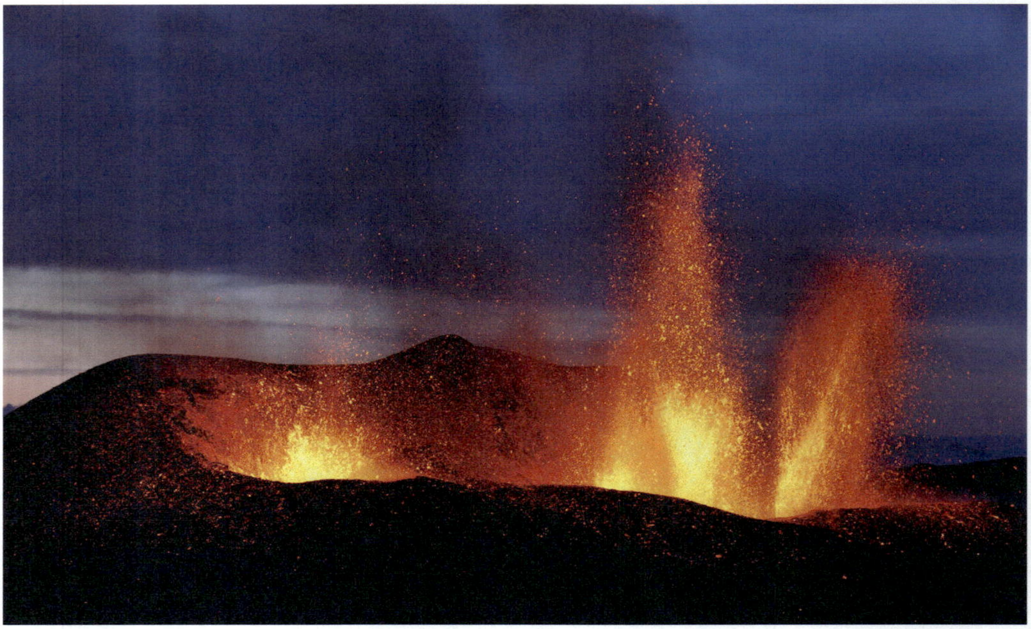

that has the potential to join your being and doing to the future good you envision. When you have done this, you can breathe more easily and put down the burden of sustaining the modern illusion of control that is fast petering out. You can put problems behind you, invent solutions that allow you to move ahead, and adjust your course iteratively as you go so that you can lead your profession toward the collective good.

With your demons behind you and the vision of a living future before you, you can harvest your remaining errors, mischances, and obstacles to hone your strategies and skills, and to transform your processes of doing as you learn of better and better ways to care for life. This entails faith, inner work, and vision, which are poor tickets to money or fame or any other evanescent reward. What they can do is to energize, enrich, guide, and fulfill the course of your life in accord with the sense that you make of it. If you engage life in this way, you will sooner or later encounter and harness new demons. You will break through the elusive and intangible barriers that divide you from your best future, which may bloody you figuratively and, at times, literally. And so you join your experiential, empirical, embodied learning to the spiritual and mythic traditions that remain, and thus enrich the shared narratives that will form the living history of the future.

Reconciling Troubling Memories

If you have primary or secondary post-traumatic stress disorder, or you harbor memories that you have never been able to put into words, take time to get counseling or to do one of the self-help workbooks that are dedicated to recovery and that have become widely available. Do not rush. Gentle persistence with breaks as needed, or perhaps low-dose hallucinogen therapy, may do the trick without destabilizing you or causing new problems.

Even if your demons are not stuck in your limbic system, take this work slowly. Reclaiming the energy that it saps from your body will provide relief. Only you will know when this has happened.

As you work with your inner burdens, stay safe and make the best use of time by remaining alert to signs that you may need help. Be prepared to go out and get it if and when you need it. Don't imagine that you should handle it on your own. Ask for help and be prepared to accept it from whatever quarter it chances to come to you—be that a wise elder, member of the clergy, therapist, or stranger—whoever holds any wisdom that illuminates your way.

WORKING QUESTIONS

Employed Physicians

- What am I feeling right now? What triggered that? Is it a skill that is working against me, and needs release or redirection?
- What is behind this fear/anger/desperation? What is it trying to tell me? How should I respond?

Self-determined Physicians

- What kinds of things hurt my feelings? What makes me angry, fearful, discouraged, disconnected, or greedy?
- What kinds of things tend to 'get on top of me' or overwhelm me? What motivations and inspirations lift me up?
- When did this—or something like it—happen most recently? Before that? And before that? Did I respond the way I want to this time? In the past? How do I want to respond in the future?

EXERCISE 1

- When a demon is active, take a time out and invite it to show itself and to speak with you. Draw or describe it in the space below.
- Treating it as a character of your subconscious, write its narrative out in such a way that you 'complete it'—that is, you resolve its unfinished business and, if the time is right, let it go.

EXERCISE 2

- Write a list of the ten life experiences that were most important in forming your character.
- Compare this list to the one you made in June. How and why do they differ? Have your efforts during this half-year of transition led to any signs of new wisdom? To the beginnings of emergence? Reflect on your efforts and write about any gains (and losses) in your journal.

Supplementary Reading

1. Mary Shelley. *Frankenstein.* Revised edition. London: Henry Colburn and Richard Bentley, 1831.
2. Robert Louis Stevenson. *The Strange Case of Dr. Jekyll and Mr. Hyde.* London: Longmans, Green & Co., 1886.
3. William Carlos Williams. "Old Doc Rivers" in *The Doctor Stories.* New York: New Directions, 1984.
4. Virginia Cornell. *Doc Susie: The True Story of a Country Physician in the Colorado Rockies.* Carpinteria, CA: Manifest Publications, 1991.

Prepatory questions for contemplation

- What demons, if any, can I now comprehend as time debts that drove me into medicine? What demons, if any, have threatened to drive me out of it?
- What demons do I feel in my flesh? In my intangible body? Around my body? Can I feel any that I have yet to face or come to know?
- Can I discern what they are trying to tell me? Are they connected with other demons whose messages I have ignored? Have I been trying to outrun them, and so made them seem much more dangerous than they are?
- Have any of my past demons faded in intensity? Have any become faint neutral memories or disappeared altogether from view?
- Are any demons dividing me from my lifework? From my legacy? What are they trying to tell me? Are they easier to face if I take it easy, or take a break?

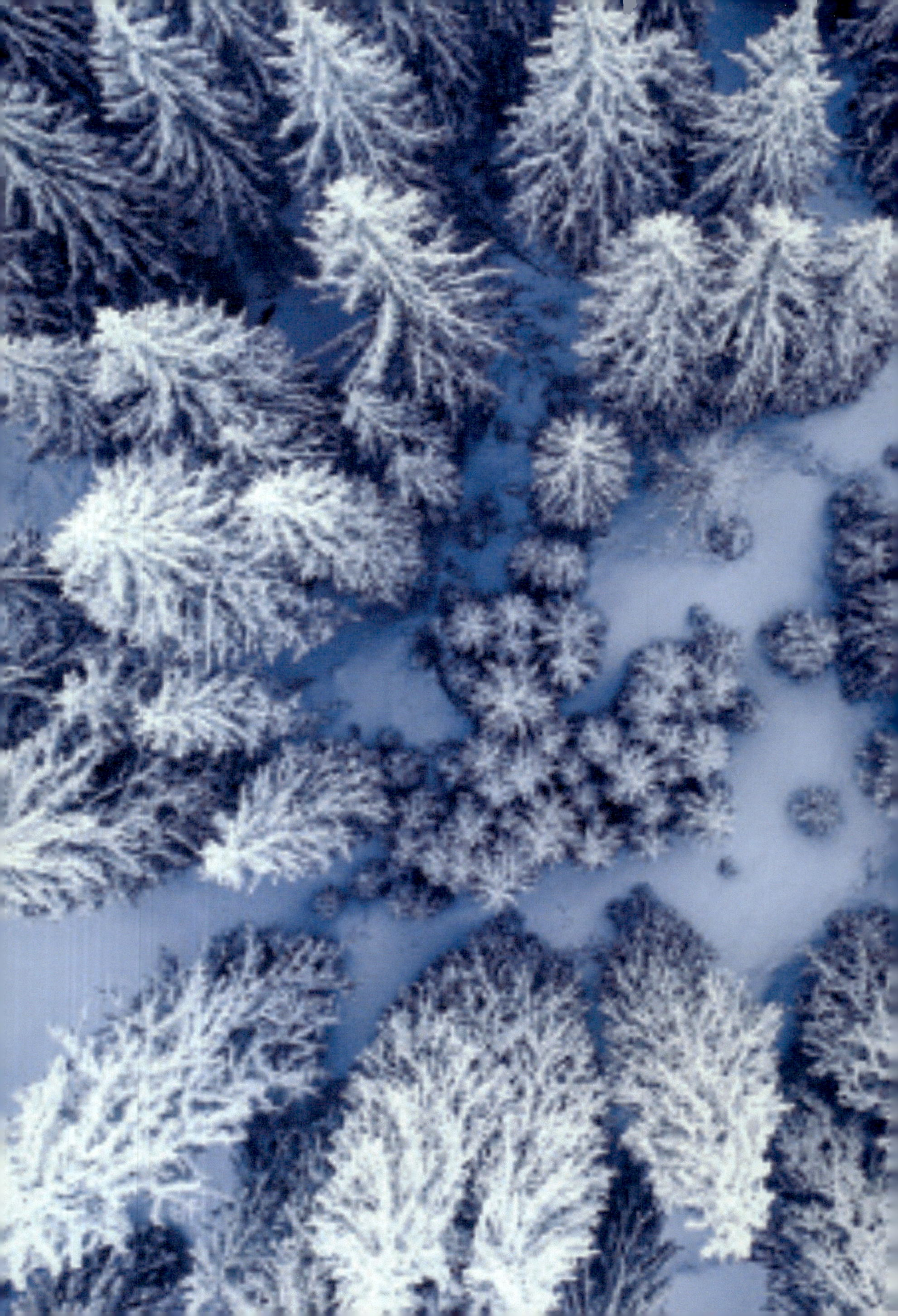

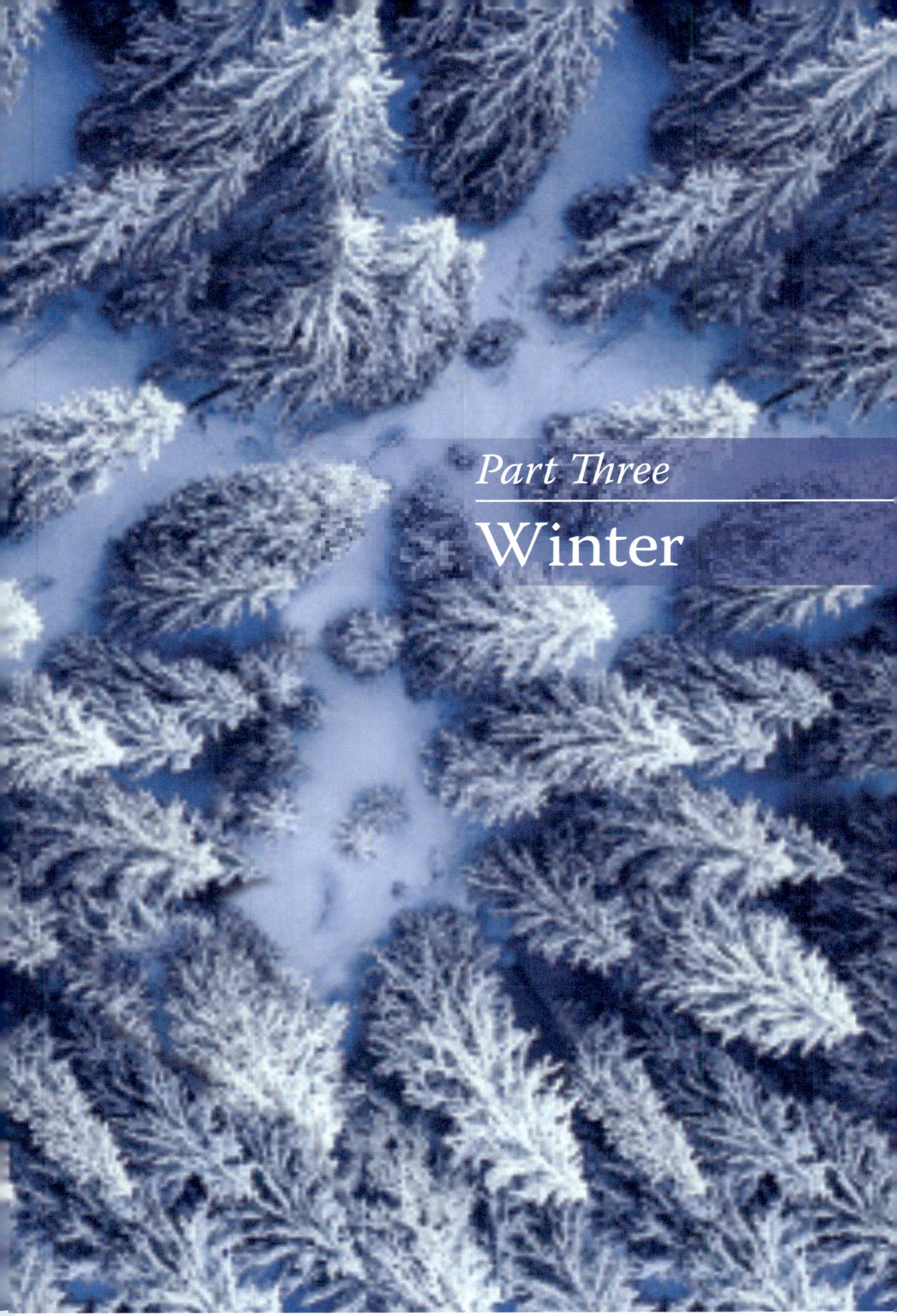

Part Three

Winter

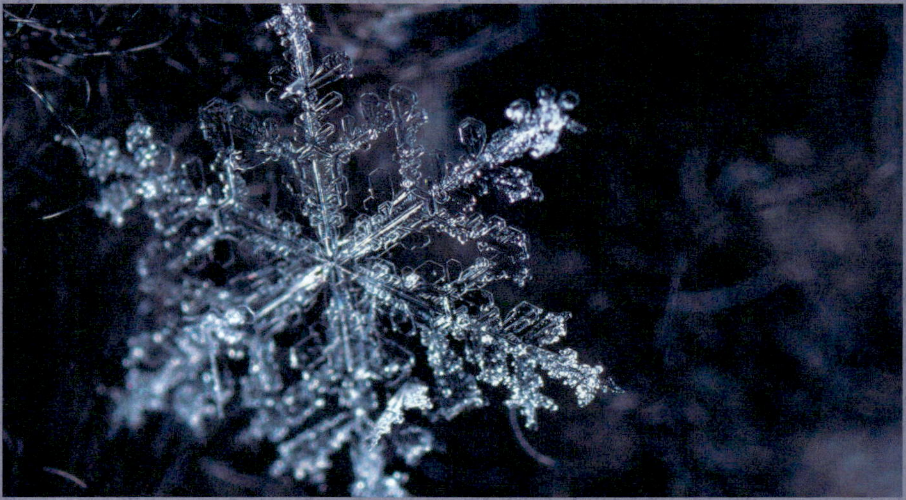

TO RESCUE LIFE ON EARTH, YOU MUST SEE THE WORLD DIFFERENTLY AND CHANGE FROM YOUR DEPTHS IN THE MANNER OF GAME-CHANGERS LIKE MAIMONIDES. AND SO YOU PREPARE FOR THE TASK AHEAD BY LETTING GO OF DESPERATE URGENCY, STEPPING BACK TO LOOK AT THE REST OF YOUR BELOVED PROFESSION AND CONTEMPLATE IT AS A WAYWORD CHILD OF LIFE. THEN YOU CAN ALLOW YOUR IMAGINATION TO ENGAGE IT; THEN YOU CAN BEGIN CARE OF THE ONE LIFE—THAT IS, THE BODIES OF INDIVIDUALS, SPECIES, HABITATS, AND THE WHOLE OF THE ANCIENT BUT ALWAYS NEW BIOME.

Repurposing Your Medical Ego

We defy augury. There is special providence in the fall of a sparrow. If it be now, 'tis not to come; if it be not to come, it will be now; if it be not now, yet it will come. The readiness is all.

— William Shakespeare in *Hamlet*

In winter, readiness becomes more and more important as you approach the extremes of cold far from the equator. In the Arctic, human life is especially fragile; elsewhere, low temperatures and icy weather remind you that careful gathering and use of resources such as food may be essential to life, health, and comfort. Winter is the ideal time to cozy up to the hearth and contemplate the darkness within and without. The illumination of inner demons that abide in recesses hidden from inner angels requires an allegorical process such as the one that Joseph Campbell framed as the Hero's Journey. Accepting this type of inner work allows you to catch up with times essential for continuation as well as for the kinds of transformation that lead to wisdom. This wintry contemplative period of your year of transition is the perfect time to take an inward journey that syncs your body with the bodies in which it nests.

Medical eldering begins when you depart from the habits you formed in the adult or middle phase of your medical life. These once supported you, but now limit you. And yet your ego—the "operating system" that you formed in your younger years—will try to hold the old ways in place. One reason for this is that moderns relate poorly to time. We do not see this moment as giving birth to all future moments. We do not see metamorphic change as necessary to ongoing growth and development. We do not welcome the death of bad old ways or the birth of better ones. We resist them. To culminate your life calling, you overcome the tendency to stasis, let go of the past, and prepare for the culmination of your lifework and the creation of your legacy. This requires a periodic journey backward and inward and to decide what to bring forward into your maturity.

In the modern era—and thus in your lifetime—our species has been exploring the limits of material aggregation without regard to the greater life within which we and our patients and descendants play a crucial role. You and we and everyone we know, ready or not, are already embarking on a new epoch that ends the reckless human experiment of modernity that has risked destroying hundreds of millions of years of evolution. Should we fail to glean the necessary and sufficient wisdom to rescue life, our profession will perpetuate its codependence with death and cease to exist.

Change requires that you enter the unknown depths of being and do what is far, far better—and harder—than anything you have done before—including the medical training that inculcated you with the neglected wisdom aspect of your tradition. To rescue life on earth, you must see the world differently and change from your depths in the manner of game-changers like Maimonides. And so you prepare for the task ahead by letting go of desperate urgency, stepping back to look at the rest of your beloved profession and contemplate it as a wayword child of life. Then you can allow your imagination to engage it; then you can begin care of the one life—that is, the bodies of individuals, species, habitats, and the whole of the ancient but always new biome.

Fortunately, your profession has a century and a half of experience in caring for the body of the species through the specialty of public health and preventive medicine, as you can see in John Snow's medical detection of the source of a cholera outbreak in 1854, the eradication of smallpox in 1977, and the ongoing rapid responses to new infectious agents such as the AIDS, Ebola, and epidemic Corona viruses. Many advances in medical hygiene have long since been incorporated into prenatal and well child care, and integrative medicine is slowly trying, weighing, and integrating into the profession some so-called complementary modalities. Before that came two and a half millennia and more of the accrual of wisdom, as well as the transformation of that wisdom with each epoch. Taking a long and broad view of your profession's history allows you to put modernity into perspective in the history of our species and of life on earth. While modernity has been breathtakingly destructive, it has taught us all we need to know to survive and thrive by loving life as ourselves.

When you look away from the modern systems that hold you back, you can prepare to realign your relation to time, make good on your personal and shared experiences, recognize life on earth as an irreplaceable resource for human life, and co-devise a sustainable form of personal medicine that cares for each as for all.

Opening Your Perceptual Filter

As soon as I got out into Heaven's light I started on another long excursion, making haste with all my heart to store my mind with the Lord's beauty and thus be ready for any fate, light or dark. And it was from this time that my long continuous wanderings may be said to have fairly commenced.

— John Muir in "Blind!" in *The Wild Muir*

Transitioning to the wisdom years is a life passage in which you relinquish old habits of bodily existence and adopt new ones. These will feel alien or uncomfortable at first, but with time they will align your passage with the epochal change that immerses you. As time passes, you—who are the protagonist of your personal narrative—may transition from conquering hero to caretaker; from world-weary, technology-dazzled striver to open-hearted, avuncular counselor; from denizen of a whirring social machine to living thread in an evolving tapestry that extends so far into the past and future as to be integrated into perennial processes of living care and cure. Your passage will require the courage and the delicacy to see the body of life in the light of humility and wonder, to perceive in it the wellspring of generative life, and to handle it with exquisite and decisive tenderness.

When you dissolve the defenses that you formed to navigate the hurly-burly of daily life, you will see how you, your profession, and your species are on a collision course with the body of life. You may begin to see how it came to be that your career defined the scope of your calling too narrowly, and to take hold of post-employment freedom to use the sum total of your lifetime of experience to form an inner guide capable of distinguishing the urgent from the important, the picayune from the essential, and the fragmented from the whole. You can then play with views, frames, and constructs that show you ways through the modern valley of shadows to the verdant field of a possible living future. There you will meet life with new senses, open your mind and heart, and fulfill your calling by patterning your care of your own life as of each and all.

In the winter of your transition year, you peer into the shadows of your life's passage and discover the roots and shoots of the third and last chapter of your life story. The winter dark holds the unprocessed events that you once put off, suppressed, or outran. It conceals jangling memories, jagged entanglements, and jumbles of unresolved desires. These may enliven the shadows that surround you and obscure the effulgence ahead. You must dispel them; there is no other way. No one can do this for you. You must process raw memories, reconcile or make amends for embodied wrongs, and share wellsprings of joy. Doing so will free your warmth and light and prime your body to create its one and only legacy.

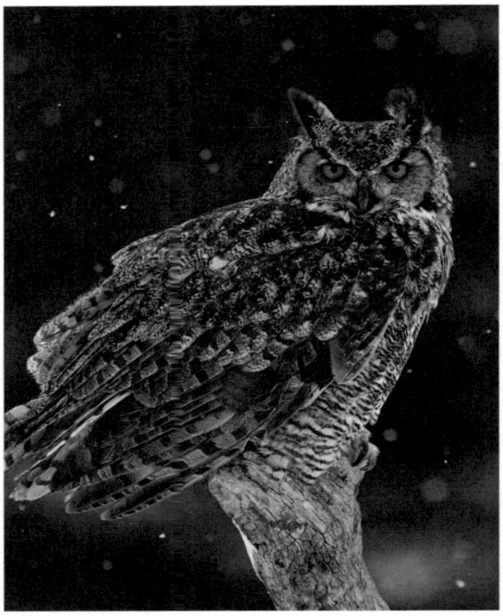

If this is your first encounter with the unfinished past, you may find the going tricky and fraught. The more expert a clinician you are—that is, the more you have been relying on the adaptive unconscious—the more trouble your aware, rational mind may face in processing and turning experience into advantage. Fortunately, countless humans have gone before you and left a trail to follow. These include the authors of myths such as the tale of Orpheus, who looked back across the River Styx and lost a life that he had reclaimed; Ovid and his early modern student Shakespeare, who redemptively transformed many historical errors and horrors; or emerging designers and artists, who give birth to the new. You may at first feel like a sculptor kneeling blindfolded at the edge of a precipice, groping for clay from which to shape a new face. You may then, like Jung and so many other doctors, discover instructive archetypes or allegories that suit the now—such as personifying our species as a baby in the birth canal of life who is emerging into a new stage of growth and development.

However you experience or articulate transitions, you will know you are ready to emerge when you have oriented your person, place, and time within the body of life and its context, and have learned to perceive your future as integral to the future of your descendants. Countless elders have preceded you: since the Axial Age at least, members of our species have been seeking spiritual rebirth through processes that clergy call dying before you die, and that New Agers called personal transformation or realizing your full potential. Unfortunately, these spiritual paths are unlikely to be of practical use to you as a doctor because they dispel the ego and allow being to reach stasis. That can stop you being part of the problem, but is not enough in your case. You are a solver of problems who, in your career, solved the bodily problems of others and their systems and who, in your elderhood, will broaden your scope and solve your own problems as you participate in solving those of your context.

The winter ahead will thus focus on repurposing your medical ego—that is, the interface between your inner and outer worlds. The aim is to prime you to move toward your place at the moving front of time, where the darkness of the unknowable is illuminated. There you can catalyze your transformation of your life and your profession. There you can then make good on the whole of your past, making the best of your present and the most of your future. You begin by orienting the whole of your past—and the cyclical light and darkness of your calling as revealed through the game-changing teaching of past eras—to the here and now. Then and only then will you be ready to reconcile with evolving biological reality and to ground your eldering in time.

ANECDOTES FROM MEDICAL LIVES

It's helpful, then, during a dark night, to constantly broaden your imagination of what is happening to you. If your only idea is that you're depressed, you will be at the mercy of the depression industry...An alternative is to see human life as a continuing invitation to be more of what it is capable, to be individual and deeply connected.

—Thomas Moore in *Dark Nights of the Soul*

In the course of medical training and experience, you learn to cull patients who will not benefit from your care. You do this by forming and maintaining a so-called perceptual filter that edits your experience to suit your needs. Some of what you edit out remains with you as a Jungian shadow—that is, as aspects of experience that you have tried to ignore, deny, project, or disown. In the film *Triage: Dr. James Orbinski's Humanitarian Dilemma,* a trauma surgeon describes his use of a well-honed filter in a time of genocide. The filter works at its heart-breaking best in such circumstances. In the course of routine primary care, which is immersed in the ambiguous, uncertain, unknown, and unseen, you are at first uncomfortably aware of problems you cannot solve and patients you cannot help, and ease this by gradually building a filter that excludes the—to you, at the time—insoluble problems in order to free you to do what you can. This filter will not be pretty or precise. It may neglect or abuse sufferers, or blame those who 'fail to read the textbooks.' It may feed a monster of regret that grows in the shadows and drives you to work faster, harder, and longer.

To free your body of regret, and to reclaim the lost experiences that you need to proactively participate in determining what comes next, you enter your wisdom years primed to review the aspects of experience that you filtered out and left by the wayside. Your intense sense of perpetual responsibility may call for gentle and ongoing relaxation of wrong expectations as well as self-compassion and self-forgiveness. When you master this, you can release the wisdom you embodied but ignored, especially that which you can now derive from past failures. This month, you will prepare to take your place on the bridge that leads from the modern era to the future, and you will look back and make sure that you have owned and brought along all that you need, including all that you may have put aside until now. Doing this will shrink your monster of regret to its proper size and prepare you to use all that you gained in real time—or on reflection—to prime your stances and form your vision. This is not easy work for anyone.

And yet, the work will be easier for you than for others. As a doctor, you have already become aware of the problems of the species and have spent the whole of your career solving them in the available way. This means that you have a wealth of experience in transforming some of the social, psychospiritual, and mortal shadows of the end of modernity. Soon you will be free to begin illuminating the rest and to use them as priming for your stances. As you do this for yourself, you will also be modeling this for your profession and your society, thereby catalyzing the game that is already afoot. Let's begin by looking back on the shadows that every modern doctor encounters and that strengthen our peer support, our gallows humor, and our ability to call on self-power and other-power.

Michaela: Better Off Dead?

While in the midst of a demanding obstetrical residency, Michaela took call in the labor suite of a large public hospital. One night, she was delivering the baby of a patient whose pannus was so large that it was difficult to judge the weight or the distress of the fetus. The baby seemed large, and the patient was a poor candidate for cesarean section. Concerned about the risks to the mother and child, the trainee decided to err on the side of safety by delivering the baby vaginally as soon as possible. The delivery did not go well. The trainee applied forceps and traction, injuring the infant's brachial plexus. The baby would grow up to be an adult with a withered arm.

Michaela was devastated by remorse. To make things worse, the infant was of normal size with good APGAR scores. There probably had been no fetal distress, which meant—in hindsight—that the forceps delivery and injury could have been avoided. While the trainee was still reeling from the impact of the event, and attempting to process it so as to discern what to do to avoid future harm, a hospital administrator came into the doctor's room and said, "Better a dead baby than an injured one. The family will sue and we'll pay for years. How will we keep our doors open?"

Michaela was shocked, and sought comfort from fellow-trainees and mentors who had passed through the awful rite of passage of doing harm to life. Now, years later, reflecting on this event, it is easy to picture an administrator toiling helplessly away behind a desk, weighed down by responsibilities that loom large to him, and imagining that economic rationalism is the best window into our human problems. It is easy to see him coming to believe that it is more important to keep the hospital doors open than to ensure that those who work within take patients and their problems as a sacred trust; form the virtuous, street-wise character to make the best high-stakes decisions at the worst moments; remember that we are a species and not a social machine; and meet people where they are—which is in a virtual reality featuring myths of rescue, all-wise and error-free information systems, risk-free technology, and the right to use up a living world that is no more than a backdrop for late modern consumerism.

Dick: Quick Karma

One night, a call team admitted an intoxicated patient to the general medical ward. This ward was in a teaching hospital that served an inner city, and that tended to draw the least among us. In other words, those who could not scrape together fifty cents or who lacked the self-respect, time or competence to take the bus elsewhere would come to this hospital rather than to another that offered more compassionate care. The faculty of the university who attended the patients were trying to draw a better class of patients by admitting fellow-faculty, staff, and students.

In this particular case, the patient was a member of the 'four hundred club'—that is, his blood alcohol level would have been in the lethal range if he were less accustomed to drinking. The emergency staff, busy with other patients, took his belongings, put them in a bag, and put them on the bottom shelf of his gurney. A member of the transport staff took the patient to his room, moved him to the bed, and left his belongings beside the bed.

In one of the beds in an adjacent room was a highly ranking member of the university administration who was suffering from gastrointestinal bleeding. He appeared to be as anxious about his admission to the ward as he was about his continuing loss of blood. His attending physician assured him that he was in good hands, then went home for the night. The resident in charge soon appeared to reassure the patient, and then went into the next room to see the new patient, who was no longer comatose, and who recognized the resident.

The patient was a regular. The staff ignored him as he lurched to a sitting position, bent unsteadily forward, and rummaged in his bag. In seconds, a shot rang out. That got everyone's attention. The man in the next bed pointed to the regular patient and reported that he had cursed the resident under his breath, extricated a loaded gun from his bag, and tried to aim it at the resident. He missed, shooting himself in the foot instead. The staff disarmed him; the resident instructed the nurse to prepare the patient for transfer to a surgical service that handled the weekend patients that some wags facetiously referred to as members of the Friday Night Friends of Bacchus, or the Saturday Night Knife and Gun Club.

The resident, his competence and gruff manner barely altered by this sad attempt on his life—or by his quick 'turfing' of this hot-potato patient—rushed to the next room to reassure the high-status patient in his care. The resident found the bed empty, the intravenous line swinging like a pendulum, and the personal effects gone. The high-status patient had sized up the risks of staying and leaving and made a run for it.

Philip and Grace: A Higher Power

You could call them a power couple. He was a cardiothoracic surgeon known for doing lengthy procedures; she was a pediatrician known for staying at home to care for her children and for working for the health of children in the community. Their family was known for being friendly, kind, and humble, especially on Thanksgiving Day, when they hosted an annual dinner in a public park. They took particular care to invite anyone they met who might be socially isolated or suffering from discouragement. This behavior was unusual at their university, and drew curiosity. However, they said very little about their motivations, which they offered as integral to the spirit of medical practice.

After a time, a story began to circulate that seemed to explain their service as well as their happiness. One day, when he was facing a time of trial in the operating room, he paused to pray aloud for aid. It turned out then when it suited the patient, or when he felt in need of the aid of a higher power, the surgeon would pray silently or with others. Some bystanders were distressed to find that their colleague appealed to a higher power, a move they may have viewed as delusional or defeatist. Other bystanders left it to the surgeon to find solace or grace in the face of responsibility in whatever way was best for his projects and his patients.

Wielding the knife is a concrete and fearsome responsibility that may prompt you to become aware that you never hold the knife alone: you hold it with the lineage of heroic surgeons who followed the enlightenment and further back, perhaps—all the way back to the shamans who devised trepanning in ancient times. As you hold the knife or otherwise take a life in your hands, you may turn to the unseen like the protagonist in the film *City of Angels* and ask who is there. The answer that suits you may derive from the foreground of your experience as embodied in a professional organization or society or from the background of your experience as abstracted in the language of mathematics or in a spirit or Godhead of theology. In these moments, you can relax into your sphere of support and shoulder your responsibility, and so avoid the error most common to surgeons—and to all doctors and moderns: the illusion of control.

BETH LOOKS BACK: Recognizing and Reconciling Neglect and Abuse

A life, a human life, is not a life until it is examined...It is a profound irony... that it is the memory man, the Mnemonist, who has in this sense lost his life, and the amnesiac, the shattered man, who gains and regains his life.

— Oliver Sacks in the Foreword to A.R. Luria's
The Man with a Shattered World

I remember the first time I had a good time. I was sixteen years old and was sitting in an ice cream parlor called the Peacock in Evanston near the college I was attending. I was with a group from the outing club, and we were talking and laughing and feeling carefree. The moment I noticed that strange feeling, I stopped and withdrew into myself. Something was wrong. I shouldn't be happy; I should be miserable. To do otherwise would betray the reality in which I had always lived. And yet when I looked around, I could see that the gathering was harmless. I felt confused. Was it wrong to take simple pleasure in life? If not, my life would change. Why and how would I live?

I grew up in the shadows. My grandmother had indulged in a love affair that was so scandalous she left Sweden and immigrated to America, where my mother grew up knowing nothing of the truth of her conception. Her stepfather must have known; when drunk and violent, he would call her a bastard. My father had survived the early death of his mother, the depression, a wartime massacre followed by three years as a prisoner of war, and discharge from the Canadian army with four hundred dollars and a severe case of PTSD, then viewed as shameful. Around the time that the British turned on Alan Turing—who arguably won the war by breaking the Enigma code—the Canadian government threw my father in military prison. Even now, there are times when the shadows of survivor's guilt and scapegoating rouse in me a state of anxiety, a response that I may harbor in some form until I die.

What I didn't know about shadow until that day in the Peacock was that it can also contain the good memories of life, and that you can release and enjoy them. That is, if you are selectively aware of the bad stuff and cache the good stuff in the closet, you can—as you become aware of it—open the door and let it out. Without forgetting the bad, you can embrace and embody the good that you can then use as time credits to offset your time debts.

Fast forward twenty years. I had worked hard, earned a Great Society scholarship, and—like many who grew up in shadow—went into medicine, then on into public health and preventive medicine. I wanted to get to the source of suffering and heal the world's ills. I was desperate for it. And then I got what I had asked for. The 'fickle finger of fate' gave me a sickness that allowed me to play the role of medical detective in my own life, and so to discover the hard way one etiology behind a major new epidemic. This new epidemic made doctors feel angry because they felt suspicious of the patients, which often triggered scapegoating. I was once again thrown away, into the depths of shadows where groups push those they fear for one reason or another, such as the fear of the unknown and obviously uncontrollable. And so I lived with pain and sorrow, but not surprise. Any child of fear or displaced blame would recognize this all-too-familiar phenomenon.

I became a seeker, looking for answers in every shadowy corner. I became an autodidact, a self-healer, and a student of shadow—including the Jungian shadow I had come to know. I cured much of my fear with courage, some of my despair with optimism, and some of my social censure by keeping to the shadows. I did what I could to cure myself and my profession. And so I gained perspective on doctors—like Semmelweiss—who take on more responsibility than is healthy, reasonable, or sustainable.

Doctors have always been immersed in and filled with shadows. We can still run from them, or into them, but we can no longer hide. We are priests of medical technology in an information age, at a time when that which we purport to control has long since gotten away from us. We are embedded in late modern ways of living that push habitat extinctions into the shadows. At the same time, the general social expectation is that errors are unacceptable, which means that these, too, are denied and pushed into the shadows. We then ignore what we cannot measure easily or uniformly, such as quality of life and rates of emerging epidemics, and push everything that we miss into the shadows. More and more reality is relegated to shadow. When we are looking for motivations and solutions we will find them where there is—as yet—no light.

COMMENT: Reconciling with Your Present Reality

I would particularly warn against imprudent planetary medication or surgery... To attempt control from outside by increasing or decreasing one feedback loop [in] multiple feedback systems is rarely successful, and carries with it the risk of dangerous and unpredictable instability.

— James Lovelock in *Healing Gaia*

We doctors are good at predicting, comprehending, and measuring death when it is near. We are not so good—as Dr. Alvan Feinstein pointed out—at seeing the hazards of daily life through which our species harms self and others, or the best ways in which to reduce that harm so as to enjoy life. These require knowledge and wisdom that fell into the shadows in the course of late modernity. Even as our species focused on heroics and fell into reductionism and fragmentation, we were learning—for the first time in history—how to act congregally so as to realize perennial dreams such as the eradication of smallpox. We took those modern experiments so far that each and every one of us is conditioned to seek out some small area of expertise and to filter out all others, thereby pushing the body of life into our shared shadows.

Modernism—most especially those aspects having to do with living systems—is untenable. It therefore falls to you to gently open your filter until you are able to become a polymath, or at least to communicate well enough with others to join in braking and reversing our species' reckless consumption of life on earth. This task will not be easy. It is important and urgent and yet will take time. To nurture wise discernment and enhance free-flowing creativity—human virtues now called out by life on earth—you can revisit your medical life and envision change. While you were dutifully trying to make the system work, and keeping faith that it did and it would, you were inadvertently taking life on earth for granted. To illuminate what you may only just now wish to learn, you can gently and groundedly open your filter and seek out new and useful views, frames, and constructs that will support your juniors in caring for life. You can explore the utility of these with emerging experts in other fields such as theology, mathematics, psychology, organic agriculture, habitat restoration, field biology, green burial practices, and so on. Together, you can create a wise medicine for a living future.

While it may not be easy for you to recall and to contemplate experiences that you disregarded in the past, you are at an advantage relative to those who are not leading medical lives. It is as if you have been preparing for bad news all your life. The fact that you are reading this now means that you have come through darkness that others can only imagine while keeping intact your love of life, your sanguine stance, your toolkit of practical strategies and skills, and your ability to improvise solutions to tenacious problems under pressure. You have an invaluable store of experience and abundant grace to share with those who follow. This places you in a position to illuminate your shadows as you have illuminated those of others, and to retrieve lost experience, knowledge and wisdom that you can use to promote the long-term survival of our stubbornly self-destructive species.

Owning the Full Spectrum of Your Past

I was probably the only man in the world dancing the tango with a partner in a straitjacket. I was in my white medical coat, and she was in a straitjacket because she had been very aggressive and was hurting people. But I danced with her, and this was bridging the gap between doctor and patient, normal and psychotic.

— Dr. Viktor Frankl via Haddon Klingberg, Jr. in *When Life Calls Out to Us*

WORKING QUESTIONS

Employed Physicians

- Is my interpretation of events accurate? What am I reading into this that isn't there? What am I failing to see that is there?
- Is my response to this event like my response to others? When and how was this response formed? When is it useful? If never, am I ready to let it go? Can I substitute one I prefer?
- What just happened? Why? What part of this is mine?
- Has this happened before? When? How did I respond? How do I want to respond next time?

Self-determined Physicians

- When I compare myself to people I admire, what do they bring to life that I don't? What do I bring to life that they don't? What do I want to bring to life that I haven't?
- Which memories of my life and work fill me with contentment? Which with unease?
- What would nourish my soul and spirit right now?
- What would make me feel content now, or by the end of the day?

EXERCISE 1

Write your top ten best and bottom ten worst memories in your journal. Whenever you like, return to your list of best memories and ask, when is the last time I did something like that? When can I do something like that again? Feel free to change the lists as you recall forgotten events.

EXERCISE 2: Opening to the Whole of Experience

Years ago I had a patient with a startling neglect of her own left side, and the left side of space, due to a stroke in the right parietal lobe. But this had not prepared me at all to find myself in a virtually identical situation.

— Oliver Sacks in *The Mind's Eye*

In this exercise, you will observe what you tend to notice or disregard; what draws or repels you; what you rule in or rule out before you think; what you choose to own or disown; and what you integrate into being, doing, and becoming—aware or not, and for good or for ill. The primary purpose of the exercise is to open your filter so as to trawl back in time and retrieve experiences that hold lost wisdom. As you learn to do this, you prepare to gain wisdom from all sources in real time, and so to turn the whole of experience to the advantage of the portion of the body of life in your care—including your own maturing body.

One of the great joys of opening your filter is that you become aware of improvising your being and becoming as motifs and leitmotifs in the symphony of creation that astonishes, drives, and inspires with intricate harmony and exquisite beauty. Your portion of catastrophe—past, present, and future—then becomes the ground from which you draw your best work, which always lies ahead of you. As you strain to hear the music to which you are contributing, you hear and see symbolic languages afresh and find new meaning in words like those of Shakespeare's Hamlet: "there are more things in heaven and earth… than are dreamt of in your philosophy."

Be aware that as you begin to care for your life in this way, you are likely at first to be a terrible patient. The reason for this is that your filter neglects your body with the idea that you are always in an emergency situation and caring for those in extremis. This presumes that you—and your patients—can stand on the outside of life looking in. This point of view—so useful in establishing objective perspectives—is founded upon a faulty premise and could easily become a fatal error. We are not outside of life; we are immersed in it. Nor are we the face that we show the world; we are ever and always our whole selves.

As you work with shadow, you may exit your care state and enter into a cure state or a hell state. The moment you notice that you no longer abide in a care state, stop and pay kind attention to your state of being. Take care of yourself to prevent needless ills or woes. Quit while you are ahhead. Any attempt to freeze, lock down, or dissociate may tide you over at the cost of reinforcing rather than dispelling your shadows. If you are carried away into a hell state, your body may become refractory. If you have come too close to a sleeping dragon, you may have to take a hiatus of days or weeks to strengthen your state before approaching it again. With practice, you will learn to rebound rapidly. You will become resilient. You will learn to feed your care states and these will benefit you and everyone you encounter.

Transfer the table below—or one like it—to your journal, leaving room to add as many rows as you please. Over the course of a week, be alert for 'blind spots' in your filter that are continuing to edit your experience automatically and that prevent you from making the best use of it. (It may help to keep in mind that if you haven't been learning from your mistakes, you probably haven't been taking enough risks to learn anything worth knowing.) When you encounter highly charged memories of events you were unprepared to process at the time, approach them gently, kindly, and inventively, like sleeping dragons that guard weak spots in your psyche. See them as Rilke did, as princesses waiting to be kissed, and invite your mature self to tame them and to care for them until they are ready to fly.

Body*		**Doing***		**The Body of Life***	
Attract	**Repel**	**Attract**	**Repel**	**Attract**	**Repel**

* Your body is your generative flesh and its manifestations, herein grouped as awareness, understanding, perceptions, sensations, energy, flesh and interbeing; your doing expresses your body as motivation, stances, states, strategies, skills, and vision; and the body of life is the aggregate of all bodies.

EXERCISE 3: Syncing with Life in Time

Many scholars began to suppose that observation could be replaced by computer simulation and mathematical models. Psychological textbooks overflowed with such models and schemas. This deluge brought a still greater danger: the reality of human conscious activity was being replaced by mechanical models.

— A.R. Luria via Jerome Bruner Foreword in *The Mind of a Mnemonist*

In these exercises, you prepare to contextualize medicine by taking time to engage fundamental developments in other fields that took place during your lifetime. These you missed because you expected to know more and more about less and less until you knew everything about nothing—in other words, because you were flooded by streams of minutiae designed to flatter the late modern illusion of control. As you gather knowledge and wisdom relevant to elderhood—especially that of seminal late modern thinkers and model elders like Daniel Kahneman and Jerome Bruner—you can bypass the fragmenting and less fundamental research that dominates late modern biomedicine and instead face practical problems that reveal modern follies.

It is easy to look back and criticize—and important to do so to the degree necessary to put modernity behind you—but the ultimate goal of looking to the past is to learn from it as you unburden your body of its weight. If this is easy for you, you may not need much—or any—of this exercise. It will be here any time you have need of it. If you do engage it seriously, you may find that you develop an aversion to some part of your adult career.

Do not worry. This is good: you are experiencing adaptive disillusionment. This is a natural stage in social evolution—especially now, when humans have become far more effective than they used to be and have thus become like the proverbial bulls in the china shop. This is the first step toward wisdom that has been delayed so long that you will have the chance to witness—and to participate in—its rebirth. You will do more than learn from your experience and the experience of your peers; you will learn from the human experience of the last five hundred years. Drawing upon that history may feel wrong to you because your expectations were formed by a period that devalued life on earth.

You begin by owning your errors. This obliges you to forgive yourself, your patients, and your context, which is a prerequisite for exploring new insights and perspectives. In doing this, you can consult the wisdom of the ages; forgiveness is a familiar and perennial process that has come down to us through religious and spiritual traditions.

A: Owning Your Errors

We know that a creative imagination—the kind of imagination that makes for great inventors—operates in a manner that is closely in touch with reality. But there is another type of imagination whose activity is not directed toward the external world, but is nourished by desire and becomes a substitute for action.

— A.R. Luria in *The Mind of the Mnemonist*

When you adopt the mindset of a late modern physician, you develop a tendency toward regret and self-punishment that you off-set with over-adjustment and creation of a perceptual filter that excludes all that you perceive as beyond your control so that you can focus on those things that do seem to be under your control. Over time, however, your filter may fill up with maladaptive heuristics and biases that have the potential to make you like the mnemonist in the quote: someone who processes reality in lieu of engaging it.

If your career was narrow or subject to invasive over-management, opening your mind is likely to take gentleness and patience. If you persevere, you will likely undergo a literal change of mind—a profound, extensive, and continuing remodeling of neural circuitry that you may recognize from scriptural passages like "the scales fell from my eyes." This will, in other words, reveal the extent of your brainwashing and enable you to reverse it so as to think freely.

B: Reconciling Errors of Commission

Surely we are provided with senses as well fitted to penetrate the spaces of the real, the substantial, the eternal, as these outward are to penetrate the material universe.

— Henry David Thoreau in *A Week on the Concord River*

Reconciling errors of commission is the work of the whole body. One reason for this is that doctors are programmed for the kind of self-neglect that prevents the heart from doing emotional work in real time and likewise prevents the brain from remodeling itself in response to experience. This means that you will have learned to shift the functions of these organs to other organs—the autonomic nervous system in particular—and will have been better adapted to respond to episodes of emergency and scarcity than to hone the skills needed for lifetime learning.

In this exercise, you try a few practices for self-transformation and so begin a gradual and comprehensive transition to eldering. You may find that you are encountering a brave new world that was hidden to you. Fortunately, you have advantages of experience and education that will make it relatively easy for you to transform medicine in collaboration with your species.

Now take a pad of paper and a pencil to a place of study—e.g. a den, library desk, or chapel—and examine your memory for a troubling error of commission. This is any action to which you were a party and that you even now wish that you could change. Choose a memory that is troubling and that you would like to put to rest, but that is not so distressing as to flood your autonomic system or to otherwise overwhelm you.

(Now comes a serious responsibility: if you recognize that you have made a malicious error in the recent past, or feel an urge to commit an intentional error, you are impaired. Accept it. If you are still practicing medicine, stop work immediately, get help, and focus on resolving your crisis. Return to eldering when you have recovered.)

When you are ready to reconcile your memory, picture your embodied emotional burden as like a complex wound and your treatment of it as a gradual debridement. Begin by identifying accessible and substantial bits and allow your body to slough them off. Imagine that while you are attending to other tasks, your wound is continuing to heal. Remember that unlike people who fear or loathe and punish the body—or simply fail to appreciate it—you see and value its miraculous, exquisite beauty and support its healing with conscientious care and whatever cure you are able to offer.

Note that this work is figurative, and yet constitutes an act of embodied imagination that can work for your good from the inside out. In this exercise, the burden of that imaginative and emotive work falls on the heart. This will—sooner or later—open you to heartache. As Buddhist teacher Rodney Smith says, "Go ahead and feel it. It isn't gonna kill you." Your heart will best be able to experience and release painful emotions when your body is equanimous and focused and you are neither distracted nor flooded. Learn to read your body. When it is—when you are—wound up, relax. Let it take whatever time it takes. Assist it with several deep sighs. Invite your heart to do this work; do not force it. When your heart is hard or numb, place one or both palms over it and support it with warm energy and kind attention. If at any time your body gets carried away and carries you away, stop and relax. Take time to find a middle way between on the one hand accepting the difficulty of the work and allowing it to proceed naturally and on the other trying to control or strongarm it.

Now, determine whether you are ready to articulate your memory. If not, repeat the first part of the exercise at will. When you are ready, write responses to the prompts below in your journal. If you want what you write to be seen by your eyes alone, write your responses to the prompts on sheets of paper and then burn them. If you like, add a blessing or prayer.

- The whole story of what happened—starting from the beginning—was...
- When I think of the mistake I made I feel...
- I am ready to forgive myself now, or I will be when...

If this exercise is productive for you—that is, if your body responds to it with relief—repeat the exercise at will until you have reconciled your emotional backlog and learned to feel new emotions in real time in your heart. If this exercise is not productive for you at present, undertake others and try this one again after some time has passed.

C: Forgiving and Preventing Errors of Omission

A preference for unbiased predictions is justified if all errors of prediction are treated alike, regardless of their direction. But there are situations in which one type of error is much worse than another.

— Daniel Kahneman in *Thinking, Fast and Slow*

Often, errors of omission are noticed in hindsight, and belong to everyone—or to most people—living in an era wherein the known is taken for all. Such errors may be recognized in hindsight when they may give rise to remorse and anguish best used to prime action to set things right before it is too late, as with medieval fatalism and modern consumerism or technoshamanism.

As a late modern, you will have—as your species has always done—shown insufficient respect for errors of omission and their catastrophic consequences. Your human exceptionalism will have lulled you into accepting human society as the be-all and end-all, and human society will in turn have encouraged you to diffuse your errors onto your profession, your managers, and your society. This will have enabled you to function without a care for the big picture.

As awareness of modern errors drives emergence, you may find that you, too, are ready for change, or that your embodiment of errors is burdening you and that you may be obliged to process and respond to them in order to release them or put them to rest. When you become aware of modern failures to care for life, and feel that it is time to own and reconcile your part in it, write in your journal in response to the following prompts:

- When I think of the consequences of human destruction of life, I think that in the future it would be better for doctors to...
- When I think of the problems that I blamed on patients and that may turn out to have been cryptic signs of chronic poisoning of the body of the species and the body of life, I think that in the future it would be better for the medical profession to...
- When I envision myself as a mentor and elder who is able to learn from the experience of my lifetime and my generation, I think of teaching young doctors to...
- When I think of people who have transitioned to elderhood and of times in history when our species has embraced change, I think of...

EXERCISE 4: Owning Your Life and Work

I have just as much hope as ever of doing something with my life, and so I don't want people to think I'm a hopeless case. I'm doing everything I can to accomplish this, and little by little use what possibilities I have.

— Zasetsy in *The Man with a Shattered World* through A.R. Luria

In a lifetime of trying to make the system work because—and in spite—of its design, you may become a white collar employee in a large organization who avoids trouble by being helpless, passive, and dependent, and who at the same time devotes your life and work to a social machine that will never respond in kind. Before you notice what you are doing, you slip into patterns that make you more and more passive and less and less responsive. You become 'frontal-lobish.'

In this exercise, you regain control of and ground your higher cortical functions, especially your tertiary processing centers and frontal lobes. You didn't intend to weaken these, but you are the only one who can take responsibility for strengthening them. Only you can glean the lessons of your life experience and use what you glean to set and hone your expectations and to give your actions direction and traction. To do this, you will be obliged to withdraw from invasive late modern medical systems and to reverse the reduction of your complex human processes into crude algorithms by systemic incentives and punishments that interfere with your intelligence.

Learning from the History of New Medical Knowledge

Taking a meaningful clinical history is similar to playing a game of chess. The patient makes a statement and, based upon its content and mode of expression, the physician asks a counterquestion. One answer stimulates yet another question until the clinician is convinced that he understands precisely all of the circumstances.

— Philip A. Tumulty in *The Effective Clinician*

In this exercise, you take responsibility for the body of medical knowledge—errors of commission and omission included, keeping in mind the inevitably of fallibility—and reimagine an incident in history when doctors were slow to respond with adaptive learning and much needless morbidity and mortality occurred in the interim. If you are a history buff, research a situation that is of interest to you and use it. Otherwise, read the real story of one of the following, which you will encapsulate according to available information—which is not the revisionism you may have learned in medical school.

Bubonic Plague. During the plagues of the early modern era, British peasants realized that rats were spreading the disease and took measures to protect themselves. Seven hundred years later, medical authorities in India sought out what they believed to be proof and obtained it, accepted it, and then responded accordingly.

Yellow Fever. Dr. Carlos Findlay, who was living and working in Cuba, noticed that mosquitos were the likely vector of yellow fever. He presented his findings at a medical meeting; doctors ignored him. Thirty years later, Dr. Walter Reed, who was out of options and desperate to control the disease, decided to test the theory but did not take the threat seriously enough to prevent deaths in the subjects or researchers. Doctors found the deaths persuasive and undertook mosquito control.

Puerperal Sepsis. Dr. Semmelweis recognized that doctors spread this often fatal infection from patient to patient in the maternity ward. He recommended hand-washing to interrupt transmission. His peers turned the ridicule and censure that they usually reserved for midwives on Semmelweis. He suicided. Eventually, his peers took responsibility for transmission and started washing their hands.

Smallpox. Dr. Jenner devised a safe vaccine made with cowpox to replace the high-risk live inoculation already in use. He was ignored. Napoleon heard of the vaccine and used it to protect his troops. Others took note and began to follow. For centuries, doctors ignored, dismissed, or abused the inhaled inoculation invented in China.

Peptic Ulcer Disease. In your lifetime, the 'nervous condition' blamed on patients and treated with rice diets in our training years was attributed to *Helicobacter pylori* by Drs. Barry Marshall and Robin Warren. They published their findings and were met with denial and ridicule. One undertook a publicity stunt in which he inoculated himself and documented the resulting ulcers. Their findings were accepted and countless individual cases cured.

When you have read up on a story, examine your memory for an error of omission that was endemic to the profession when you trained and that your elders or peers corrected in your lifetime. Remember how it felt to note and accept the error, or to read about and reflect on it. Take some time to observe any patterns in your behavior with respect to new knowledge. When you have recollected your personal acceptance and adoption of useful new medical knowledge, write responses to the following prompts in your journal:

- When I think of that breakthrough, I can see that I have been best able to consider new knowledge when it comes from.....or is disseminated by....or is mandated by....
- When I consider new knowledge, I have been able to open my mind to it if...and to change my ways if...
- When I think of how to reduce the delay between obtaining and acting on new medical knowledge, and how to account for the risks of denying true findings on the one hand or accepting false ones on the other, I think that it would be better if doctors were to... if I were to...

Now, write a fictional paragraph or story in which you are the protagonist and you discover the cause of a new or existing chronic illness and devise a way to cure it simultaneously in the bodies of individuals and in the bodies of the species, the habitat, and life on earth. Write it as speculative fiction—and yet take care to ground your speculations in your knowledge base and in the realities of your life as it is now. If you are ready to imagine your future, use the exercise to support you in thinking through the consequences of a single possible choice. Once you are grounded in life and time, allow your imagination to run free and your words to create a new world of possibilities infused by your growing sanguine strength. Allow yourself to try on a new worldview; to introduce elements of whimsy; or to use any exalted or extravagant or erotic language that elevates the part of you between your ears and above your crown. Write three sentences in your journal at least—and add as many paragraphs or pages as you please.

Making Plans

This overcoming of all the usual barriers between the individual and the Absolute is the great mystic achievement. In mystic states we both become one with the Absolute and we become aware of our oneness.

— Dr. William James in *The Varieties of Religious Experience*

Once again, prepare for this exercise by going to a quiet place where you can be alone and think, perhaps a library or park or sanctuary. When you are ready, close your eyes and envision yourself walking out the door of the system that embedded you and throwing out all of your devices and every single one of the useless or counterproductive procedures you were obliged to—and agreed to—carry out while there. Then imagine that you are finally free of the manipulations that programmed you and that thereby limited and warped your judgment and prevented you from providing the care and cure that you believed to be conscientious and optimal. See yourself going to a place where you can think, speak, and act freely and use your many years of experience to do all of these things wisely. Then contemplate the questions that follow and write brief responses in your journal:

- The meaning of my view of my personal life hinges on...of my medical life hinges on...of my species' life hinges on...of life on earth hinges on...
- The purpose of my personal life from now on is...
- The purpose of my medical life from now on is...
- My top ten goals for the rest of my life are...

In your journal, draw a timeline that extends from now to the hour of your death. On it, pencil in the steps you want to take and so begin a working plan for elderhood.

Supplementary Reading

1. Amos Tversky and Daniel Kahneman. *Judgment under Uncertainty: Heuristics and Biases.* Science, New Series, Vol. 155, No. 4157 (Sept 27, 1974), pp. 1124-31.
2. Michael Lewis. *The Undoing Project: A Friendship that Changed Our Minds.* New York: W. W. Norton & Company, 2017.
3. Daniel Kahneman. *Thinking Fast and Slow.* New York: Farrar, Straus and Giroux, 2013.
4. Malcolm Gladwell. *Blink: The Power of Thinking without Thinking.* New York: Back Bay Books, 2007.
5. A. R. Luria. *The Mind of a Mnemonist: A Little Book About a Vast Memory.* Translated by Lynn Solotaroff. Cambridge: Harvard University Press, 1968, 1987 (recommended).
6. A. R. Luria. *The Man with a Shattered World: The History of a Brain Wound.* Translated by Lynn Solotaroff. Cambridge: Harvard University Press, 1972 / 1987 (recommended).
7. Alvan R. Feinstein. *Clinical Judgment.* Baltimore: Williams & Wilkins, 1967.
8. Oliver Sacks. *The Mind's Eye.* New York: Alfred A. Knopf, 2010.

Rewriting Your Personal Narrative

A self is probably the most impressive work of art we ever produce, surely the most intricate. For we create not just one self-making story but many...the job is to get them all into one identity, and to get them lined up over time.

— Jerome Bruner in *Making Stories: Law, Literature and Life*

If you worked too hard for too long, you may emerge from employment in need of respite and recuperation. You may have to rally your body before you will know whether medicine was only a job or remains your calling. If the latter, and if it is your highest priority at present, you will discover your post-employment years as your last and best chance to complete your unique lifework and legacy. A key element of this is the meaning of your unfolding life as represented in your evolving and passionately motivating life story. This narrative will alternately guide and follow you through a landscape of treacherous and beautiful possibilities to your denouement. If medicine was only a job for you, it will still be the beginning of the continuum that includes the vision that supports the extension and resolution of your personal narrative.

Whatever role medicine comes to play in the rest of your life, you will make the best use of it when you draw from the full spectrum of your experience—that is, on every event of your past, ranging from those you valued and viewed as defining to those you have ignored to those you rejected, neglected, or abused. All experience forms the raw material that you use to form your character arc, to define transformative events, to make sense of your context, and to own your choices and consequences. The more you exclude experience—consciously or unconsciously—the less you interpret and resolve via your life story. The unexamined life leads to a thin and useless narrative. And, as no one else can know your story for you and no artifice can compensate for your loss of real raw material, any unclaimed experience will detract from the meaning and purpose of your final chapters. Only you will know when you have made the most of your trash and treasure.

Meanwhile, your context will change radically—and to your benefit. You will be able to see your role in late modern complex systems of care with new eyes. As you emerge from these, you will find that you may have given over the writing of your personal narrative to others and that your ability to own your story has thus become deeply buried by drudgery. If you followed the late modern herd into the role of economic tool, your social expectations may have become so concrete and intrusive as to make it impossible for you to form core values or integrity, compose your own being or doing, or to author your own life story. You may have been conditioned by industrial design to function as if working in a defunct form of production. In the medical context, this production will have been 'tweaked' to serve the pervasive psycho-social myth of the last-minute rescue; to sustain the biology-blind monetary economy; and to mediate a fixed belief in technology. This belief—reinforced intermittently by successes both real and perceived—is beginning to fail along with all late modern systems, which we are gradually recognizing as destructive to the biocentric view needed to reverse the sixth extinction. For the purposes of this book, we call this medical idée fixe technoshamanism.

The context of your transition—which you must engage one way or another—is thus part of the perilous transition of your profession, through which you have the chance to lead your patients, peers, and the life on earth that is your kindred. Rather than try to swim upstream against the currents of time, or to go fast or into an ungrounded future by abandoning the successes of modernity, or to deny or delay change, you—like an improviser—say yes to what is given, and go with the flow. You will have plenty of raw material for your improvisation if you receive all of the lessons that life has tried to teach you through the sum total of your experience—including the experiences you put aside because you were too busy doing the wrong thing as fast as possible to enrich your life or your profession.

To do this, you may have to pass through a time when you see modern systems as a Frankenstein's monster of massive proportions. These were set in motion by good intentions that we must finally revise and realize or else betray the whole course of evolution. In this dark passage, you will see that humanity's well-intentioned social processes became too big, too complicated, and too robotic not to fail. In accepting the modern and premodern expectations that landed on your shoulders, you accepted conditioning that made you a product rather than a fully human keeper of an essential art of living. Even if you practiced psychiatry or some other field in which you were free to encounter the unseen and unknown, you will have accepted given algorithms—regardless of their worth—and so fed the illusion of control as you allowed your problem-solving capacity to atrophy.

As you begin to revise your personal narrative to suit your full self in your chosen context, you will discover the value of taking in the full spectrum of experience from best to worst and valuing it according to its long-term, sustained, and sustainable utility. You will find then that you cannot turn back to the fatalistic narratives that preceded the Scottish Enlightenment, in which human failures were projected onto God, or to more recent narratives in which using all available resources to intervene in a dying patient was thought sufficient to ensure the best care of life in each and every instance from now into the indefinite future.

The good news is that the profession cared for the whole of the human body and for the species and its context from the very beginning. Even as centralization was being taken to excess and dividing decisions from their necessary personal context, we were beginning to practice preventive care. Some of this was aggregated—as with shared systems of hygiene—and some disseminated—as with well-child and prenatal care. To set things right as you retire, you can reflect on the personal and congregal lessons you as a doctor can draw from your experiences. Then look for ways in which these may help restore life, before the damage becomes irreversible and your hard-won experiences come to naught.

ANECDOTES FROM MEDICAL LIVES

Sue's letter continued in this lyrical vein, describing experiences utterly novel for her, beyond anything she could have imagined or inferred before. She had discovered for herself that there is no substitute for experience, that there is an unbridgeable gulf between what Bertrand Russell called "knowledge by description" and "knowledge by acquaintance," and no way of going from one to the other.

— Dr. Oliver Sacks in *The Mind's Eye*

You may have heard that truth is stranger than fiction. The reason that this seems true is that you are always editing your life story, always cutting out bits that don't seem to fit and splicing in others that do. This is how you make sense of your life. This is how you form threads of action that you extend as events unfold. This transformation of your experience into your life story is—teleologically, perhaps—the reason that existence begins to leave impressions in your body even before you are born. When you learn to write your story well in the emerging context, you ground your life in the body of life as it differentiates and allow your sequences of thought, word, and deed to cohere as your story

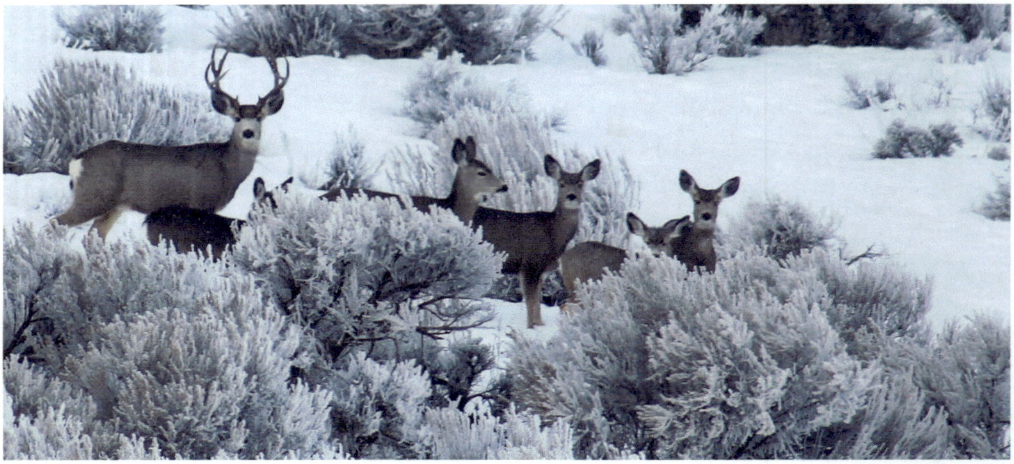

within the body of life. Done right, this narrative can sustain your faith in the future, and in your ability to continue supporting life by adapting to context and circumstance.

As you transition to elderhood, you begin to create your last and best life story. This story should have traction in existence and give your life—and the lives entangled with yours—the potential to craft a way of living that allows your nesting bodies—your womb—to survive and thrive. That story is worth your life, the life that you will soon have spent. That story is already written on your flesh, but your editing has been imperfect and has hidden your truest story from your view. You—as a member of the human species that evolved over eons in response to life—have exactly the skills you need to decode, enrich, and propagate your life story as a contribution to the survival and thriving of life on earth.

As a late modern, you may have wished to be an ersatz human—to be a robot that has enough data processing capacity to take in the whole of your experience every moment. This is nonsensical. Think for a minute. If you could comprehend your flesh one molecule at a time, what would you gain, and could you distinguish it from psychosis? No. You are human; it is your destiny to make sense of your experience and to express it through the life story you are about to complete, which includes carefully-chosen instances of all that you thought, said, and did and all that those things added up to. Your story will go on after you pass its consequences to other lives and to life as a whole. Only you will know how best to draw on the whole of your experience to make the most of this precious story.

Joseph

Like many physicians in public service, Joseph became eligible for a pension while still relatively young—at sixty years of age. While physicians of the previous century worked themselves to death—or, as described by William Carlos Williams in *Old Doc Rivers,* to the point of bolting, burning out, or courting banishment through drug addiction or sexual misconduct—Joseph belonged to the late modern cohort of doctors who accepted the role of employee and gained benefits such as retirement pay. He decided to take the opportunity to leave his previous employment and to make his own way in life.

Having been overtaken by junior colleagues whose master's degrees had given them up-to-date skills in developing fields such as epidemiology, statistics, and bioinformatics, Joseph had felt himself at a disadvantage. He decided to use his newfound freedom to gain expertise in those fields and to see how they might advance his skills and revive and redirect his motivation. He might then refurbish his curriculum vitae and seek out a new career in some area of public health or public administration. He could then harness the full range of his existing skills and take them in a new and engaging direction.

Luckily for his young teachers, Joseph grew wise before he grew old. He took his exit from employment as a chance to enjoy family life and his explorations of recent ideas and methods while he got to know other mid- or late-career professionals who had chosen careers unlike his own. He found the material familiar enough to be fun and relatively easy; didn't under- or over-achieve; and took note of what he was doing and how he was feeling about it. When his training was finished, he decided that his medical life was complete, and that his heart's desire was to move on to create another kind of life with his wife and extended family.

Kim

Kim was among the first family doctors to be grandfathered into the new specialty of emergency medicine. His career grew with this specialty. He took a position on the staff of a big city hospital and continued upward and outward to the culmination of his career as director of emergency services at a regional referral center surrounded by cattle ranching and by farming. As his children grew up and had children of their own, he began to relax and to feel the high toll that his work was taking on his family. He moved to a small city and stepped down from the heavy responsibilities of his most demanding position.

Then he decided to return to family medicine. He took a position at a public clinic that served migrant workers. Kim began to study Spanish. He delayed telling his colleagues of his plans. He had become accustomed to a high-status administrative position in a well-regarded specialty that commanded a high salary, and now he was returning to primary care. He would be serving patients in great need who propped up the economy and yet were not always welcome, and he would be returning to the specialty of family medicine, which had been new when he entered it and which was still disrespected by elite peers. He expected his choice to draw disapproval or disrespect—perhaps even censure or ridicule. He prepared himself to feel the sting of shame.

To his surprise, his choice drew admiration from people who appreciated service; it gave inspiration to doctors and peers in search of more meaningful work. He took new interest in stories of doctors who were leaving the profession and choosing work that drew on creativity, ingenuity, independence, and other virtues construed as problems by complex systems designed to impose uniformity and conformity to pre-set—and often low or ill-fitting—standards. Over dinner, he said, "This has to be the only place in the country where people would respond positively to my choice." I doubt it, but I can tell why he would think so: many doctors identify so closely with their location in the medical hierarchy that they seem to value little else.

Matthew

After high school, Matthew studied engineering and secured a well-paying job in the aerospace industry. For years, he designed bombs. Over time, he became dispirited and disillusioned; eventually, he saw that it was time for him to make a change. He wanted to stop working for death and to start working for life. He applied to medical school, earned prestigious training positions, married, and moved to a city where he and his wife could join a faculty of medicine.

Not long after, the hospital where he worked implemented—and became increasingly dependent on—an electronic medical record system. Each stage of implementation and each change ran into unexpected glitches. The record system drew more and more resources from the institution and expended them on a virtual reality that was beginning to eclipse real patient care.

Worse—from a regulatory standpoint—the billing system worked poorly and failed to compensate for the increased expense. It seemed to administrators that doctors were failing to bill for services, and that the doctors were

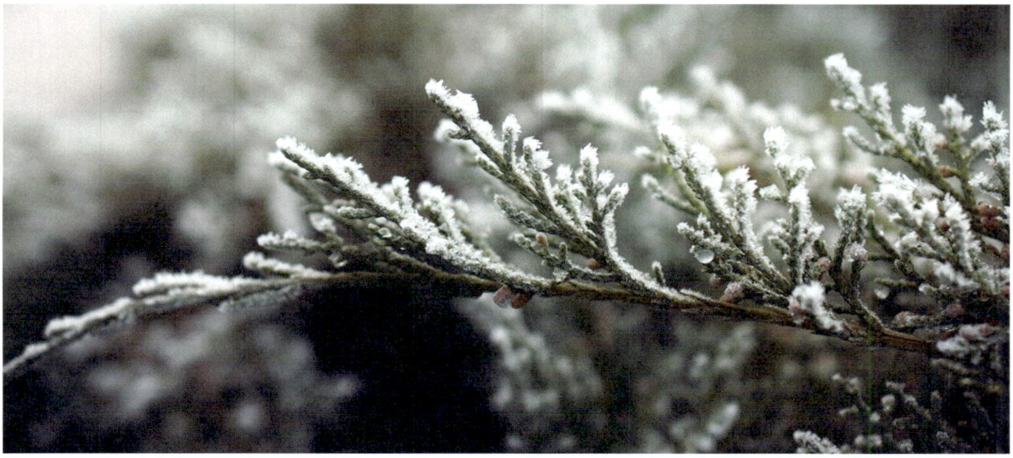

unreasonably curt when questioned. The chief of staff—aware of Matthew's expertise in engineering—asked for help. Matthew wrote programs to flag services that hadn't been billed, screened the clinic notes personally, and notified doctors who had neglected to bill for services. The system began to function effectively. His careers converged.

Tragically, his wife developed a rare cancer and died. Her colleagues were bereft. As Matthew took care of her, he developed a strong inclination to leave the city so as to live closer to surviving family members and to start life anew. He began to extricate himself from his second career. He hired three people to take his place and cut back to part time. He was financially independent and in need of respite, but felt too young to be sidelined or to enjoy idleness or desultory pleasures. Like many who experience a life-changing loss, Matthew began to look for a third career that would welcome his gifts without dominating his life or his impending elderhood.

BETH LOOKS BACK:
The Emergence of the New Paradigm

Natural selection, for Darwin, did not forbid cultural and individual developments on a timescale hundreds of thousands of times faster than evolutionary development—on the contrary, it prepared the ground for them.

— Oliver Sacks in *The Mind's Eye*

Like others born in the shadow of war, I seemed to emerge from the womb aware that our species and its constructs—however real or enchanting they might seem—were inherently frail, deeply flawed, and liable to collapse. Many who were similarly aware disappeared into drugs or desensitization or into forms of social change like the human rights movement that began to mend our modern and pre-modern failings from the center, often inadvertently adding to social complexity and increasing the inertia of the status quo.

Like others who entered medicine around the time of the Vietnam War, I came with the aim of changing myself, my profession, and my world. I was prepared to work as smart and as hard as I could to define the modern problems that were making us sick and to solve them. Unlike most of my peers, I chose to do it the hard way. I went against the grain. It was, in retrospect, ludicrous. My protagonist looks like she is attempting to dog-paddle up a whitewater stream broken up by level-three rapids.

This swim began with an independent study course in medical school that several of us students instigated to focus on the topic of public health. The professor, an expert in infectious disease with experience in disease control, took us through the Epidemiology Intelligence Service training manual. This prepared us to act as medical detectives in real-life situations in which an epidemic might take lives en masse. The manual did not view failure as an option, nor lionize or fetishize academic methods that might or might not prove useful in real life.

None of this was to the liking of the Dean of Students, who was a soldier rather than a doctor by training. He called wayward students interested in public health or family medicine into his office one by one to inform them that the university did not believe in public health and that molecular biology was the way of the future. Students who could should subspecialize in high-status fields and do bench research of the kind that might one day earn a Nobel Prize. Fortunately, his 1950s crew cut tipped us off to the fact that he was not cool.

Eager to do what I thought was right and best according to my own conscience, I tried to go directly into preventive medicine. Fortunately for me—in hindsight—the system made that impossible. I would have to do an internship in a general field such as internal medicine and then seek out a preventive medicine residency. During my clinical year, I could find no funded PGY2 position in prevention. I defied social incentives and censures and applied for an unfunded one. When I arrived and met with the program head, he asked me about my background, looked at my file, regarded me with annoyance, and asked, "What the hell are you doing here?"

I could have provided the Blues Brothers riposte: I'm on a mission from God. Or, in my own language, I'm doing the best I can with all the dimensions of my reality; or, the status quo is always a bad hack to be bettered.

The program head's advice was followed by stern advice from the other program head that I should get more clinical training and go to the Centers for Disease Control or leave the field. It was good advice for someone in search of money and status, but it wasn't right for me. Luckily for me, I had inadvertently heeded a disapproving uncle's advice to marry a rich man to avoid starving. My husband wasn't rich, but he did exceed expectations and eventually achieved a degree of status and level of income that made his mentors proud. His ambition made it possible for me to follow my conscience without joining a fringe group or sleeping on the streets and eating dog food out of a can.

After residency, during which I learned to do epidemiology research, I got an offer for a relatively low-paying but otherwise desirable faculty position that I was happy to take. By the time I arrived, the chairmen of the three big clinical departments had taken half the budget of my new department and also positioned themselves to receive the prevention funds that were becoming available just then. The chair of my department responded by taking a terminal sabbatical; I dined with him during my job interview and never saw him again. The senior faculty were not accustomed to applying for grants. They looked to us new faculty to do our part in gaining funds, but didn't have the funds to give us the tools that we needed to do so. I bought a computer that I could use to seek funds for research. All I needed was a fundable idea that might do some good.

One night, while listening to the news, I heard about an outbreak of a rare birth defect. This was just the kind of thing I was primed to investigate. My mentors cautioned me that it was risky, and therefore a poor career move. I would be researching a real problem to which I didn't already know the answer. Doctors at the local health department, on the other hand, welcomed me and offered critical support. Because there was no one else to receive funding, a private foundation that had decided to offer financial support on the q.t. gave the funds to me. The project went forward. I found myself in a position to investigate a real problem in a free-living population. I knew how to do—and dared to do—what I was trained to do: face a real problem, contemplate it, and try to solve it.

You may recognize how rare this was and recognize my good fortune; or you may have helped bring it about, in which case I thank you from the bottom of my heart. The most pressing problem—overtreatment—was solved by a team from the Centers for Disease Control. This swept the original cluster under the rug, and as the case number was too small to support statistical analysis, my work was at an end. I noticed then that our methods were designed to fail.

Thus prepared, I was not as devastated as I might have been when I developed myalgic encephalomyelitis and lost my medical life, and with it all that I had worked for from a very young age. One colleague said quietly, "I thought doctors didn't get that." Others said that they didn't 'believe in' my problem—as if they were high priests of medical ideology, rather than investigators of biomedical reality. Those I consulted formally often turned me away. The few who tried to do what the situation required generally kept a low profile while patients complained or suffered in silence.

I had been looking at mainstream medicine from the outside for some time; it was my job to try and do better. I resolved to step up and do what I could. This illness put me in a box seat from which I could see the worst failings of the late modern, overmanaged, unresponsive care delivery system, as well as those of the new gray market in health care. I learned the hard way that doctors were the only ones who could mend our present health problems or metamorphose the profession, so I had to try and do it myself. I had already watched as modern and early modern habits of care were grandfathered into the system as usual, customary, and reasonable; as basic scientists and information technologists quashed clinical science and diverted resources from the core functions of the profession; and as the "treat the chart" pearl of my medical education eliminated what little remained of clinical knowledge and wisdom. I did what I could to pick up the broken threads and to weave them together.

Lucky for me, I was able to access every available kind of inventive care and to use my many years of formal and informal education as a polymath to aid my ailing body and the body of my profession. I worked with doctors who were willing to try and help, but who were also preoccupied and ultimately unable to collaborate. One of these observed patients carefully and collaborated with them in empirically devising an effective elimination diet. This freed me to experiment with the best local organic food and so to free my brain of neurotoxicity. If I wasn't so aware of the many millions suffering in similar ways, and if I didn't know that bad human habits are threatening the future of my children and the whole of evolved life on earth, I would have relaxed into being content with my isolated, fragile safety.

COMMENT

This was for me a very personal way of dealing with this story, but I didn't want to tell [Shakespeare's Titus Andronicus] story if I didn't have that one sliver of hope. We can tell all these nasty, horrific, barbaric stories, but what do you do with them?

— Julie Taymor at Columbia University on her film *Titus*

When you look at life through what some facetiously call the restrospectoscope, you may feel as if you have 20/20 vision. At the threshold of elderhood, you can take advantage of this clarity and discover patterns that escaped your notice in the past and that you do—or don't—want to perpetuate or improve on. As you take stock, you may become aware that the whole of your life experience is written on your body and had been guiding your becoming. You may see the imprints left by nature and nurture that motivated you, shaped your course, and transformed your views again and again—especially in times that forced discovery or change.

As you enter your post-employment years, you can release your responsibilities to the status quo and become productively disillusioned with the virtual reality created by late modern systems. You can then examine black boxes—e.g. computers, statistics, and jargon—that mediate present-day medical care and project wishful thinking onto large, overmanaged systems. They are only magic in that they make time and effort disappear and delay the emergence of grassroots biocentric solutions. You may recognize that you, too, have been suffering from blind belief in technoshamanism. You can then view the past and your profession with skepticism and take modern problems as experiences that can still teach you to evolve your profession—and through it, society. You can observe, diagnose and treat the ills of the species as you would a patient who is in critical condition.

You will be best prepared to do this when you are open to seeing the errors of your ways—and those of your profession. You may have adopted a modern managerial or regulatory perspective embedded in proxies that present a picture of safety and control even as they undermine your ability to face, define, and solve real problems. If you sensed this, you may have taken refuge in denial and dissociation. You may have been encouraged in this by any or all of the following: 'sponge' learning habits that suited students of the past but that undermine clinical skills and strategies in times of deep change; immersive systems that oblige you to behave like a predictable bundle of algorithms; economic rationalism that precludes biocentric thinking; molecularism that fragments knowledge and confuses everyone; looking good by excluding from your care anyone who might make the medical database look bad; and, last but not least, the monoculture created by industry, technology, and the information age—especially data processing.

However you coped with the blessings and curses of late modernity, you will leave your employment years primed to turn experience into wisdom. As you do this, it may help to recognize that our ancestors always did the best that they could and that we are all standing on the shoulders of giants. The course of history was thus neither needless or accidental; it is exactly as it needed to be to prepare you to make the best choices in your last and best moment of unprecedented freedom. From now on you will make choices that cast the die that will mold your remaining time on earth and take your life narrative toward its denouement. You, like all before you, will change the world—but this time those who follow will not become moderns; they will—they must—become what they need to be to enable the survival of evolved life.

You may find it useful, as you embark on the final phase of your narrative, to note that the late modern medical ego is a cause of the end of modernity. It allowed us to lollygag in the poppy field—or, rather, the hospital—in which we were anesthetized by the illusion of control and enjoyed—and overvalued—the quick fix and last-minute save rather than the long, slow, comprehensive, incremental work of deep systemic change on which human survival depends. The latter is emerging medicine, the medicine that treats individuals with their context and has a time horizon that lies far beyond this call night, this training year, and this career. As spiritual teachers point out, this is like lifting the plank that you are standing on, a task that becomes possible only when you leave your career behind and contemplate your legacy—and your mortality.

Unfortunately, the stories that journalists, artists, and almost all moderns and premoderns favor sound an alarm bell that signals one problem or another. They do this over and over again until those who would respond have been desensitized. They push many into defeat and despair aggravated by pervasive sources of neurotoxicity. To counter these stories requires you to develop a robust, resilient, evolving personal narrative. If you choose to look, you will find plenty of stories that offer good news and good templates for sanguine—perhaps even interventionist—narratives. For example, you can emulate Mohandas

Gandhi, who showed that hate cannot be ended by hate, or Martin Luther King Jr., whose vision showed us a society in which the content of character can be valued and nourished, or Deitrich Bonhoeffer, who distinguished death from a bad ending, and so echoed ancient tales like Beowulf and sci-fi tales of Klingons.

While modern and pre-modern narratives back to Shakespeare and ancient Greece disturb their audiences by threatening the status quo and then relieve them by restoring it, we must do more. As you consider how your life could become a tale of inspiration or transformation, you can choose from an endless array of possibilities. You can create a life narrative that turns experience into the wisdom needed to solve systemic problems that imperil life on earth. If you play your cards right, you may be able to divert your life and your profession from its collision with the body of life and counter modern stories of sterilization with emerging ones of cultivation. At this point in history, the stories of our lives must be true ones of love that enable timely congregal accord and action: they must lead to optimism and joy.

As you emerge from mechanical systems that disconnect and decontextualize flesh and being, you can begin to reclaim your life and to move forward. Chances are good that doing this will require you to undergo a process like the stages of grieving. These will intervene between your present habits and the future that you choose to create, and will require you to meet your life experiences as they appeared to you when they happened and also as they appear to you in hindsight. This passage is like the Hero's Journey: you must encounter those errors that are written on your body and that reside in your being so that you can put them to rest and repurpose your energies. This is the only way for you to turn stories of problems into stories of solutions.

Fortunately, as is often the case in history, you will find when you look around that many elders are already creating constructive narratives for their final years in which they envision what they would like to do and set about doing what they can. As you hold the working questions of this month, feel free to turn to historical and contemporary examples of elders whose lives and stories you would like to emulate.

Rewriting Your Personal Narrative

From my earliest childhood my zeal to serve suffering humanity with my art was never content with any kind of a subterfuge; and no other reward is needed than the internal satisfaction which always accompanies such a deed."

— Ludwig von Beethoven to the Director of the Court Theater via Freidrich Kerst

WORKING QUESTIONS

All Physicians

- What is the ultimate purpose of the life that I have been creating? What do I want my life purpose to be from now on? What do I want it to become as my life reaches its fulfillment?
- What meaning can I draw from my personal past? From the pasts of my kindred, of my community, of my profession, of my species, of my habitats, and of life on earth?
- What meanings can I glean from the recorded history of my profession? Of my species in the context of the body of life and its context—that is, from the dynamic conditions of the earth and from the evolving human response to those conditions?
- What would make a happy ending for me now? In ten years? When dying of old age?
- What is more important to me than life?
- Do I value quality of life over quantity of years lived? Or vice versa?

Self-determined Physicians

- How can I create a grounded personal narrative in which I solve the problems that life has put to me, and so succeed from now until my end?
- What unforeseen change can I bring about to transform my flesh and being?
- How can I live so as to care for the body of life?

- What I am doing to choose the happy ending of living for meaning and purpose, and to recognize death as natural and neutral—that is, as inherent to each instance of life, and avoidable in the aggregates that continue forward for the foreseeable future?
- What can I do to care for my life as integral to life on earth? What can I do to envision cure in the context of each and every life?

EXERCISES

I know your spiel about tragedy. It's true, most stories do feed on misery. But when you find happiness, there's nothing more to say. So it's time to stop.

— Xavier in Cédric Klapisch's film *Chinese Puzzle*

Now and then life obliges you to pause and put it all together—that is, to integrate and update the whole of your experience so as to be free to renew your life story. Even if you believe that you continuously edited your life story so as to glean life lessons and turn experience into wisdom along the way, hindsight will reveal experiences that you missed and that may prove useful at present. These will have slipped your notice or your memory because you were focused on something else, you didn't comprehend them, you were poorly grounded, you had a blind spot, or you could not have foreseen what would matter later. When you leave the employment years, you will discover that the systems that you were embedded in wrote much of your narrative; to reclaim it for your own, you will have to use hindsight to own and update your story.

EXERCISE 1: Owning Your Past

In your journal, write a list of ten experiences that are alive in you, that you recall vividly, and that are set to die with you. Below the list write about each event with the aim of immersing a reader in the experience as you convey its impact on you. Write them in first, second, or third person as you wish.

Now, list ten times in your life when experience shut you down—that is, when you flooded with emotion or your awareness contracted or your understanding failed you. Select one that did not switch on your "automatic pilot" (e.g. a medical emergency that was routine in that you had a ready and appropriate response)—that is, one in which you were aware, even at the time, that you were missing some of what was going on because you were overwhelmed with delight or horror or anything in between. Record each event and its context in as much detail as you can.

EXERCISE 2: Owning Your Word Flow

Take two hours a day to write about your past on blank sheets of paper. Don't think about what you write before or after a session; just write without pause in the way of 'automatic writing' in the 1800s. The purpose is to cut through the craft of technical writing and to establish the neural pathways between the work of creation in the mind ant the articulation of that work on paper—to not overthink or have to overthink in order to be clear. While craft is important, it is flow that matters here, because it patterns you to be able to communicate experience as a storyteller or writer should do easily through practice. Don't worry if it doesn't make sense at first, and don't keep it. Just keep at it.

EXERCISE 3: Writing Your Future

In this exercise, draw on the sum total of your experiences and the life stories that you know to outline a speculative narrative of the final purpose of your life story. As you write down this outline in your journal, consider your present purpose and meaning. When you have finished, analyze your story as follows:

1. List the characters with their themes and arcs.
2. Diagram your completion of a lifework and creation of a legacy.
3. Write an epilogue that includes a short obituary and one-sentence epitaph.

Do not share this exercise at first; keep it to yourself. Take whatever time you need to rethink your life and to revise the outline accordingly. Repeat as desired. When you are ready, share it with a soul friend and listen to how that individual reflects it back to you. Take time to ponder what these remarks say about both their life and yours. Journal to support your growth and development as an elder.

Return to this exercise whenever you feel confused about the meaning and purpose of your life going forward, or about what you should be doing now to shape your story.

EXERCISE 4

If you are interested in writing your story for your children as Darwin did, or for posterity as Oliver Sacks did, or for science and spirit as Thoreau did in his journals, begin to keep notes in a blank book, or on post-its that you put on pieces of paper, or on notepad sheets that you keep in a shoebox—whatever best suits the way that your thoughts arise. You may find that you need to keep a fieldbook or black book with you as you go through your day, and at your bedside at night. Over the course of a week or so, create a sustainable method and keep it up as long as you like. The more notes you write and don't use, the better your book is likely to be—unless you are already a skilled and experienced writer of long narratives.

NARRATIVES

Expert

1. Hope Jahren. *Lab Girl.* New York: Alfred A. Knopf, 2016.
2. Oliver Sacks. *Seeing Voices.* Berkeley: University of California Press, 1989/1990.
3. Oliver Sacks. *An Anthropologist on Mars.* New York: Alfred A. Knopf, 1995.
4. Stephen Levine. *A Year to Live: How to Live This Year as if it Were Your Last.* New York: Harmony, 1997.
5. Rachel Naomi Remen. *Kitchen Table Wisdom: Stories that Heal.* New York: Riverhead Books, 1996.
6. Charles Darwin. *The Autobiography of Charles Darwin.* Edited by Nora Barlow. London: Collins, 1958.

Grassroots

1. Jacques Lusseyran. *And There Was Light.* Boston: Little, Brown, 1963 / New York: Parabola Books, 1998.
2. Phillip Campbell. *Zioncheck for President: A True Story of Idealism and Madness in American Politics.* New York: Nation Books, 2005.
3. Studs Terkel. *Hope Dies Last: Keeping the Faith in Troubled Times.* New York: The New Press, 2003.
4. Eric Metaxas. *Bonhoeffer: Pastor, Martyr, Prophet, Spy.* Nashville: Thomas Nelson, 2010.

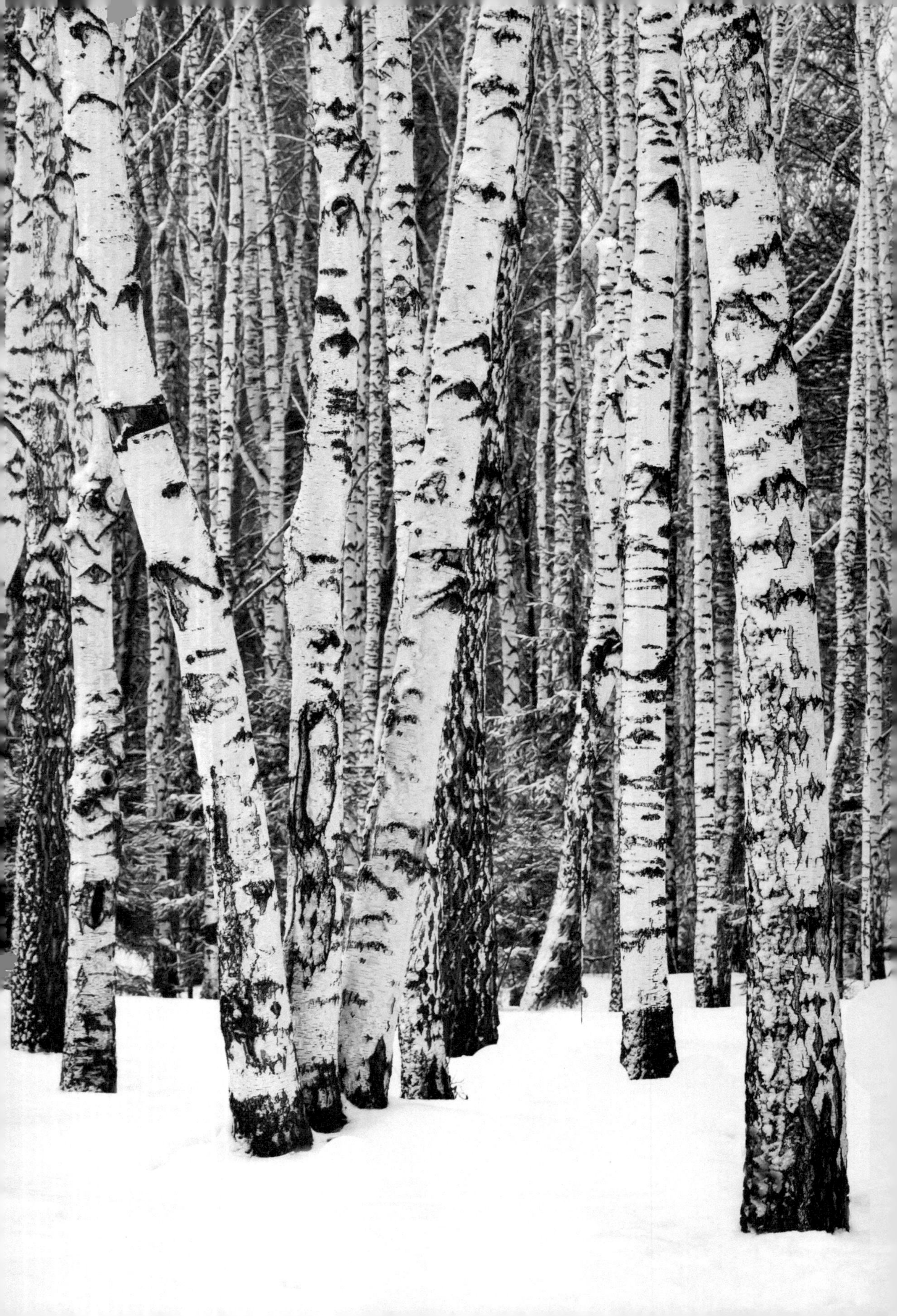

Constructing Emergence

For so I think the whole art has been set forth, by observing some part of the final end in each of many particulars, and then combining all into a single whole.

— Hippocrates in *Precepts II* via W.H.S. Jones in the Loeb Classical Library

To delve into the task of devising what is emerging now, immerse yourself in the constructs offered by this first version of medical emergence. During the first month of summer, you encountered integrative and comprehensive constructs for the human body, the nested bodies of your living context, and a process of self-patterning for being and doing. You also gained knowledge of care states and continuing self-care. Go back and ponder those now that you are orienting to biological time and place, opening your perceptual filter, rewriting your personal narrative, and jettisoning or repurposing the memorabilia that have been languishing in your mental attic.

Then, while you begin to disembody a late modern life and embody a new one, visualize caring for life from the core of your flesh and being until you yourself become a source of care and cure, and you are once again able to use your tools rather than allow your tools to use you. In this you are returning to the perennial archetype of physicians like St. Damien and Maimonides. You may quickly realize that you would like to brush up on your clinical skills, to be a little more like Sherlock and the doctors of the Scottish Enlightenment who inspired him and a little less like the doctor in Frank Herbert's *Dune*.

Now imagine yourself curing life from your core with the most careful thinking and delicate touch. The pelvic extenteration that gives the patient a few more months of suffering may appear as it is: a costly Pyrrhic victory. The possibility of detecting causes of illness and thwarting them may appear as it is: thoughtful, kind, compassionate, and worthy of time and effort and partnership with the able patient. It may not be terribly exciting, but the adrenaline high clouds judgment and precludes wisdom. The value is in the life, the being, becoming, and doing, and in the love. In doing the right thing rather than the expensive, last-minute desperate thing, you develop the ability to be exquisitely happy and effective in your work. You become care and cure that you share.

In this paradigm, the archetypal setting for care and cure is the residential habitat restoration clinic and community. This clinic is formed by a group of retiring physicians who pool their resources, buy a ranch, and put up a purpose-built living structure or an array of tiny structures on wheels. The care team comprises a physician, body-worker, counselor, and habitat restorer who have access to local experts in public health, veterinary medicine, plant pathology, ecology, arboriculture, limnology, organic farming, toxic cleanup, and the like (see Construct 7 below).

The clinic invites the local or regional medical community to refer patients whom they diagnose with chronic ambient poisoning—that is, toxicity due to chemical or radiation exposures in daily life (see Construct 6 below). Those who live at the clinic aim to devise a set of local best practices for renewing the body of life in their area, including humans who care for and cure all life as one. The aim is to evolve ways of life that culminate in survival and thriving.

Residents share non-fiction case studies or biofiction narratives featuring views, frames, and constructs that are new or in development. In biofiction, authors assume that humans save evolved life from modern ways of living and describe how we do it. Grounded in life and biologically plausible, speculative biofiction worlds can serve as templates for living that suit all manner of habitats and histories. Rather than propagate modern blindspots by catering to errors of thought such as human exceptionalism, fatalism, idolatry of technology, and so on, biofiction aims to open the perceptual filter and narrative mind so as to end the late modern war on life by modeling habitat restoration and integration.

As noted above, medicine and its narratives—including your medical life story—cut across the full range of the human experience, from the earthiest to the most ethereal. When you pursue medicine as a calling, your story becomes a part of the story of that calling. When you step up and become a co-keeper and co-developer of the larger story, you integrate memoir and history. You can then discern patterns in clinical research and practice as you might in a piece of music, in which life, its ailments, and the human response are like music featuring call and response.

From time to time, you may catch glimpses of the psycholinguistic processes through which you define and diagnose ailments. These are like the keys, chords, and clefs that support musical composition, or the equations that mediate mathematics. These may revive your curiosity. They may lead you to a deeper appreciation of your medical life and of your ability to expand the scope of your care and cure by taking an interest in related but as-yet disconnected fields such as ecology and theosophy.

Such moments of insight may open views that engage human ways of living dating back long before the industrial and computational models that have been feeding our human illusion of control. Through these views, you may glimpse the extreme nature of the habits that we presently hold, such as wasting resources and creating mental monocultures in each walk of life. You can become aware that late modernity has destabilized the profession. You can then come into sync with biological reality and participate in designing the medical tools of the future—which may or may not remind you of the ones that wow you now.

ANECDOTES FROM MEDICAL LIVES

There is no map and a compass wouldn't help at all.

— Björk in *Human Behavior*

As integrative medicine draws together the best of our species' responses to ailments from around the globe, individual doctors are delving into the healing arts to explore those dynamic and protean ailments that have modern causes but lack modern solutions. The syncretic and creative efforts of these individuals and of boundary-crossers in other fields are setting the example for emerging boundary-breaking in medicine so as to cull any useful abstractions that derive from other academic niches such as field biology, religion, and psychology. In exploring these newly-opened borderlands, doctors will meet the unknown, define new ailments, and discover or devise cures for them.

The task before the medical profession is to note gaps in thinking between various human endeavors and take them as the best places to discover new ways of apprehending and comprehending the new. By crafting views, frames, and constructs that turn old obstacles into new opportunities, doctors will see and solve problems caused by modernity and develop a new design for living free of its dire consequences. Success therefore requires you to develop new breadth; that is, to nurture your latent abilities as a polymath and the creative streak that you can awaken as you enjoy the freedom of elderhood.

Jolie

As her pediatric patients became more and more obese, primary care provider Jolie became more and more aware that nothing she could do in the course of well child care would counter their social conditioning to eat and sit too much, nor could she provide them with the skills they needed to thrive and to avoid chronic ailments. Their parents were fully absorbed by the monetary economy; their peers were preoccupied with social media devices and platforms that cause anxiety, depression, screen addiction, and sedentary living; and both were driven by a commercial culture pushing future-blind, self-destructive consumption. Worse, medical programs supported by the new funds for health promotion and disease prevention were having little or no effect.

Unwilling to fail her patients, Jolie decided to step up and do what she could to alter the status quo. She searched for people who shared her views and who were trying to define and solve the problems faced by all children. She found many amongst those practitioners who were driving the local gray markets in medicine that were mushrooming alongside rigid institutional systems of care. These markets drew on folk practices from around the globe; on patent medicines like those once banned for reasons good and bad; and on innovative modalities arbitrarily rejected by the mainstream, such as chiropractic and osteopathic hands-on treatments. These practitioners were engaged in wild and wooly exploration and experiment, supported by patients who were determined to get help and to help themselves. They had already gone far beyond the limits of accepted brands such as self-help, health promotion, healthy living, wellness, and active aging.

Jolie learned what she could through encounters with this gray market and then moved on with her ongoing self-education. While exploring the local community, she discovered the social creatives working to develop the emerging field of early childhood education. She opened a dialogue with local teachers who were also aware that personal habits form very early in life, and that social forces were working to inculcate maladaptive and destructive ones. She and the teachers devised a curriculum to support children in forming strong habits of self-care that might enable them to detect, oppose, and transformdestructive influences and inculcate skills and strategies for prevention through self-care.

Delaney Ruston

Delaney was born to a father suffering from mental illness. This personal experience motivated her to work hard and to go into medicine. Training galvanized her desire to prevent and ameliorate mental illness, but prevailing systems of classification did little to support it. Existing definitions of mental illness address social complaints about people deemed troublesome by their family and friends. Doctors can suppress signs and symptoms to mend the social fabric—or, as in Bethlehem or Bedlam Hospital—to drug, shock, operate on, or confine patients until there are no complaints. The diagnoses of today lack the biomedical traction that doctors might use to identify and remove an underlying cause of neurotoxicity or other dysfunction. The physical environment is generally regarded as irrelevant to disease definition, while pop psychology provides ungrounded rationalizations for undefined ailments.

As she matured as a practitioner and had children, Delaney began to process her early experiences with mental illness and recognized that this would do little to benefit her family or peers. She would have to create some kind of open social dialogue. She turned to the arts to find ways to expose and explore new ailments and to engage others through interactive learning. She applied to film school to learn to write, direct, and craft multimedia stories that focus on phenomena that are causing suffering in the young. Her first film, which was grounded in personal experience and biomedicine, met with a favorable reception and positioned her to win local funding for filmmakers ready to inform and engage the community.

Like Jolie, Delaney connected with educators and made a full-length feature film designed to draw attention to the shadow side of social media that was captivating—and also tyrannizing and seeding maladaptation in—local teens. The film *Screenagers* is now available to groups to catalyze congregal action. Unlike standard documentary films such as Werner Herzog's *Lo and Behold*, Delaney's release is enabling her to harness her art to her vision, and so to effect the purpose and meaning that continue to inspire her life practice.

Dawn Dewitt-Talbot

Dawn's desire to excel in her medical career arose from a profound desire to put her faith into action. Her zeal took her into competitive sports as a student and then on to medical training programs and faculty positions at prestigious institutions in several countries. As she rose and sought positions of greater responsibility and wider leadership, she explored ways to heal and learn with her patients and students, practicing spiritual healing through means such as prayer and preaching.

While developing a rural medical education program, Dawn joined a congregation that enabled her to develop skills in ministry and to combine these with her growing skills as a medical practitioner, educator, and researcher. Over time, her expression of faith and her success as a spiritual healer both met with obstacles. While her medical skills were universal and available to all without distinction, and she viewed her spiritual care similarly, patients received her medical care and her ministry differently.

The social consensus regarding the role of patient was at odds with that of spiritual or religious seeker; that is, patients came to her for medicine and medicine alone. While patients who also visited practitioners of traditions such as Daoist or Ayurvedic or indigenous medicine might welcome new forms of religious or spiritual healing, patients who sought care from mainstream doctors seeemed to want scientific healing—and to seek out any religious or spiritual aid on their own. In other words, patients who might or might not care for—or cure—themselves would look to doctors for scientific 'other-power' and then look elsewhere for any other desired forms of 'other-power.'

In modern medicine, it is important to recognize that patients who come to doctors for 'other-power' have not read the textbooks and may be motivated by a blind faith in science that resembles the blind faith that may be expressed in religious contexts. These patients may come to you for the 'other-power' that moderns buried in the shadow side of medicine. That is, patients who share the late modern blind faith in the mystical 'other-power' of technology and medical hierarchy may look to you for 'other-powers' that you might label as transference, pastoral care, shamanism, psycho-spiritual factors, or the like. If you engage clergy and field biologists in deep dialogue, you will create the chance to see yourself and your species from unfamiliar angles that prepare you to ground your eldering in robust perceptions of reality, and of care and cure.

BETH LOOKS BACK: Turning Data into Wisdom

Statistics offers correlations, not explanations.

— Joel D. Howell in *Technology in the Hospital*

Like many physicians who choose academia, I exited medical training and entered an educational job. In my new department, the most essential courses were introductory and therefore forced on students and fobbed off on junior faculty with no experience. These classes tended to be unpopular amongst students and unrewarding for faculty; you will recall their like from your first year in medical school. Some faculty appreciated this kind of teaching, recognized it as theater, and had the aptitude, motivation, and training to do it well;

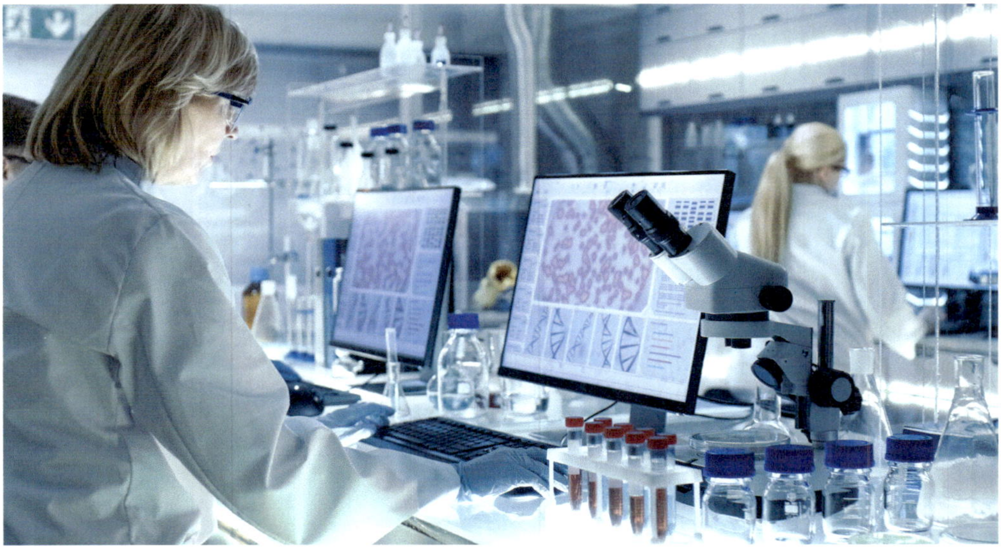

these managed to transcend the status quo. Most faculty were motivated to bring enough fame or fortune to the department so as to put themselves in the position to say no to such teaching and still do well.

Being green and enthusiastic on arriving at my new job, I was mystified and horrified by those 'deadwood colleagues' who had adapted to 'institutionalization' by learning to keep their heads down and their mouths shut. Those in the burn-out phase knew to disappoint their colleagues enough to be met with enthusiasm when they did anything at all well. I still had the can-do attitude fostered by training, and I expected to see one, do one, and teach one. I was a bit concerned about having little experience in my field. I knew that it was overly-simplistic and under-developed, but thought I could revise my part of the course by grounding it in biomedicine and new constructs.

Though I did not succeed, I learned from the effort. As a colleague and I prepared our course materials, we learned the most from a manual that had been prepared by experts in education. The department required us to use the manual so that we would create the paper trail it had to provide to higher-ups, who would in turn use that trail to satisfy accreditors as well as students who expected us to spell everything out. This surprised me. My education had been fundamentally Socratic; I expected students to encounter primary sources such as real cases and to work things out for themselves. On the other hand, we were happy to shift from competitive to competency-based learning, and so came up with a syllabus that featured pertinent points and pre-set questions with 'right' answers.

Luckily for me, the educational experts who prepared the manual did their best to pass on their basic knowledge of pedagogy. Buried in the manual was a simple but arresting diagram that proposed a hierarchy for intellectual material. I had gathered, analyzed, and interpreted data related to clinical and population-based epidemiology studies, and concluded that some data were better than others. I had also intuited that most published data analyses mattered little if at all, and were more likely to propagate irrelevant threads of investigation than to make a difference in clinical or public health medicine. And now I could see why: intellectual material could be viewed as progressing from data to information to knowledge to wisdom, and most people never got beyond the data or asked the question inevitably posed by our senior colleague Mim Orleans: "So you got some results. So what?"

At the present time, late modern systems reward physicians for complying with fixed algorithms and punish them for "deviations" that might either derive from applications of knowledge and wisdom or from error and incompetence. In other words, data and managerial metrics push out higher-order thinking and obstruct the development of new clinical knowledge and wisdom. This is the shadow side of the information age; this is the sketchy origin of all that we view as true. As medical elders, we have the chance to develop the kind of higher-order thinking that is desperately needed at present and that evolves in real time through experiential learning. We have the chance to sift through the dross of a lifetime and find the few pearls that will be ours to contribute to the tradition that will serve future patients in their hours of need.

COMMENT

Information processing cannot deal with anything beyond well-defined and arbitrary entries that can enter into specific relationships that are strictly governed by a program of elementary operations...meaning and the processes that create it are surprisingly remote from what is conventionally called information processing.

— Jerome Bruner in *Acts of Meaning*

Many physicians mentioned in this section are women; this is no coincidence. As decreasing family sizes motivated male physicians to send daughters to medical school and mid-century rights movements spilled into the profession, doctors opened to the women and minority candidates historically excluded in the wake of the Flexner report. In those days, the patent medicine market alarmed doctors with its ill-founded claims. To guard patients against dangerous forms of quackery, the profession raised standards and circled the wagons: They protected patients at the cost of elitism and exclusion.

As the profession re-opened to women, one third of the positions in medical school classes were taken by women. Had candidates been judged on merit alone, they would have taken two-thirds. In other words, women had to outperform their male counterparts, who were expected to be late bloomers. Women had to overcome so many hurdles that they did not tend to enter medicine for what Jane Austen called prudential reasons; they pursued it as a calling. Even before entering medical school, they had their eyes on outcomes; while there, they kept their sights on the big picture. Many had no need to learn to go big-picture—they did that before they began, and so perplexed the pragmatic alpha males among their peers and faculty.

This is not true only of those women; everyone who trains as a physician partakes of its esprit de corps, finds its heart, and sooner or later takes it as a calling. And, having arrived at the threshold of your wisdom years, you have seen the costs of excessive pragmatism. You have been immersed in the social dynamics that define quality as conformity and that enforce it with peer pressure, and that impose the role of employee and the logic of technology on 'experts.' You may have seen that the resulting approximations to reality run counter to biology and that their effects are now so adverse and so strong as to put all life at risk. You may be ready to accept responsibility both as an individual and as a member of your profession for the fact that doctors relinquished the heart of their calling to people who were not doctors and who could not comprehend it or care for it.

In your wisdom years, you are free to do better. You are free to revise systemic errors that you previously enabled by meeting foolish legal and social expectations that divide doctors from patients and their essential habitats. You can step out of your role as a function in a system that turns both doctors and patients into functions; you can return to the role of integral and specialized member of a living community. You can step back and see the big picture—including the modern innovations that are constantly imperiling our health and safety and degrading the habitats into which living humans and sustainable innovations must be integrated. Only then can you see what to do to enable those who belong to your calling to respond to real problems in real time and to continue doing so over the long term for the good of all lives. Only then

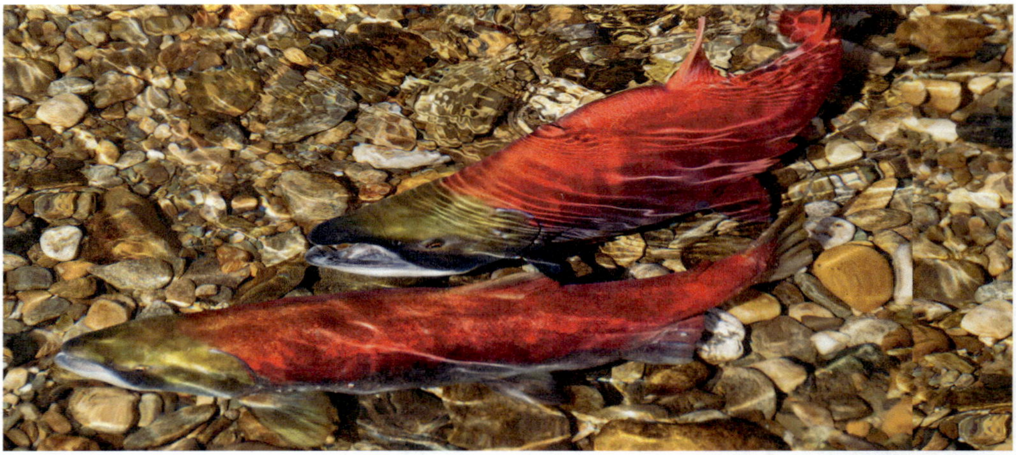

will you find the new simplicity that will support the necessary complexity.

When you have done this, you can connect with experts in fields such as counseling, body work, habitat restoration, organic agriculture, communications, and design. These hold experiential learning that is essential to the present evolution of medicine, and that will enable it to emerge from the vast radical experiment of the modern age. With this emergence, you will become able to take the body of life as your ultimate patient and to use technology as a tool to support life rather than as an idol that feeds on it. As you transition, remember to put on your oxygen mask first—that is, to care for yourself as you would wish to care for others and so prepare to do so.

CONSTRUCT 5

Alderman Syndrome

Occurrence of chronic diseases is escalating and new "silent" epidemics are appearing and growing. At the same time, toxins are becoming ubiquitous as habitat and species damage accelerates toward the sixth extinction. The diagnosis labelled Alderman syndrome, or chronic ambient poisoning, links the emerging epidemics with habitat poisoning.

Modern Methodological Problems

Modern methods are inadequate to link these consequences and causes because statistical modeling is useless when exposures are low-dose, ubiquitous, and unprecedented; exposures cannot be defined or assessed, and are likely to be additive, multiplicative, and cumulative over a lifetime; outcomes are protean, lack gold standards, and are likely best modeled by continuous rather than discrete variables; and key aspects of impact are excluded or truncated because outcomes arise from multiple intersecting causal webs and countless primary sources. Most importantly from the point of view of statistical methods, everyone is exposed, meaning that there is no unexposed comparison group. Moreover, results of exposure depend on countless genes, and outcomes are generally reversible before the formation of one or more distinct final common pathway diseases. Fortunately, the N-of-1 study design promoted by Dr. David Sackett, the father of evidence-based medicine, enables doctors and patietns to investigate individual cases.

Other obstacles to linking cause and consequence come from the modern perceptual filter that in doctors limits the basic human self-knowledge of the body, the living context, and patterns of actions. These modern problems are paired with solutions in the form of the emerging constructs presented in months one and three.

Need for Change

Recall here that the 'corpse' paradigm—the material gold standard of modernity—and the pendulum swing toward generalism have led medical science to exclude particularism, subjectivisim, the intangible, and aggregated bodies. This has warped the modern view of flesh and being. For example, our awareness contracted around the concrete; our perceptions excluded the inner life, the as-yet unknown, and the unknowable; our understanding was fragmented by excessive analysis, reductionism, and molecularism; our sensory skills were neglected; our consideration of energy was restricted to EEG, EKG, or EMG results; our conception of flesh was reduced to a limitless array of dynamic molecules assessed by limited laboratory metrics; and our interbeing was noted and then—with exceptions such as asthma, occupational ailments, and allergy—disregarded.

To expand on modern medical neglect of the human context—especially the living context on which all lives depend as one—consider that urban institutional medicine naturally views oxygen as coming from air rather than from plants, and finds it difficult to pay attention to habitats as sources of climate, clean water, soil, and other essentials. Space colonization fantasies may seem reasonable to you; this can be catastrophic as your species is relying on you to sound the alarm when human health is threatened by loss of context. Hence the nested bodies construct.

With respect to self-patterning, the modern medical relation to time and the patterns that depend on it fall fatally short of the mark. They are not suited to a biocentric view, which has its own timetables, as mentioned above: lifetimes, generations, and evolutionary time—as well as extinction times, which relate to the modern reckoning of time by the nanosecond, minute, hour, financial quarter, and earning year or years. Indigenous people considered in their thinking the next seven to twenty generations; those who work with habitats today look ahead 500 years or more. If humans were manufactured, modern time-reckoning would work well, except that everyone would be dead. Hence the need for biocentric views and self-patterning for survival and thriving.

Epidemic of Exposure

As a doctor-patient with a broad education, trained in clinical epidemiology and cognitive psychology, I have observed my case and my exposures and outcomes over a long period of time. I used this N-of-1 study to define the etiopathogenesis of my case as Alderman syndrome and to match it to solutions that seed emergence.

In modern thinking, chemicals and money are innocent until proven guilty and patients are guilty until proven innocent—a process that is far too slow to protect life. Solutions to clinical mysteries come from close clinical observation and years of clinical study. 'Aha' moments come from thought and experience rather than technology. Ultimately, they come from patients who live the science of everyday life in close collaboration with astute expert clinicians. Relative to physicians who do procedures, thinkers are poorly paid. Even so, the only way for me to afford such care was to provide it myself, and to get help from another doctor maverick. The end result is the definition of an actionable diagnosis called Alderman syndrome, which is summarized in the following figures from *Medical Detective: Chronic Ambient Poisoning,* available at FutureMedicine.us. More information is available on EvolveMedicine.us.

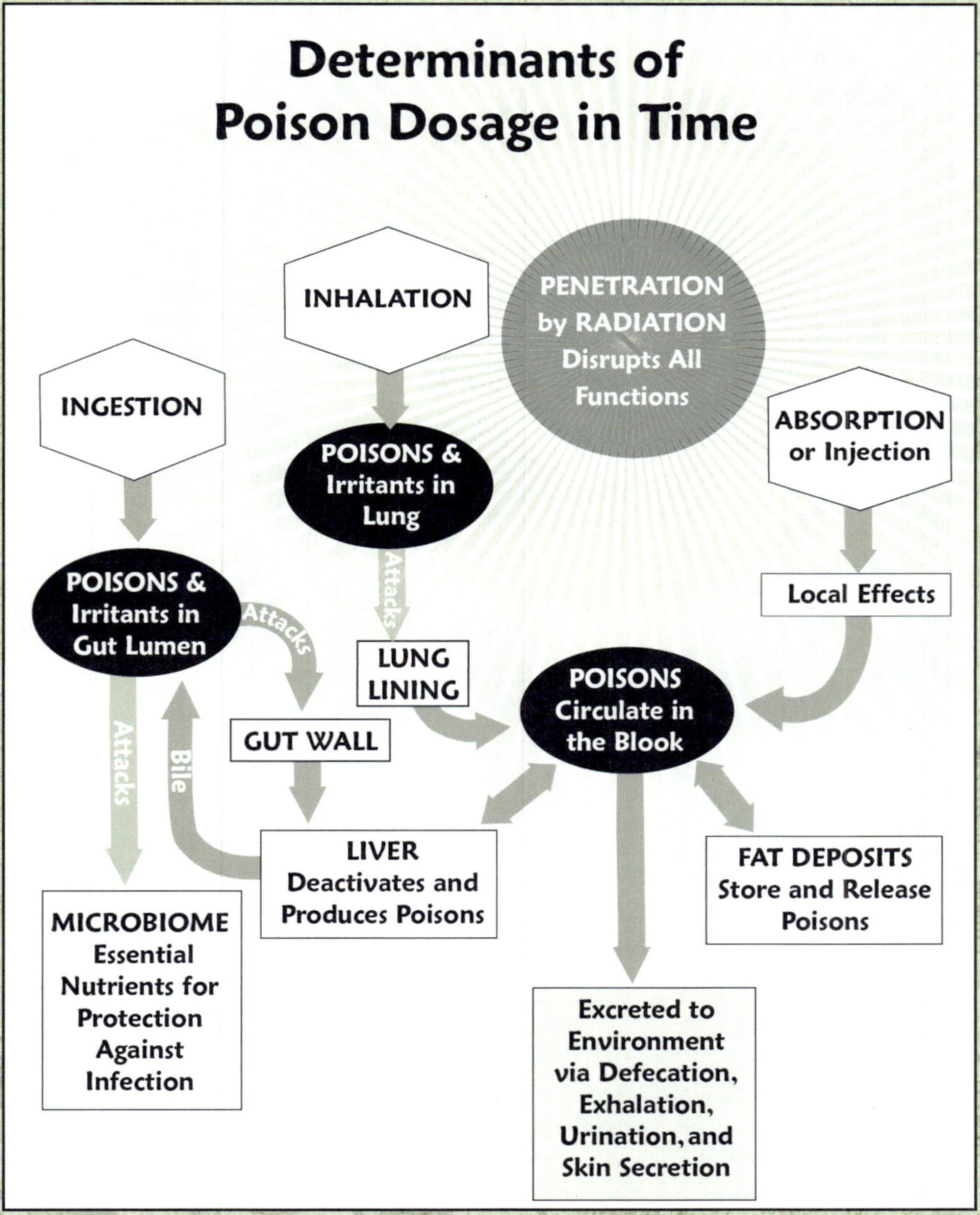

Consequences of Chronic Ambient Poisoning Over Time

Compensated by Tolerance

Causes Reversible Damage to Systems

Neuro-psychological

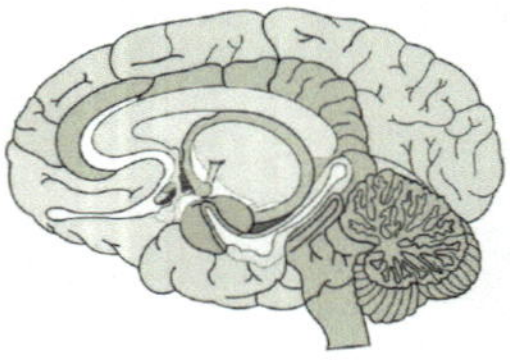

Gastrointestinal Microbiome

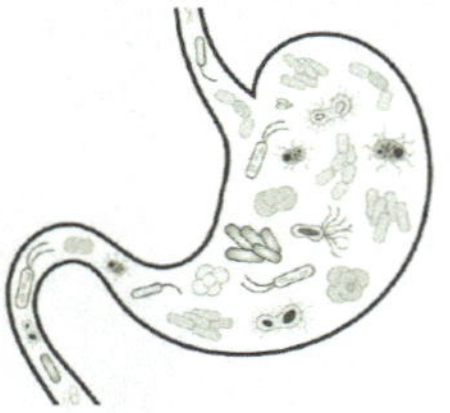

Musculoskeletal

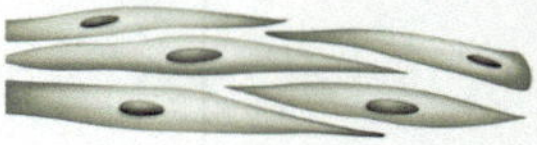

Endocrine/ Metabolic

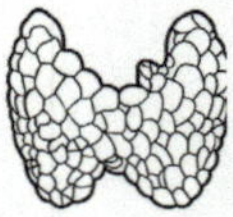

Genitourinary

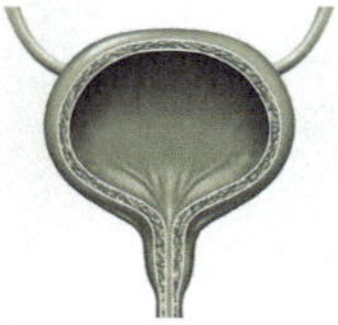

Ear, Nose, and Throat

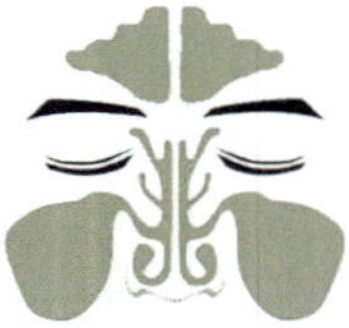

Allergic/ Immunological

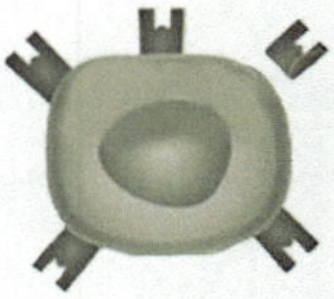

Other

Tolerance Fails

Provisional Diagnoses such as Chronic Fatigue Syndrome, Fibromyalgia, "Sensitivity" to Electromagnetic Radiation or Chemicals, or Neurotoxicity often Misdiagnosed as Mental Illness.

Organ Damage and Irreversible Disease, and Depression or Suicide

Habitat Restoration and Integration

Modern Problem

Now, during the Anthropocene era, when humans have denuded over three-quarters of the surface of the planet, and consequent climate change is accelerating extinction of species and habitats, humans need to work with rather than against their own evolution—and the last 300 million years of evolution. This may solve all of the problems that we are causing, including Alderman syndrome. To turn our species from liability to asset in choosing life, you can see each human as a potential habitat restorer who can adapt to coexist with or enhance the habitat until it is healthy—and safe—enough to restore to full biomass potential.

Emerging Solution

Fortunately, solutions are underway, as the members of the Society for Ecological Restoration and similar local groups can attest. Medical input could catalyze these efforts by providing new views of fertility as multiplying life on earth (see the Evolve Fertility series on FutureMedicine.us). Habitat integration work is less formal and may be undocumented, like the young people who are bringing foraged foods to market; who are reviving indigenous ways (as with shellfish farming in the Salish Sea); and living wild in forests. Physicians can experiment with habitat restoration clinics and communities with particular attention to preventing wildfires exacerbated by higher daily minimum temperatures in summer.

Residential Habitat Restoration Clinics and Communities

These recontextualize doctors and patients in habitats in need of gentle restoration to pattern emerging medical care of one as all. Initially, groups of retiring doctors would pool resources and purchase a range or other spread; construct living building to suit the local habitat; and invite the local community to refer patients with Alderman syndrome. Over time, with fee for service funding, it could become economically sustainable. At first, the consent form would be long; cash/work charges would take time to price out, as would the development of curricula for training, and networking with volunteer or paid consultants such as organic farmers, veterinarians, arborists, habitat restorers. It

CONSTRUCT 6

might take five years to start-up the first one, and continue beyond my lifetime and yours. Incorporating as a non-profit with covenants to define scope of work and protect land legally would be advisable.

CONSTRUCT 7

The Science of Everyday Life

Biographer Laura Dassou Walls views Henry David Thoreau's journal, which recorded his daily observations of the habitat of Concord, MA, as his greatest work of art and of science. His contemporary, Charles Darwin, lived science in an analogous way, but with more formal experiments. They did not profit by it, but their species did. Autobiographer and botanist Hope Jahren is now participating in hundred-year forest experiments in Norway. Doctors once lived science in these ways—especially during the Scottish Enlightenment—and doing so again will place doctors and their collaborating patients in a position to pattern ways in which patient and habitat restoration become one.

CONSTRUCT 8

Biofiction

In biofiction, biomedically literate authors begin with the assumption that humans will succeed in rescuing the body of life and write long case studies or speculative fiction detailing or imagining how this might have been accomplished (see FutureMedicine.us for more). If you are a doctor who looks forward to writing post-employment, please consider submitting a manuscript.

PLAYWORK

Recontextualizing a Lifetime of Learning

Can there be any greater reproach than an idle learning? Learn to split wood, at least.

— Henry David Thoreau in *A Week on the Concord River*

WORKING QUESTIONS

This month, use the questions below as a starting point for creating questions that are real for you in this moment and that reveal more and more of the big picture. In other words, refresh your awareness of your present place in biological time, take it as your starting point, and devise questions that enable you to take the next step in your transition to the elder years. As you compose questions, note that you are patterning a process of evolution that you will be able to use for the rest of your life.

- How do I embody my childhood? My calling? My relation to the bodies of my species, other species, my habitats, and life as a whole?
- What key experiences did the most to form the purpose and meaning that guide, cohere, and harmonize my being?
- When I look ahead to the future what do I see? What do I want to see? What can I do to accord my way of life with my vision of the future? How can I bring it into being on my own and in collaboration with others?
- Write questions of your own in your journal—or wherever you would like.

All of the research that you need to do to emerge is stored in your body as experience. In revisiting and re-encountering this now, you follow through on the experiential learning you began even before you were born. You filter it through the growing wisdom of years and epochal change so as to read and decode its teachings and to use them for the work of the wisdom years.

EXERCISE 1: Contextualizing Your Experiential Learning

To speak of wilderness is to speak of wholeness. Human beings came out of the wholeness, and to consider the possibility of reactivating membership in the Assembly of All Beings is in no way regressive.

— Gary Snyder in "The Etiquette of Freedom" in *The Practice of the Wild*

In your journal—or wherever you wish—draw a picture that places your body in the bodies of your profession, species, habitats, and of life. Then, express your vision of these bodies in a descriptive paragraph or 'SOAP' (i.e. subjective, objective, assessment, plan) for care of the body of life as of your body, taking care to be especially mindful of each nested body.

EXERCISE 2: Checking In

A living being is a temporary combination of various elements, always changing, just as a river is composed of uncountable drops of water, never remaining static even for the smallest imaginable moment of time. The sense of continuity we have from day to day, which we experience as a static state of being, is really a dynamic process, a continuous flow.

— Francesca Fremantle in *Luminous Emptiness*

Introduction

When you can read your body—that is, assess your state of being—you can more easily enter into and sustain care states. In this exercise, you learn to read your sevenfold state of relaxation and to use this reading to enhance your state. Do this exercise every morning and evening until you finish the book.

Purpose

This exercise is to assess and enhance your sensory awareness and to use it for sevenfold relaxation.

Instructions

Preparation. Prepare by defining sensations in the context of your flesh. Include your conventional senses of sight, hearing, taste, smell, and orientation with respect to gravity that are mediated by cranial nerves. Also include the light touch, pressure, and body position mediated by somatic nerves; and the satiety, distension and other visceral senses mediated by autonomic nerves.

Also consider sensation in the context of the sevenfold body—that is, include the less tangible senses that may be mediated by energy and interbeing, as when you realize that someone is looking at you, or is angry with you, or is in distress. Recollect that the levels of the sevenfold body are conceptual rather than actual, and that anything that affects your sensations may affect the whole of your flesh and being.

Practice. Assume a favorable posture, refresh your care state of alert relaxation, and call on your present sources of confidence in life. Now assess your overall state of relaxation. If you find that you are tense and constricted, do Sufi Square Breathing for five minutes or longer to deepen and broaden your care state. Now assess your present sevenfold strength by considering the following questions.

- Can my awareness extend to any subject, however near or distant and tangible or intangible?
- Can my understanding penetrate everyday problems with ease?
- Can my perceptions accommodate the new and unexpected while sustaining care, courage, and confidence?
- Are my sensations providing the information required for daily activities?
- Is my energy feeding my purpose and vision and my efforts to be and become healing?
- Can my flesh carry out the usual physical tasks with ease?
- Is my interbeing sustaining a vital connection to time and eternity and to the web of life?

If the answer to any question is no, contemplate your weakness and its source and possible remedy. For example, if you lack physical strength or energy due to sedentary living, overeating, or lack of sleep, physical activity may restore you. If you lack fleshly vitality, you can seek help from a consulting doctor or bodyworker. If pain is sapping your strength, you can construct your own placebo (see Care course, Woodpecker level, on EvolveMedicine.us). If you cannot discern the problem or its remedy, make a note of what you sensed and try to discern your problem and its remedy at a later time. Now explore any limitations to your care state by considering the following questions.

- Is my awareness contracted around a subject or restricted by denial or avoidance?
- Is my understanding limited by confusion or fragmentation or obstructed by useless or harmful thoughts?
- Are my perceptions constricted by pessimism or obstructed by automatic actions or reactions?
- Are my sensations limited by physical loss or by undeveloped or maladaptive sense awareness?
- Is the axis of energy in front of my spine weak, or is it unevenly distributed?
- Is my flesh affected by new or unusual symptoms or signs of illness or injury?
- Am I freely connected with sources of care in the web of life in time and eternity?

If the answer to any questions is yes, use your relaxed, alert focus to locate the part of your flesh that corresponds to your obstacle or obstacles. Do this by bringing your relaxed, alert focus to your crown and moving your focus very slowly and gradually toward your feet, as if you are using your awareness as a scanner to take a series of cross-sectional images of your body. As you do this, explore your sensations and read your state. Where you detect ease, offer it your enjoyment. Where you detect unease, offer it lovingkindness and compassion. When you have finished, make a note of any obstacles you detected and use a comfort practice to gain relief. If you note no obstacle, close your practice and dedicate it to knowing your body.

EXERCISE 3: More on Grounding Your Being in Your Flesh and in Life in Time

Mother Nature is Boss. That's why we follow her lead!

— Vital Farms, Inc.

Plan ahead so that you can do the exercise at least two hours after a meal, to avoid indigestion with gastroesophageal reflux. When you begin, assume a good position, enhance your alignment, and ground your energy via gravity. Take several deep, slow breaths and assume the stance of a lover who keenly appreciates life and is disposed to complement it, to cooperate with it, and to share its wellbeing as well as the travails that the love would erase or reverse. Next, enter a care state in which your imagination can reconnect your being with your flesh and with the body of life.

Bring your focus to your crown; if you have difficulty with focus, place a palm in the place where your anterior fontanelle was at birth and allow it to stabilize your focus. Then return your hand to its position of ease and recollect the nature of awareness for several cycles of breath or longer. Now, trace a thread of awareness out from your crown into shared interbeing. Take it as far as you can without losing your embodiment of it, and then picture rather than embody it as you extend it to a distant point in space or time with which you would like to connect. For example, you may extend your embodied awareness to a nearby plant, and then your awareness alone on to the healthy Amazonian rain forest of 1491 that is producing abundant oxygen and life energy. Once you have embodied or imagined your awareness connecting with a local and then a distant habitat, imagine it extending into space and time, perhaps into the upper atmosphere in a future time of abundant life. Allowing your picture to stabilize, and then return it to the limits of embodiment in your crown and allow it to stabilize again. Then trace the connection all the way back to a place where your flesh is making contact with the earth, and back through your body to your crown again.

Now use a like process to visualize the grounding of each level of your being in your body and then in interbeing, first with embodied awareness and then with imagination alone. At the level of understanding, trace your being to your central nervous system, then back to an experience of care and cure that inspired you. Next, move your understanding outward through your imagination into a future form of care and cure such as an emerging clinic in a lovingly restored habitat that you love and would wish to know better. Then return your imagination to the limits of your embodied understanding and back in to your central nervous system. Finally, relax your focus into your being as it is in the present moment.

At the level of perceptions, bring your focus into your anatomical heart and rest it there until you feel your emotions. If you feel distressed or depleted, allow your state to return to baseline or better before continuing. Now, look through the eye of the heart in the light of love and contemplate the beauty of the body of life. When you see beauty, trace your perceptions outward to the limits of your embodiment and allow your imagination to continue on to the network of hearts with which your embodied perceptions will connect more and more strongly as your perceptions grow brighter and more loving.

Now bring your imagination back to the limits of embodied perceptions and on into your anatomical heart. Allow your focus to rest there as long as you like, perhaps as long as it takes to sense the movement of your heart—which, when you become more aware of it, may feel like a dryer that is spinning your circulation by propelling blood from veins to arteries.

At the level of sensations, expand your focus to encompass your skin and other sense organs. While your focus is expanded, relax it and allow it to become fuzzy, then enlarge it by allowing it to expand outward from your flesh to the limits of embodiment and beyond through your imagination. Expand it further and further until it reaches the closest healthy parts of your present habitat. Now imagine yourself exchanging matter and energy with your habitat in care of your body and its body.

Rest your imagined sensations in your habitat for as long as you like in order to draw inspiration, and then allow your focus to draw in again to the limits of your embodiment of it, and next on into your skin. Allow it to gather and rest in your solar plexus, which is below and behind the pit of your stomach, below your ribs. Use your palm as a guide for focusing on your visceral sensations. Note that you can sense the subtle, internal, and small as well as the coarse, external, and immense. After a reasonable interval, return your focus to your skin and rest it there.

For energy, bring your focus to your secret energy center, which is deep inside your pelvis, in front of your spine between your navel and pubis. Allow your focus to expand to include the ovaries or testes on either side of your generative center. Thus grounded in your flesh, extend your imagination back in time through your lineal ancestry as you conceive of it. In times past, as many as ten percent of Americans did not know the identities of their biological fathers. You may therefore ground your energy in your forebears, culture of nurture, or habitat. Rest your imagination in this personal history for long enough to enrich your conception of it in support of your present care and cure, and then let it move into the real future that you are working to create. Now allow your imagination to move into the personal future of care and cure that you envision and intend to bring into being.

For flesh, relax and expand your focus until it encompasses all of the bones between your scalp and your soles. Rest your awareness there, and then gather it and move it gradually from your scalp to your soles, dwelling on and wondering at the strength of the bones that protect and support your organs as you go. Now gather your focus and rest in inside your nostrils, and note the breath that is passing in and out as it carries gaseous matter from the atmosphere to your lungs and back again. Now move your point of focus to your throat and note that food passes through it with every meal. Do not move your focus to your anus or perirectal area as this can cause circulatory problems—that is, hemorrhoids. When ready, move your focus to your bladder and note that excess solutes are continually gathering there with water in preparation for elimination.

At the level of interbeing, ground your being in the linings of your lungs and gut where the inner surface of your tangible flesh meets the matter of your interbeing inside your flesh. Bring your relaxed, expanded focus to the lining of your lungs. Contemplate the cells inside the tiny sacs in your lung tissue—your alveoli—as they allow gases to flow in and out of your bloodstream while excluding larger molecules such as allergenic proteins. Marvel at the inherited evolved wisdom of the tiny cells that form your inner boundary with the atmosphere. After several cycles of breath, during which you relax into the generosity of the atmosphere that is still rich in oxygen, move your point of focus outward to the limits of embodiment and then extend your imagination to the closest source of oxygen in your outdoor habitat, such as a tree, a shrub, or a lawn or meadow. Then return your imagination and your focus to your gut; contemplate the microbiome that resides in your gut and the gut lining that absorbs just as much of the available nutrients as you need. Marvel at the complexity of this ordinary process, and at the relative clumsiness of engineered systems in comparison with evolved ones. Take a moment to extend compassion to humans who suffer from the modern illusion that engineered systems are preferable. Finally, release your awareness and bring your exercise to a close.

Simplify, elaborate, or replace this visualization as you please in keeping with your circumstances. If you wish to deepen your connections with friends, family, mentors, communities, animals, plants, or habitats, include them in your embodiments or imaginings. Feel free to do likewise with sources of inspiration for care and cure or connections to any and all regions of space and time. I like to work with care states while walking in nature and to use my arms to trace arcs of embodied awareness. You may enjoy that too.

Supplementary Reading

1. David Wallace-Wells. *The Uninhabitable Earth: Life After Warming.* New York: Tim Duggan Books, 2019.
2. Paul Hawken. *Blessed Unrest.* New York: Viking, 2007.
3. Juliana Birnbaum and Louis Fox, eds. *Sustainable [R]evolution.* Berkeley: North Atlantic Books, 2014.
4. Scott Freeman. *Restoring Tarboo Creek: One Family's Quest to Heal the Land.* Portland: Timber Press, Inc., 2018.
5. Charles Darwin. *The Autobiography of Charles Darwin.* Edited by Nora Barlow. London: Collins, 1958.
6. Laura Dassow Walls. *Henry David Thoreau: a Life.* Chicago: The University of Chicago Press, 2017.
7. Virginia Cornell. *Doc Susie: The True Story of a Country Physician in the Colorado Rockies.* Carpinteria, CA: Manifest Publications, 1991.
8. Hope Jahren. *Lab Girl.* New York: Alfred A. Knopf, 2016.
9. Tara Womersley and Dorothy Crawford. *Bodysnatchers to Lifesavers: Three Centuries of Medicine in Edinburgh.* Edinburgh: Luath Press, 2010.

Physician Cure Thyself

Our entire much-praised technological progress, and civilization generally, could be compared to an axe in the hand of a pathological criminal.

— Albert Einstein via Wikiquote

The admonition that doctors cure themselves—ironic in its time—invoked the ancient shamanic habit of treating patients as separate and other, as if from behind a curtain like that which hid the Wizard of Oz—or like the canvas top of the wagon that concealed his alter ego's patent medicines. Because insight and perspective were discouraged in the tradition, and its memory has become too short and too crammed with trivia, doctors lack perspective on technoshamanism—and are not allowed to use it wittingly or objectively. Like me, they can only use it on themselves. Now, in the age of objective science—especially the science of ecology—all such curtains have been lifted and we have the change to engage the patient's magic—beginning with teaching them to own their own placebos. You must see and do this—probably many times over a long period of time—before you can teach it.

Emergence is revealing to our species its historical imposition of a hierarchy of nested tyrannies in which the human species lorded over all and were lorded over by projected versions of itself; these tyrannies eventually allowed life on earth no rights and no value. We can look around and see that none of us is able to do exercise for someone else or to wean another from drug or device dependency, or to do and have what is essential and no more. It is up to you to take personal responsibility for caring for, curing, and enhancing your own flesh and being and for cultivating your own becoming. As you leave the role of employee, you relinquish the myriads of petty tasks that made it difficult for you to discern what was important and essential and to ignore the rest. As you age, your decline will show you how to use and share your resources wisely. Then you can model the process of discovery, care, and cure.

So it is time now to take to heart the admonition to cure yourself. When you are able to do this, you will be able to safeguard the life that nests in your body and in the bodies in which yours must nest. You can then join with other doctors in contextualizing the care, cure, and enhancement of the species in the context of the bodies of all species, all habitats, and life on earth. You and

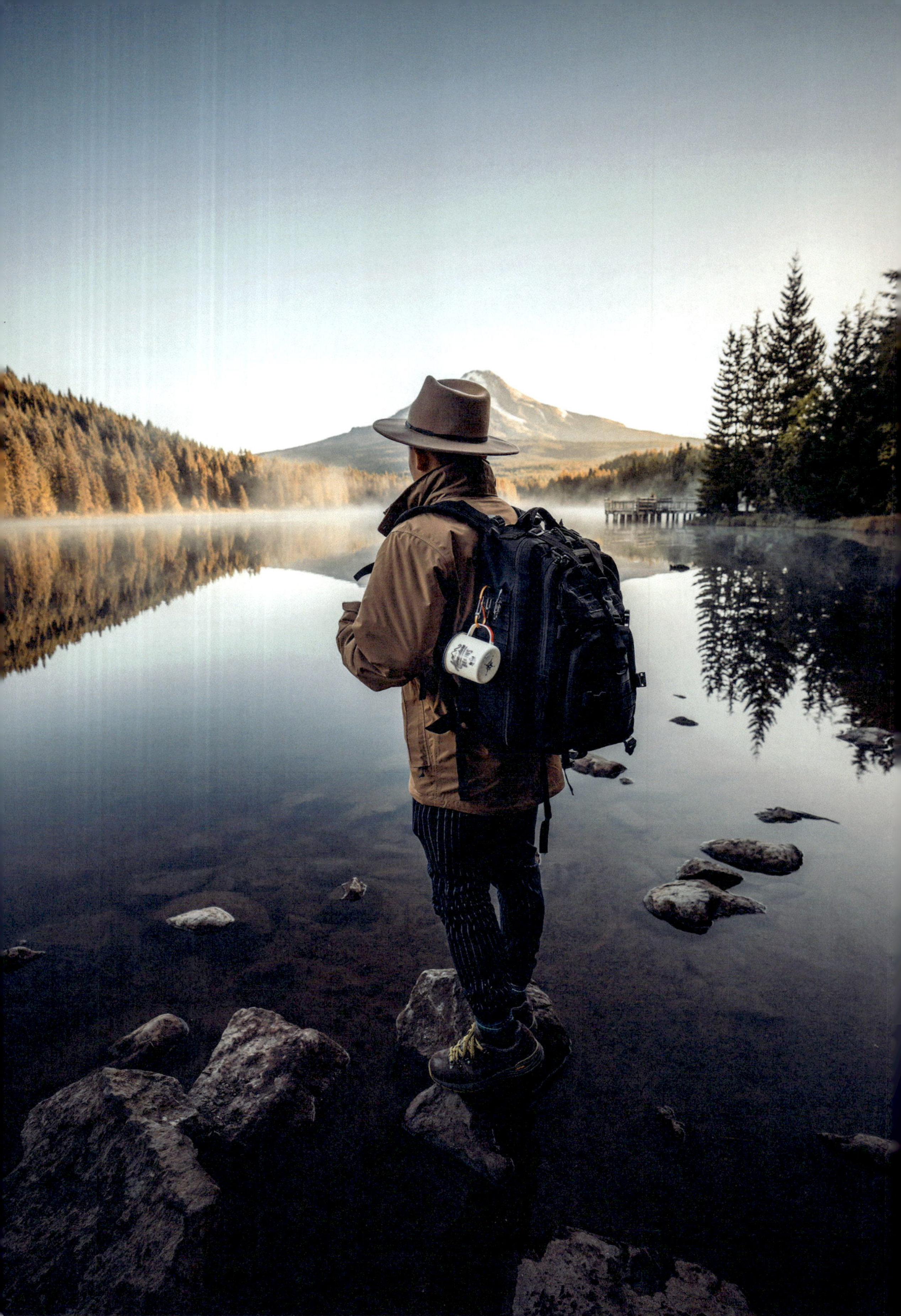

they can then diagnose the afflictions of life that do not limit themselves to one body, one species, or one habitat, and discern how best to treat one as all. You and they can then construct a new view of the big picture in which you mediate harmony as you intervene on the side of life, instead of battling death and destruction.

ANECDOTES FROM MEDICAL LIVES

Space was once a hospitable, deep realm in which I could locate myself and wander at will. I could enter it, I lived in it, I had a spatial relationship to everything I could see. That sort of space no longer exists for me visually—or mentally.

— Oliver Sacks in *The Mind's Eye*

The skills you will need to care for and cure your body in its present social context are like those developed by Dr. Viktor Frankl when he remained sane in a late modern insane asylum in Vienna, and then in a series of concentration camps. While it may be true that the best who were sent to the camps died, and that survival was a matter of chance and not choice, Frankl's resilience arose from that which he developed as a physician, held as an inner light in his time of trials, and articulated and shared as a survivor of the deathliest human impulses. Like Rafael Lemkin, Gandhi, King, and so many other peacemakers, Frankl left a legacy that illuminates the way forward. It shows us that personal construction of meaning, purpose, and responsibility can enable us to make good on experience.

You are free now to follow that light—and many others. You can find it in the ecstatic religious poetry of Walt Whitman, whose prophetic voice was one with leaves of grass; in the wisdom of habitat-integrated peoples, who lived well in and with the body of life; in the legacies of conscientious dissenters, who saw the right thing to do and did it; and in the sparks ignited by original thinkers like Jonathan Edwards, Elizabeth Peabody, Henry Thoreau, and Dr. William James. All of these show you some of what it takes to diagnose the body of life, to cure its ills, and—in the distant living future when our descendants have far more wisdom that humans do now—to enhance life on earth.

To help carry the profession over the threshold between late modernity and what comes next, you recognize that life is and always has been a vast material and ethereal experiment in which our species played a hitherto small—and dynamic—part. To play a salutary role in the future, you must learn to care for and cure yourself as you would others—that is, to follow the golden rule in regard to self as well as others. It would be pointless to sacrifice your life for this in the way of old Christian saints. You must do something more difficult: sacrifice your past errors and habits continuously as you evolve and share a better way of living and working in the world. To begin, you and your peers can own and share stories of caring wisely for—and curing—yourselves.

Lena

Lena is part of a group practice in obstetrics and gynecology that runs a busy clinic on the campus of a large university-affiliated hospital. When her practice was small and still forming, her use of prenatal technologies increased sharply and changed rapidly. Her percentage of forceps births plummeted while her percentage of Cesarean sections climbed from single digit figures to thirty percent—and kept climbing. As first-time mothers grew older, she prescribed more and different hormones to induce conception and did more and more amniocenteses.

As American society came to view medical outcomes as sure things, and doctors tried to push the rates of adverse outcomes to zero through heroic medicine, the standards of care of Lena's practice—and other American practices—diverged sharply from those of large public hospitals in other countries that had lower surgical rates and better prenatal outcomes. In her practice, surgical delivery became routine. Patients began to request earlier and more invasive interventions. When large practices in other cities began to report good outcomes after chorionic villus sampling, one of Lena's partners went to learn the procedure. Soon Lena and the others had learned it too, and were offering it to those who demanded it.

Lena had mixed feelings about the procedure. The fetus and placenta were tiny and the amount of tissue required was significant. She wondered about rare adverse outcomes that might not be detected for years, if at all. She shared these concerns with patients; few took her concerns to heart. Months later, a patient miscarried not long after Lena did the procedure. She discussed this with a partner who said that she, too, had observed a loss but attributed it to spontaneous abortion.

Lena's practice moved up the annual date on which they evaluated their statistics. They discovered that several patients had lost their pregnancies soon after chorionic villus sampling. They had not associated the loss with the procedure, but could find no other explanation. The numbers were low; so was their threshold for concern. They decided to discontinue their use of the procedure and to rely on a tried and true one in which they had full confidence: amniocentesis. And so, through careful and objective observation, Lena and her partners took note of patients' concerns and their own experience and kept pace with the now.

Jessie

Jessie's practice offered obstetrical services to a wide range of patients seeking care at a well-heeled urban hospital located on the boundary of an affluent neighborhood and an indigent one. Because the hospital was generously supported by patrons, she was in a position to give to all of her patients—both low-risk and high—the best prenatal care that love or money could offer. As the practice grew and evolved, she did very little obstetrical care but continued to offer gynecological care and to keep up with new developments in women's care, including new means for preventing fetal loss.

During her training, she had met and married a man and made plans with him to start a family after her practice was established and he would be free to work less and to look after the children. As she began to feel that she could take time, and as they felt pressure from both families to have children as soon as possible, she discontinued her birth control. She expected to conceive quickly, and did. She and her husband were thrilled—but a few weeks into the pregnancy, she lost it. They were devastated but hopeful that they would conceive again soon. They did. They lost the pregnancy again, and soon lost two more.

Jessie could not pinpoint a cause. While adverse outcomes had been linked to operating room exposures, she had not been spending time in surgery—or in any intensive, pre-op, or post-op care unit. While immune factors could cause loss in the second trimester, she was losing pregnancies at varying gestational ages. While her family feared job stress, she could discern no particular psychological risk factors for any—much less all—of the losses. Her colleagues could give her no useful advice. She was on her own, with no help from her profession, her family, or her colleagues; the few who knew oppressed her with sympathetic worry and looked to her for comfort.

She decided to rely on common sense. She restricted her work time to necessary tasks. She asked a few colleagues and support staff to help her avoid potential hazards by doing tasks such as using synthetic chemicals and lifting heavy objects. She researched promising medications for the sustenance of pregnancy and took them. She gave her husband a task list so that he could help—and to relieve his worry. The next time they conceived, she carried the pregnancy to term.

Sue

Sue trained as an anesthesiologist and secured a position in a regional hospital in a large town in a river valley dominated by chemically-intensive agriculture and a large canning plant. She and her small group of specialists supported all of the local surgeons and their patients through a call schedule that enabled them to provide high-quality care around the clock and also to sustain it over the long haul by allowing for personal and family time. Sue took the further precaution of buying all of her food at a local co-op where she could get chemical-free, fresh foods. Having grown up on a family farm and become responsible and independent at an early age, she was appalled by corporate farming methods and prepared to lend a hand at the co-op.

While working at the co-op, she met one of the organizers, a man with whom she joined a guru-led spiritual group that preached mind over matter. Both of them had been grounded at a young age in self-sufficiency, cooperation, and teamwork. Both had traveled the world and gained experience in esoteric methods that supported intentional personal and congregal change. They were living in a strong, dynamic, and supportive community. They moved in together, married, and started a family with every expectation that they would be able to negotiate whatever gender and family roles might be needed to raise a strong family.

Things did not go as easily as expected. As Sue continued to meet her responsibilities at the hospital, he cut back on work at the co-op to care for the children. She noticed that he played with the children and kept them busy but did not cook or clean. He paid little heed to safety, encouraged physical risks, and seemed unwilling—or unable—to change. She did her best to accept his limitations. The children suffered allergies and injuries, some serious. He became more heedful, but stopped working altogether.

Sue and the family continued as they were until she developed new onset pain in her hands and weakening of her grip. She feared that her wrist might fail when she had to intubate a patient, and that this possibility might make her unable to continue working in her area of specialty. She suspected rheumatoid arthritis, and sought and took treatments that stabilized her hand function but failed to ease the nocturnal pain that was keeping her up at night. Her husband cared for her through her waking hours, but soon stopped his home carpentry projects. She was cook, mother, patient—and bread-winner. It seemed likely that she would have to hire a caretaker for him and to take responsibility for everything else. Not long after, they divorced; she remarried and grounded her altered family in matter as well as mind.

BETH LOOKS BACK: Renewing Your Love of Life

Fears of every sort are rushing through my mind, mixed with (futile) regrets and recriminations that the tumor was not diagnosed earlier...I could, should have paid attention, questioned, sought clarification months ago...but I must not think on this; must focus instead on how fortunate I am that the thing has been caught now.

— Oliver Sacks in *The Mind's Eye*

When I fell ill, and had to view care, cure, and thriving as a patient, I began to see care states as one point in a continuum of being ranging from hell states to states of relief to improvement in baseline states to near normal to yet better and better states that ascend a kind of Jacob's ladder up into bliss and beyond. I even wondered whether self-care might open the door to spontaneous cure. As time passed, I came to see that self-care could enable the creation of a new and better life. This counted as a cure to the patient in me, as it was better for me than meeting medical expectations. Even so, I wanted whatever was eating away at my flesh to stop doing so, and sought a fleshly cure as well.

I had tried many simple forms of meditation and prayer, and had moved on to difficult esoteric methods that were as risky and invasive as many medical interventions. These drew on the energy body to create a strong core and intense focus that the mind could use to bypass neurological dysfunction. They also drew attention to ancient cautionary tales in which such practices led to insanity and death, as with Rabbinic stories of the dangers of Merkavah mysticism, and newer tales of psychotic breaks in Westerners practicing tantra. Such anecdotes emphasize the need to sustain a relaxed field of awareness and to ground flesh in the earth in the way of a home electrical system. Personally, I found this grounding insufficient. I felt it key to remain grounded in the bodies of the species and habitat, and in stable human communities like congregations or sanghas that remain mindful of the big picture in all its aspects, including spiritual practice and sustainability. I also found it essential to create an environment free of chronic exposure to harmful chemicals, of electrical and electronic devices that emit non-ionizing radiation, and of excess body fat that may have stored chemicals. When practicing independently, it is wise to do what is simple and safe with the support of ethics as well as old-fashioned virtues such as prudence and caution.

One sweet practice that can pattern the whole of your body and that can be done at any time is lovingkindness (metta) meditation. As with the Judaic path of blessing, it can ease your being into a state that shifts the body and its processes toward the heavenly—that is, toward the healing. I once practiced it for almost an entire day in a high-ceilinged, high-windowed sanctuary in which a hundred or so retreatants had gathered to share in the meditative practices of a well-known teacher. We students sat on cushions that supported good alignment of the flesh through the Burmese position or seven-point posture of Vairocana. The teacher sat facing us, speaking gently and easily and telling humorous anecdotes to illustrate her teaching points. These put me in mind of the traditional teaching anecdotes once told to young physicians by elder ones.

She guided us through a series of meditations that offered blessings to loved ones, to self, and to strangers. Then, when we had reached a strong and robust state of lovingkindness, we thought of those whom we found most difficult to bless, such as the tyrants of the past, and then blessed those whom we could freely bless in our hearts without forcing it, which would both both create new problems and weaken our states. After a time, as all present entered states of greater love and happiness, the atmosphere in the room became blissful. Each person's state supported those nearby. Those whose baseline states were heavenly or who could hold strong states of blessing lifted the group, while the rest of us contributed what energies and skills we could.

The day was wonderful, and yet the doctor in me saw that while spiritual healing was a wonderful element of care, it was no more able to do all than was molecular care. One glance at the teacher was enough to illustrate this. She glowed with a healing state that came of great art applied to the easing of early psychic wounds, but she was morbidly obese. Unlike the ascetics of old who starved themselves and retreated to huts or caves as if desirous of living as disembodied or dead, this teacher ate modern food, lived with central heating, and otherwise accumulated more calories than she spent. One glance from her might be enough to tell her that my state of being was hellish; once glance from me would reveal that hers was poorly grounded in present reality. Together, we showed that to enhance old ways of care, I must glean and interweave the best of old and new, distant and near, material and ethereal. She might become a source of spiritual light yet still be unaware of the gifts of enlightenment thinkers and their philosophical descendants—or of the gifts of Hippocrates and Maimonides and all who draw on or add to the spirit of their arts and sciences today.

COMMENT: Nesting Self-Cure in Self-Care

The wisdom of Thomas Aquinas, the logic of Newman, and the clinical genius of Osler will not be effective in making well a patient who does not fully understand why he is sick, or what he must do to get well. A first-rate clinician trains himself to do two things exceedingly well: to talk to his patients, and to listen to them.

— Philip A. Tumulty in *The Effective Clinician*

Chances are good that you have the skills you need to help patients define an illness and discover a cure. In your education, you developed the intellectual chops to solve any number of problems. You are able to focus, to concentrate, and to work things through step by step with the aid of discipline and passion. These skills enabled you to walk through walls of ignorance and incomprehension. As you matured, you learned to grasp complex etiopathogeneses, to reconcile the wishes of an individual with particular cultural and biological contexts, and to advise patients to live well and to value the time that they had.

What you may not have learned is self-care, and this may have limited your ability to create, sustain, and strengthen care states to share with patients and to model self-care for them. To recover those personal and interpersonal abilities that support and share care and cure will require you to repattern many ingrained habits of observation and response—especially the deeply buried, lightning-fast ones that you have long since ceased to notice. In the post-employment years, when you are free to think and act, you can learn or relearn states of contemplation that favor the solution of the intangible, systemic problems of your profession, and that allow you to read your body and recognize, enhance, and hold the care states that support you in solving personal and interpersonal problems in the context of the big picture as we humans know it today. You will then find it easier to frame problems in a way that is accessible to the light of kind, compassionate wisdom, and to respond to them with newly primed sequences of stances, states, strategies, skills, and dynamic, evolving vision.

As a late modern doctor, you will be good at helping to detect and solve familiar problems such as infectious epidemics. These pass through filters that may exclude and reject all that has defeated you in the past. When you relax that filter in the elder years, you have a chance to reconsider chronic epidemic and endemic ailments. You will doubt the judgment of those orthopedists who pursue thrills through extreme sports and replace the body parts of daring young athletes who abuse their bodies. You may wonder at obese, smoking cardiologists who say one thing and demonstrate another. You will see how a whole generation was swept up into unhealthy worklives that incentivize the maladaptive habits of late modernity, and recognize that you have more to offer yourself and others than you have been allowed to contribute.

As you become aware that late modern doctors are complicit in the destructive economy, and that idolatry of technology has been leading us to cut off the roots and shoots of the tree of life, you will gain perspective on the complex systems in which you have been embedded. You will recognize that to allow managerial data to supplant professional acumen is to ignore the warning 'garbage in, garbage out' and to reverse alchemy by turning gold into lead. Medical wisdom comes of the sense born of personal and lineal experience. As an elder, you will have time to process the radical experiments of late modernity and to turn your early experiential learning into personal wisdom. When you share this wisdom with your colleagues, you may be able to guide your juniors in transforming premodern desires for control and modern possessive individualism into an emerging way of life in which they can care wisely for each as all.

Blessing and Delight

In the 1930s, [Dr. Viktor] Frankl was unique in his intentional use of humor with patients as a way to help them put some distance between themselves and their problems…using defiant humor can bring enormous relief [of] phobias and anxiety.

— Haddon Klingberg, Jr. in *When Life Calls Out to Us*

The word blessing can mean many things to many people. For those who have lived outside a religious tradition, the word blessing may be free of any sense of obligation or manipulation and so be taken to mean a spontaneous—or voluntary—gift of being that is intangible and inestimable. The word delight is less common and thus less likely to be abused or devalued. For the purposes of this book, the words blessing and delight are intended to evoke states that support care, cure, or enhancement of flesh or being. If these words carry troubling connotations for you, use others that inspire you to strengthen your equanimous faith in life, in cure, and in the prospect of abundant wellbeing now and into the indefinite future.

When you have found the right words, use them to inspire your faith in the future, to strengthen your care states, and to connect with the motivations that inspired you to pursue your calling and that are now inspiring your transition to elderhood. When your care states grow strong, they will support you in gleaning meaning, purpose, and wisdom from the sum total of your life experience.

EXERCISE 1: Crafting Blessings

Use the question below—or ones you create—to develop the skills you need to recognize, return to, deepen, and sustain care states inspired by blessing and delight.

Sit in a favorite chair or other place of comfort and close your eyes. Visualize several individuals—including yourself—and offer each and all well-wishes such as health, happiness, and joy. Do this until you are offering blessings to a dozen individuals. When you have been doing so for ten minutes, ask, "Which of these well-wishes (blessings) is (are) inspiring a state of delight in my body right now?" Repeat those as long—and as often—as you like.

As the days pass and you learn to delight in blessing, expand your well-wishes and include more individuals. Allow your state to be sweet and restorative and to grow in strength and length until you feel a shift in your baseline state of being. Yes, this is esoteric work, but it is not abstruse, baffling, ascetic, or useless! It is simple and can change your life for the better.

However, it may be unfamiliar and therefore tricky. It may take time to get the knack of allowing blessings to flow naturally and so to enhance and express care. Old habits may intrude. One is the competitive striving that may be useful for cure but that can undermine care and faith in the future while also wasting energy. Another is the set of inner prima donnas that typically dominate your inner life and your personal narrative: your preconceived views, ideas, expectations, and reactions; and habitual hell states of dislike, blame, guilt, shame, regret, sulking, fatalism, nihilism, frustration, catastrophizing, self-punishment, or the like. Should these stop or commandeer the easy flow of blessing, take time to relax and recover your ease and then begin again. Note that to begin again is to learn, not to fail. You may have much learning to do. As a doctor, you will have used force and been subject to all kinds of forces that tyrannized and warped the professional maturation that you are now learning to nurture. If you are not sure that you have got the hang of it, use pre- and post-exercise check-ins to guide your subjective success.

EXERCISE 2: Transitioning to a More Life-Affirming Reality

I pull away. And then, pulling away too far, an astronaut floating in an enormously lonely outer space, I know that I cannot sustain my sense of a separate reality forever, for after all, the only reality is a shared reality, situated within a common ground.

— Eva Hoffman in *Lost in Translation: Life in a New Language*

In medicine, patients consult you for problems that you interpret in medical terms and address through differentials and treatments. As in the early days of the doctors of the Scottish Enlightenment who gave birth to interventionist medicine, you will have learned to stand sentinel at the threshold of death and pull people back from the brink. As at the dawn of disease control and prevention, you will have learned to report potentially epidemic diseases and to identify risk states amenable to modification. With the push toward health promotion and wellness, you may have balked at moving up into the no man's lands between disease and absence of disease, health and supreme health. You may have noticed that in this brave new world of anticipatory intervention, your attitude may have shifted to the point of losing its grounding in the gold standard of anatomic and histologic diagnosis and floating away into a disorienting ocean of molecularism.

You were not trained for this. Your training emphasized problemizing as the gateway to analyzing and then sterilizing or eradicating or easing. If you thought of synergy, you did so in the context of enzymes and cofactors, not lives or ecosystems. You didn't dwell on the big picture, or think of turning evil consequences into good ones. Your elders didn't think that way, and you may not have thought to try.

In this exercise, try and reframe your own problems in such a way as to allow you to experiment with repatterning and regrounding your flesh and being so as to become able to share any salubrious patterns that might benefit others. As you revise your intuitive methods of framing problems, you become free to try new ways of resolving them, and of articulating, enumerating, and harmonizing or integrating your problem-solving.

1. Take ten minutes to think about your life as it is and as you would like it to be. Take as long as you like to ponder how to get from here to there. Consider any new stances, states, strategies, or skills that might be of use, or any new means of priming (motivating) or inspiring (envisioning) your transition. Take as many days as you wish to come up with a list of five solutions that you like, and record them. Then think through and list the problems that each solution might obviate. Enrich this list as much as possible. If you reach a new level of insight, redo the exercise in reverse until you have a list of problems matched to solutions that you intend to implement. Record all your lists in your journal.
2. Repeat the solutions exercise for the life of the species both as it is and as you would like it to be. This time, allow yourself to envision a better world and to come up with solutions and problems that you cannot implement on your own. Record these lists in your journal.
3. Compare your lists. See where your changes harmonize with and could catalyze the larger salutary changes that are underway in the world. Write a paragraph about how you might be the change you want to see in the

world, and another about how you might change with the world. As you do this, presume that any change you make in yourself might fill you with blessing and delight and overflow to create a ripple effect.

EXERCISE 3: Change as Personal Narrative

Write a list of the ten life experiences that were most important in forming your character.

Compare this list to the one you made in June. How and why do they differ? Have your efforts during these months of transition led to any signs of new wisdom? To the beginnings of emergence? Reflect on your efforts and write 1000 words about any gains (and losses) in your journal.

Part Four

Spring

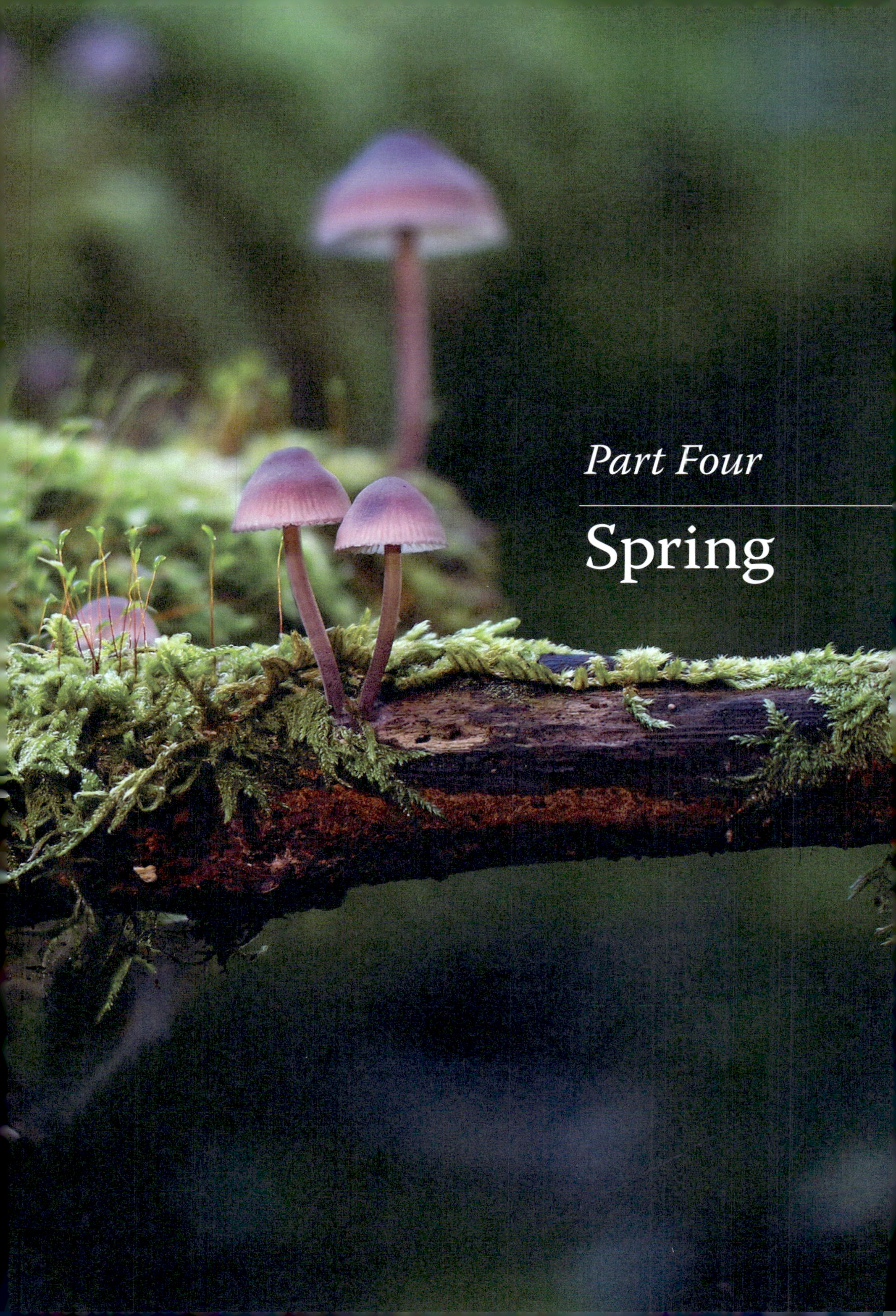

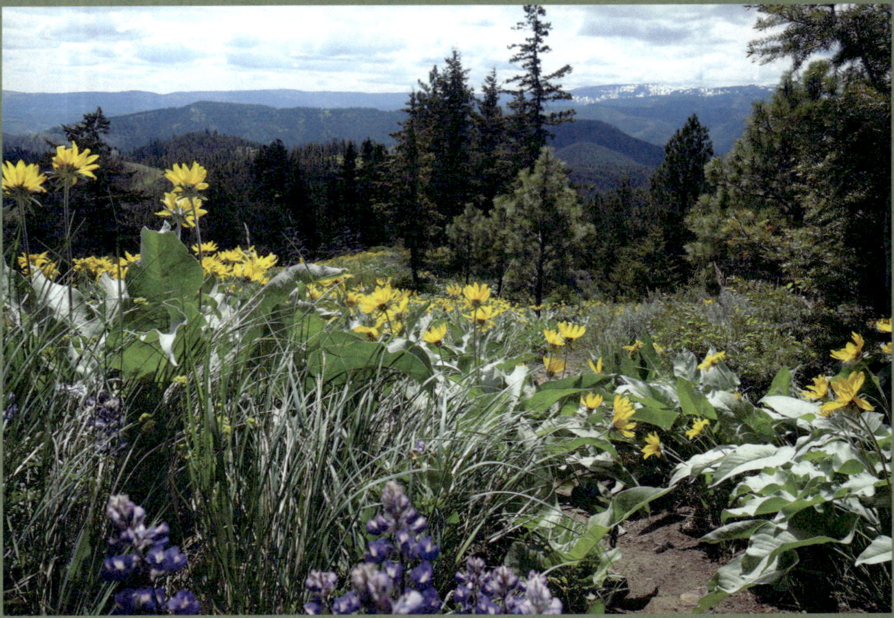

IN THE SPRING, YOU ARE LIKE THE PRUNED TRUNK OF AN OLD GRAPE VINE THAT, WITHOUT FOLIAGE, IS NO MORE THAN A SPUR. BUT BENEATH THE SOIL LIE THE ROOTS THAT GIVE RISE TO YOUR NEW FRUITS. OTHERS MAY BE UNABLE TO IMAGINE THE SPLENDOR THAT IS ABOUT TO EMERGE IN YOU.

Cultivating Wild Roots and Shoots

Sweet are the uses of adversity, Which, like the toad, ugly and venomous Wears yet a precious jewel in his head; And this our life, exempt from public haunt, Finds tongues in trees, books in the running brooks, Sermons in stones, and good in everything.

— William Shakespeare as Duke Senior in *As You Like It*

The sap begins to flow. Things look different. With every spring comes a rebirth that you feel even in the depths of the inner city. With budburst, you recall seasons of rebirth in which the vitality of your body took over. You may have felt exhilarated or restless, lifted and brightened, or thrown into disarray. Now, as you emerge into your elderhood in this, the last season of your transition, you begin to contemplate a specific capstone and legacy that will survive you. Life on earth is in critical condition, and as you come to terms with its mortality, you will also be coming to terms with your own, and with your destiny, which is to restore the future of life for the sake of all patients born and unborn.

In the spring, you are like the pruned trunk of an old grape vine that, without foliage, is no more than a spur. But beneath the soil lie the roots that give rise to your new fruits. Others may be unable to imagine the splendor that is about to emerge in you. You may have doubts. You may be tempted to sit on the sidelines and say that you did your part. You may underestimate the value of the personal growth and development that awaits you in your last great metamorphosis: the exciting and perilous passage that will take all you've got, render you unfamiliar to yourself, and be productive of the last and best fruits of your life.

This is a time in life when you may turn to Shakespeare, who took Ovid's metamorphoses and made them modern. It is up to you and your peers to resurrect their forgotten wisdom so as to help doctors emerge from the modern era and to once again come into sync with life. This is an act of imaginative, creative vision that is lying dormant in your body, and which you are now free to restore so as to release its last fruits into the dying world where they can nourish a living future.

With this spring's rebirth, you can begin to make the most of every moment by adapting and changing as you navigate the currents of time. In this way, you become ready to meet whatever may come your way by reading and responding to the moment. As you decide whether you wish to create a capstone, and how to develop and pursue a vision of your legacy, you may—perhaps when you are least expecting it—find all of your experience in adaptation and change coming together with your budding faith in the future of life. I invite you to consider your rebirth in light of the forming constructs below. Take them as elements of an outline, a rough draft of human rebirth, or as a foreword to the chapters in your life that will meld your golden years with the first years of the next era.

As you do this, let spring revive the love and passion that blossom in your upper and lower heart centers. If you love new life—of grandchildren or of species wild or tame—linger on the first month of spring, which looks at fertility in a new light. If you love gardening or forestry, you may enjoy the second month, which explores habitat integration. If you wish to develop the fertility of your whole body, try the third month. If you love numbers and mathematical abstractions, linger on the extra month, which introduces the possibility of macrobiology. If you are not sure, keep your eyes and ears open for the inspirations of spring and rebirth. And in addition to thinking about what you want to do, think about what you want to have done.

REDEFINING FERTILITY

There are children to consider! Children born of your sexual energy shared with another are entities in the invisible world. They have form and speech. They are crying to you now. You have forgotten us. Come back!

— RUMI through Coleman Barks in *Rumi: The Book of Love*

CHANGES IN FERTILITY are integral to secular trends in birth control, sexual mores, and reinterpretations of the old scriptural admonition to go forth and multiply, the latter of which is become—when taken in the old way in the present context—a prescription for destruction of the universe of life. Following old narratives without thought renders them—and the teller—foolish, and invites a return to barbarity and bestiality. New narratives in which fertile creativity is expressed for the good of life as a whole are now essential, and no one can tell such narratives better than wise elders with extensive experience of truth and error—and the time to process all that and put it to good use.

Moderns generally frame issues of fertility in terms of exponential increase, carrying capacity of the planet, and other concepts that have modest efficacy. Young leaders of emergence are imagining and testing out alternative ways of expressing fertility, like couples who choose organic farming over childbearing with the intention of feeding a community. In this first budding of medical emergence, I propose that two problems solve each other: the old and unsustainable view of human fertility on one hand and the dire need for humans to adopt, restore, and integrate into habitats on the other. What better and more just solution than for humans who have imperiled life on earth by their disregard for it to choose to tenderly rescue it along with the species, and so create a living future for evolved life?

Medical elders who desire to live in nature in retirement can catalyze that rescue by creating action groups that found residential habitat restoration clinics and communities that both train the young in caring for patients with their habitats and support them to create and disseminate education programs. These intergenerational communities could, for example, divert resources from institutions to habitats while collaborating with habitat restorers and advocates of active aging. Many building blocks and resources exist that wise elders could

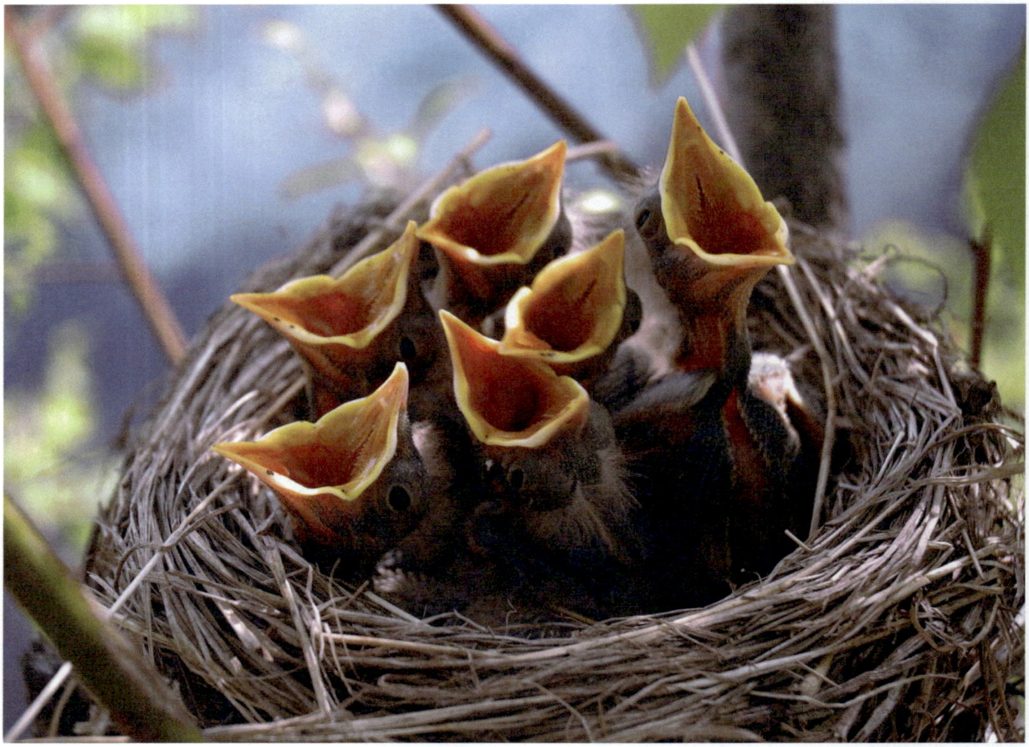

bring together creatively and experimentally, and so take America's history of intentional community—from the pilgrims to the Ebenezer colony to the Mormons to the organic farming movement—into a living, scientifically- and spiritually-informed future. The do-it-yourself movement has prepared the public for this.

In my Fertility and Restoration series, a first saga of speculative biofiction, I feature characters who fertilize the future via continuation of the species, solving of medical ailments, birthing brain and spirit children, and devising ways of life that sync humans with the body of life and thereby restore evolution. This kind of creativity draws on the historic creation of Christian communities after the fall of Rome in what is now France; it draws on the New Monasticism movement; and it envisions a way of enjoying intentional decrease. If you like, delve more deeply into new constructs of fertility and catalyze discussion of them by posting long and instructive case studies in the Doctors of Life International discussion group of the Evolve Medicine website, or by submitting biofiction to the Future Medicine website, and so lead the formation of a critical mass of transformational reading material for your peers and juniors.

ANECDOTES FROM MEDICAL LIVES

If people are on the brink of a dangerous precipice, shall they not be told of their danger? –shall they be permitted to pursue their course of destruction, for fear of exciting their alarm? Is not a knowledge of their condition their only safety?

— Dr. Lemuel Shattuck in *The Report of the Sanitary Commission of Massachusetts* 1850

As you transition to elderhood, you revive your fertility and contextualize it in the timeline of your medical and personal life as well as in your body and the bodies in which you nest. This frees you to reflect on your life and to discern what you—and only you—can do to cap the fertile lifework that is your own and to complete the process of turning the raw material of your life experience into a last and best legacy to life on earth. As you do this, you can become aware that your species is like a fetus that has grown so large as to compress the mother's lungs and consume her nourishment. If it does not slim down, it will kill her and so kill itself before it is fully formed. For you and your species to mature and emerge, you view your fertility biocentrically, as the fruits of a passion for creation that you—or your juniors—use to enhance life as a whole. In this way, your fertility is only just beginning.

Some of our peers have created legacies in time-honored ways such as creating aphorisms, writing up case series, or teaching and mentoring. These have changed again and again throughout history in response to need. Now, in the era of the pill and means of personal cure and congregal control of sexually transmitted diseases, fertility has become a matter of personal choice. This change has yet to play out. Most of us can remember a time when women had few choices: reclusion in a cloistral community; participation in procreation and family formation; dedication to a caring profession like teaching or nursing, perhaps substituting for an improvident or absent male; and use as a sexual toilet and repository of disavowed male fertility.

Amongst those women who went into medicine in the interval between the Flexner report and the rights movement that returned women to medicine in the 1970s were some who became teachers and leaders. We all saw them, those mentors who—for one reason or another—chose to enter the profession and to take responsibility for the perpetuation of its intangible essence by sustaining and advancing the field through teaching, research, administration, mentoring, or eldering. These women generally lived as solitary careerists and yet supported their juniors in claiming the human rights of kinship and community as well as those of earning professional credentials and practicing alongside male peers.

The women of our time could look to historical figures who expressed upward as well as downward fertility—that is, who gave birth to brain children as well as to physical offspring. Some of these possessed high status by birth and were wealthy in their own right, as with Lord Byron's daughter Ada Lovelace, who invented the computer, or Voltaire's consort Émilie du Châtelet, whose work catalyzed that of Lagrange and Laplace. Some women of history were visionaries whose lives have been rediscovered by the biographers of today, such as Hildegard of Bingen, Anne Hutchinson, and Elizabeth Peabody. These women were able to contribute significantly to the work of their time and to avoid or delay the hazards of fertility, which ranged from death in pregnancy or childbirth to lasting genitourinary difficulties to early death from a wide range of disregarded or poorly-comprehended consequences of childbearing. Rather than take all, they gave all, and we who follow are ripe to glean their and our life lessons and to use what we learn to inform emergence.

Emma

Emma was strong, tall, kind, confident, and charismatic. She stood out in medical school as the kind of woman that her elders saw as being worth their while. There would have been many more had her entering class admitted on merit. It didn't; the admissions committee limited the proportion of females to one third for fear that they would snap up desirable husbands immediately and drop out as soon as they conceived children. That view reveals much about gender stereotypes and male medical egos of that time—which is still your time.

The most tenacious of the proverbial old habits that die hard are those that form the basic structures of family, such as gender roles, sexual mores, and family size. Even so, those changed rapidly in the wake of late modern developments such as birth control and control of sexually-transmitted diseases. The human rights movements of the past century increased the rapidity of change by incentivizing the admission of women and minorities to professional schools; those changes began to enter the workplace, and the faculties of professional schools watched them closely. Emma eased their fears, especially when she kept her feelings to herself and voiced her preference for one of the traditional roles open to women: that of dedicated careerist who would not marry or bear children and would thus remain free to give her all to her work.

Their ease evaporated, however, when she expressed her admiration for the new specialty of family medicine and for the possibility of entering that field and earning a leadership position that would enable her to help people by improving primary care. In the eyes of the faculty, she had failed to understand her duty to the school. They intended her for a high-status specialty that would position her to pursue an academic career, one featuring the kind of bench research that could lead to a Nobel Prize in medicine. She could see patients and do procedures and get rich if she pleased—as long as it did not limit her scramble to secure as much prestige as possible. They did not see their views as she did: as a failure of learning and vision and leadership. She pursued her intended path and formed, before the end of her adult career, an inspiring lifework and legacy.

Robert

Robert and his husband remained untroubled by the intense paternal feelings that overtook many of their peers when it was illegal or too late to act on them. He was happy to work intensively, and his husband was happy to enjoy creative work that enhanced their lives together. Unlike the closeted faculty of the prior generation, they did this openly and went out of their way to host gatherings and to enhance the social life of the clinic group of which Robert was a part.

They did, however, sense that something was missing. They had not given birth to a brain child. They had not sought answers to the big questions or formed a spiritual life that nourished their souls. Robert had worked in a helping profession, participated in the ongoing human rights movements of his youth, and secured a loving partner with whom to creatively explore, define, and share a desirable way of life; he had earned many advantages, and had the good fortune to enjoy them. Even so, he had not quenched the thirst for meaning and purpose that was driving him to go deeper.

He and his partner went to India for several months. There, they traveled, got to know the land and people, and began—as some spiritual seekers put it—to know its fragrance. They had traveled extensively before, and were soon able to get about easily, to begin to taste its exquisite spiritual fruits, and to experience in new ways the feminine and masculine aspects of being free of outside constraints; they began to gently enter into the transformational aspect of the culture. When their journey was over, they longed to remain. Robert ended his adult career and they moved to India to begin their third life chapter.

George

When George had reached a place in his career where he felt professionally secure and financially well set, and had secured a wife who looked forward to caring for him and raising his family as he advanced his career, he decided that it would be optimal to have children as soon as possible. They tried to conceive a child; they did not succeed. Two years went by. They consulted an infertility specialist, who offered a series of increasingly invasive and eventually toxic algorithms of care. As they became disappointed, and then ashamed, and then bleak, they decided to give up.

Their marriage held. They realized that they were still determined to pursue the plan they had in mind when they married. The problem—as they saw it—was that doctors were not devising good enough infertility interventions. The rising rates of infertility were getting ahead of them. He was an internist, and accepted rather than questioned the chronic illness. They did not think to find and remove a cause of infertility or to right an imbalance or to re-imagine their lives. They tried every medical intervention they could access. The only option they could see now was to adopt.

Several years later, they had created the lives that they had planned for themselves. Their children looked more or less like them. They were taken for what they had intended to become: a biological family. They had considered no other options. And yet they were pioneering something unfamiliar to most: an aggregated family of choice, bound by intention, desire, and love and supported by a caring and cohesive and—to some degree—self-sufficient community.

BETH LOOKS BACK: Nurturing the Fertility of the Whole

"The departure of so many people has seriously weakened rural communities and economies all over the country. And that our farmland no longer has enough caretakers is implied by the fact that, as the farming people have departed from the land, the land itself has departed. Our soil erosion rates are now higher than they were in the time of the dust bowl."

—Wendell Berry in *What are People For?*

In the late 1980s, our family moved to Bainbridge, one of the southernmost islands in the Salish Sea. It was exurban and still supported farms and forests, a situation we hoped would last due to the three-hour daily commute to Seattle. Unfortunately, the population—and the forest-annihilating development that

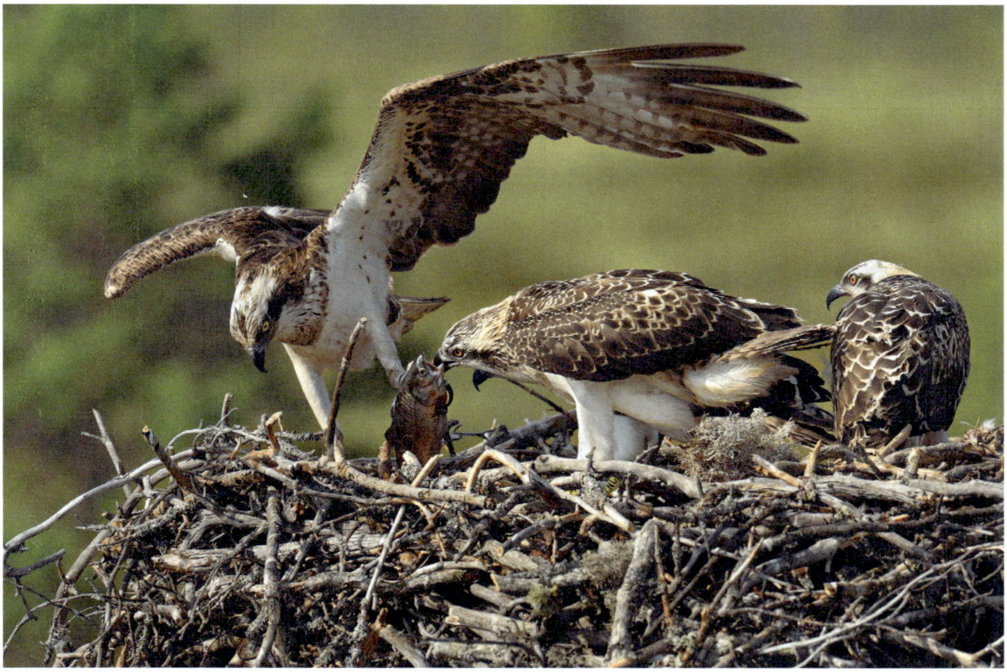

went with the bloated single-family home—seemed to mushroom. Traffic increased. Grumbling rumbled. The paper published complaints. There were incidents of vandalism against new homes built in the wake of clear-cutting carried out in defiance of restrictions.

While we were all still in a snit over the dead trees, the paper published an article pointing out that the population of the island was exactly as would have been projected on the basis of expected increase. Many children born on the island moved away to the city, culling the population and slowing the erasure of priceless—but cash-poor—farms and forests. Those who moved to the island to bring children into the world of a suburban paradise had the chance to think again.

According to family lore, I am descended from Jonathan Edwards, the sometimes-unpopular minister who catalyzed America's First Great Awakening. This was the fruit of the Puritan tradition that gave rise eventually to Transcendentalism and then to new forms of spirituality and religion unique to North America. Edwards and his congregation transformed the early Puritan practice of journaling for spiritual discernment into introspection for personal responsibility and right living. This transformed the self-fulfilling belief in original sin into other ideas such as healthy-mindedness that evolved into more recent ideas such as original blessing.

These and other popular movements inspired ephemeral or enduring communities such as Shakers, Quakers, Amish, or Orthodoxies that transformed society in countless positive ways: rule by representation rather than by tyranny, use of price tags to enable ethical commerce, abolition of the slave trade, protection of women and children, support for human rights, and international understanding and cooperation with successful rule by love and law rather than incipient chaos suppressed by force and punctuated by war. These rapid changes have been accompanied by education of women and reduction in family sizes. Many of these have unfolded within our lifetimes.

To succeed in reframing human fertility richly, satisfyingly, and quickly so as to bring it into accord with the fertility of the body of life requires us to 'catch up' to biological reality, and to wisely mentor and elder the transformation that is already underway. This entails adoption of new ways of aging that engage elders in 'pulling their weight' by doing the work of the wisdom years, instead of following social cues rooted in economic rationalism that block maturation and stymie self-guidance and independent thinking. Wisdom work includes the psychospiritual work of expressing human fertility in a practical way in the context of life in time. I therefore propose an emerging paradigm that gives birth to a legacy of residential habitat restoration clinics and communities that care for and cure the individual and aggregated bodies that bear us from dust to dust.

COMMENT: Human Fertility as Conception of a Third

There is nothing so practical as a good idea.

—Dr. Pekka Puska during the Anthropocene

The human transition that is imminent is different from all others: this one comes at a time when we are not only well able to destroy the body of life but are doing so. This means that the stakes are different—many times higher—than those we faced in the past. We have no choice but to learn from the past and to act wisely and expeditiously. We must each determine how to fill our world with life rather than with the fantasies of robots and virtual technologies that comedian Rick Mercer calls 'digital crack.' To do this, we must give up the errors of the past, one of which is controlling our fertility rather than taking responsibility for it. If we are responsible, we do not take for granted our ability to save many maternal and infant lives at the last minute; we recognize that life is in control and that it is up to us to accord our fertility with its ways so as to enrich each and every life as all.

Though we are old and infertile according to medical definitions, we have never been as fertile as we are now, nor as able—thanks to the wisdom born of experience—to be the 'change we wish to see in the world.' Because we are the keepers of the profession that is most enduringly and effectively responsible for life, we have the opportunity to do more than others can. We have the chance to lead personal and social adaptation and transformation. We have the chance to leave this life blessed by what others have prepared us to attempt, and by what we dare to accomplish.

For the purposes of this first version of an emerging paradigm, I frame fertility as the creation of a third. Some practitioners of Eastern religions—which include the three major Abrahamic traditions—recognize that there is always a spirit result of sexual union, whether physical or transcendental. We in late modern society are not accustomed to paying attention to this, and therefore ignore what we here call the third, that is, the intangible and ineffable entity or entities that come into being between two people who are able to serve as consorts—physical or spiritual—to one another or to a group such as a congregation that creates and shares a more fruitful state of being which could be harnessed to enhance and increase life on earth.

Those who do join being and doing for the good of life can access 'original blessing,' a theological alternative to original sin, and thereby catalyze what is rapidly becoming the third Great Awakening—which is this time ready to join spirit with actions such as caring for and curing the body of life. Doctors who are religious seek out and collaborate with theologians who have already chosen to support the evolving syntheses of constructs relating to the big picture of life such as Care of Creation and Earth Ministries.

The good news is that doctors have persevered through times of transition to new fruition, as you know from the work of thinkers and leaders like Hippocrates and Maimonides. It will, in the long run, be a great relief when we come to realize that most of the ephemeral and dubious technical data that crams our late modern brains is trivial or erroneous, not worthy of our time or attention. You may find it a pleasure to set aside the uniformity and conformity that preclude problem-solving, and to think and attend to and revive the living heart of the profession, which is key to creating a living future.

THE VARIETIES OF CONCEPTUAL EXPERIENCE

For Elizabeth, the movement from crisis to resolution, chaos to revelation, was a way of life—was life itself...If Sophia and Mary wished her to be married, perhaps they were hoping for the wrong kind of consummation [or] were wrong in hoping for any sort of consummation, when Elizabeth so reveled in the search itself.

— MEGAN MARSHALL in *The Peabody Sisters*

In times of renascence, old frames and constructs fail under the weight of their accumulated errors, and humans create fresh syntheses that make new sense of eternal complexities and support new ways of life that promote survival and thriving. In this season of rebirth, you have the chance to encounter naked reality and to grapple with the possibility of devising new callings that are analogous to the new methods that moderns developed as late modern science. This science is no longer sufficient to support life and must therefore change or give way to new methods that enable our species to conceive of—and to rapidly develop—new chains of being and doing that use past lessons as fuel for creating new ways of succeeding.

EXERCISE 1: The Consequences of Limiting Conception to Procreation

Margaret herself provided the best model of all. When she felt her students weren't striving for original thought in their journals, she started one herself and read passages aloud...In the end, all her students learned that 'we must think as well as study, and talk as well as recite.'

— MEGAN MARSHALL in *Margaret Fuller: A New American Life*

In your journal, draw three Venn diagrams to represent the universe of life on earth. Use the first to depict the universe of life at the present time as a finite set of mutually exclusive and exhaustive habitats, including artificial ones. Within habitats where humans abide, draw circles that represent the proportion of the habitat comprised by humans by numbers or by weight. Shade in those habitats that produce the most oxygen and are therefore essential to the future of life—including the sum total of humanity. Now, use the second diagram to depict the universe of life as it will be in the year 2100 should human fertility rates remain unchanged. Use the third to depict the universe of life as it would be in the year 2100 should the fertility rate fall at a rate chosen by the species.

EXERCISE 2: The Creation of Solutions as New—or Renewed—Vocations

[I started out as an animator.] When I got into farming, it challenged me in all kinds of different ways. I felt like I was becoming human, like I was learning to use my head, and my heart, and my hands all at the same time. It was making me into a whole person, and I didn't realize that I was so fragmented before I started farming.

— Nathan Carey in Steven Suderman's film *To Make a Farm*

For the purposes of this book, we use the words vocation and calling to emphasize the motivation rather than the methods that pertain to a line of work. For the species to survive and thrive, and with it the entangled lives which together comprise the body of life, doctors must become what they have never yet contemplated: a group of individuals dedicated to caring for and curing each and every life as one, beginning with the individual humans already in our care and extending to include the body of life and other meta-patients that are in danger of flatlining as a result of our neglect.

Doctors can then collaborate with a variety of colleagues who pursue lines of work that have yet to be developed. Two of these may be habitat integration and medical communications. The former would develop sequences of being and doing that enable late moderns to transition to ways of life in which they integrate into and enhance rather than detract from their habitats; it is a calling that will undoubtedly involve habitat restoration. The latter would shift the responsibilities for technology and information flow to an expert who is able to support experiential learning in real time and to limit the amount of extraneous data and disinformation that would otherwise mislead and overburden a care team dedicated to providing and evolving hands-on care and cure.

Imagine that you are part of a residential community with a clinic, and that this community runs on a variety of currencies—e.g. time, love, tools, expertise, and so on—that enable it to care for and cure life as guided by its vision, ethics, and values. As a member of the council of elders, you volunteer to write a job description for a habitat integrator or a communicator. In your journal, create this job description and detail suitable qualifications.

EXERCISE 3

Plant a new garden or tree in a place of your choosing. Record your process in your journal as one of fertility—of going forth and multiplying life.

Word Associations, Thoughts, and Lists

Unseen buds, infinite, hidden well,
Under the snow and ice, under the darkness, in every square or cubic inch,
Germinal, exquisite, in delicate lace, microscopic, unborn,
Like babes in wombs, latent, folded, compact, sleeping...
Waiting ever more, forever more behind.

— Walt Whitman in *Leaves of Grass* through Gay Wilson Allen

Preparation

Transfer the following table to your journal and fill it in. For each of the words in the table, write the first word or phrase that comes to mind in the association column. Now take as much time as you like to return to each word, to think of how you would like your mentees and juniors to respond to it, and to make a note of these things in the suggestion column. Are there are important differences between the association and suggestion columns? If so, do you detect a pattern in what you take for granted and what you envision for the future?

Word	Association	Suggestion
Asexuality		
Celibacy		
Self-pleasuring		
Monasticism		
Consort Practice		
Monogamy		
Serial Monogamy		
Polyamory		
Fecundity		
Birth Control		
Desire		
Sterilization		
Meno- or Andro-pause		
Fertility		

In your journal, write a few sentences or a paragraph about the most important epiphany you have had about fertility in the course of your medical life to date.

Take time to recall people with whom you have shared an exchange of ideas, that is, people with whom you 'brainstormed,' puzzled through projects, or sustained an ongoing passionate and productive interaction whether erotic or platonic. List them in your journal as they occur to you. When you have finished, add a column and record each of the 'thirds' that you created together. Include tangible and intangible products of conception—as broadly defined in these pages.

Ignoring feasibility and plausibility, think of an exchange you would like to enjoy with one or more of the people listed above—or someone else—and describe it in your journal, along with the third or thirds you would hope to create.

Writing Prompts

Use the following questions to write fertility questions in your journal that you keep in mind and write responses to for some portion of this month.

- How do my assumptions and expectations regarding human fertility impact my daily life? My plans for my future? My thoughts about the future of life?
- What can I do to cultivate a fruitful exchange with the people in my life? What can I do to ease our shared fears and strengthen our shared hopes for renewal?
- What issues related to fertility and the future of life would I like to discuss with others? What impact would I like to have on the larger dialogues amongst my peers and juniors?
- Is this fertility?
- Is this a chance to create a living legacy?

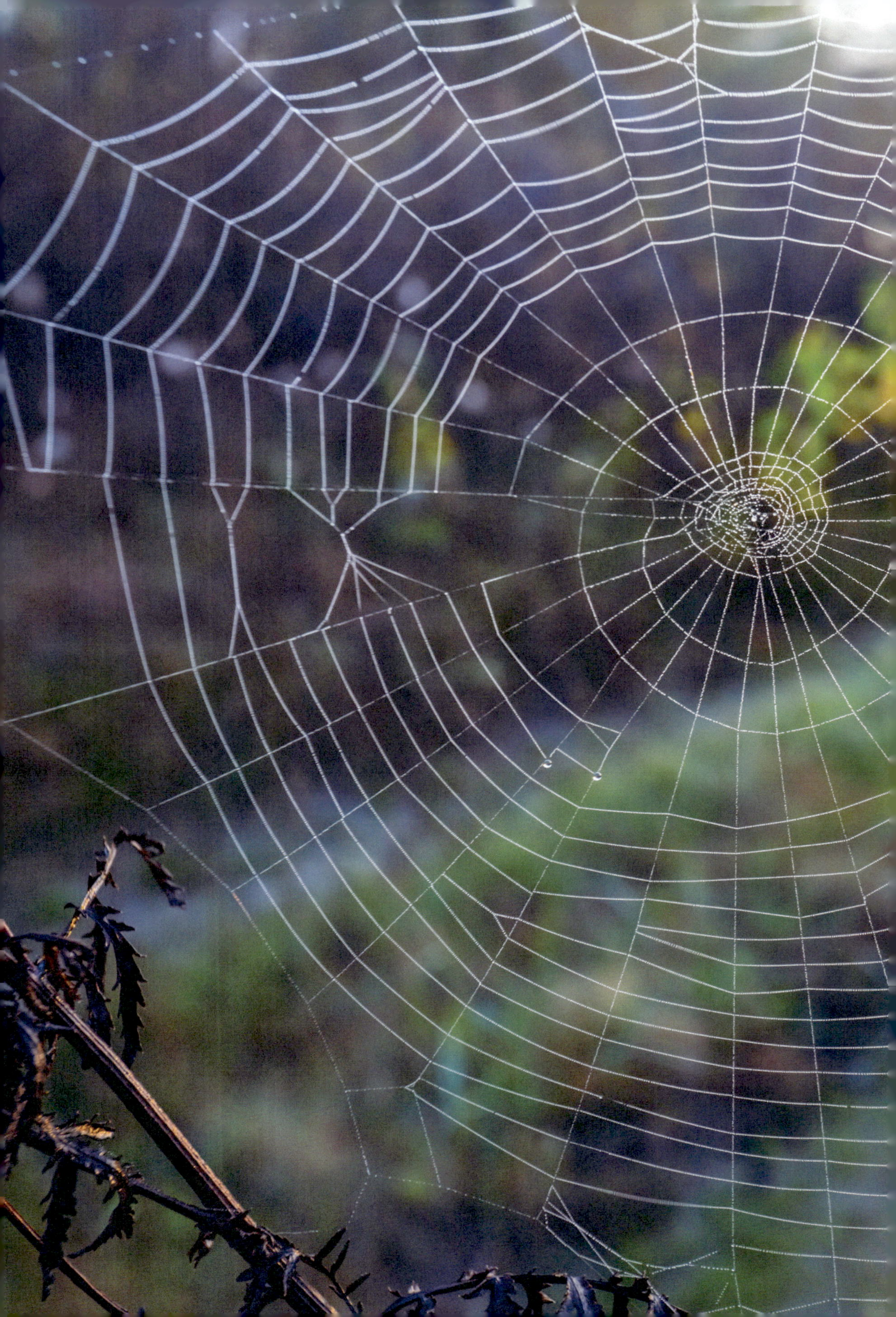

Habitat Integration

During the first half of the [nineteenth] century medical experts clashed over whether treating symptoms, rather than investigating the cause of disease, was paramount in ensuring the best patient care.

— Tara Womersley and Dorothy Crawford in *Bodysnatchers to Lifesavers*

With the rise of heroic medicine, our doctor forebears put fatalism to rest—or rather, they aimed to do so, and appeared—in company with society—to succeed. The results have been mixed, however, perhaps because the follow-through has met with real world snags that preclude intentional change from being rational or effective. At present, doctors may intervene bluntly or aggressively and realize diminishing returns, or they may remain blind to causes and consequences and lapse into complacency. We are—along with the rest of late modern societies—faddish; we are like the crowd on the deck of a boat running from one side to the other, careless of tipping it or losing sight of the destination.

The trick now, as the juggernaut of late modernity grinds along its decline and as post-industrial social machinery decays along with the great metal hulks that brood over the earth in the world's rust belts, is to replace the old fatalism with visionary realism—and not with the fractious messages of media that reiterate problems and blame and fail to deliver solutions. This is—without a doubt—easier said than done, but our profession and our species have done it many times before—and as doctors have of late rushed to the rescue at the last minute, this is our time to do the same for the body of life for the sake of a living future.

Oddly enough, the save of life on earth begins with theory. We cannot act sensibly without useful views, frames, and constructs. One of these is macrobiology; another is the n-way cure that comes of restoring habitat. When we come to grips with biology as it is now, and also with the impact that our species is having at present, we can recognize that to restore the universe of life on earth is to restore each and every congregal and individual body that lies within it and relies on it for life. To continue to treat the symptoms of the impending death of life is, clearly, ridiculous. It is time to reverse the cause: the falsely efficient, large-scale, consumptive-destructive human mores of late modernity.

It is time to cure endemic human ailments through the body of life. This is our greatest challenge; to meet it, we must learn to care for our bodies and then to care for all bodies as one.

ANECDOTES FROM THE GRASSROOTS

Mark taught us two important lessons: A grass-roots effort could make a difference, and degraded habitat could, with effort be restored...We began to make regular donations to smaller groups working to save or restore habitat, rather than give the money to large NGOs with big staffs, overheads, and corporate connections.

— Yvon Chouinard in *Let My People Go Surfing*

In this section, I usually tell stories from medical lives, but no doctor I either know or know of has participated actively in habitat restoration—at least not to my knowledge. Many pursue or cheer on extreme sports, go to the mountains to get their glad tidings, or give money to various environmental organizations that promise to right one or another wrong. But amongst doctors I know who love the outdoors, the barrier between medical and ecological thinking seems to be holding fast.

Earthcorps

While walking through a park near my home, I ran into a group of young and vigorous people who were talking sustainability and digging up invasive blackberry plants. They were wearing branded T-shirts advertising the Earthcorps. Some time later, while looking into habitat restoration efforts in my area, I found their website. Over the next few years, I tracked the group's growth and development and the maturation of its activities. Like members of the Society for Ecological Restoration, members of Earthcorps were working through definitions of terms like sustainability and experimenting with the optimal allocation of resources for habitat restoration. The general cultural dialogue favored removal of Mongolian thistle, which could rapidly sterilize large sectors of the soil in eastern Washington, but there was less agreement regarding remediation of toxics and use of public monies or unpaid volunteers to remove ectopic plants such as holly trees and blackberries from public lands.

Earthcorps decided to remove all invasive species from the habitat that they were restoring in my neighborhood park—Magnuson Park in Seattle. The federal government had recently given this land to the city, which had split it into areas for indoor activities, outdoor playing fields, and natural habitat. I decided to volunteer to help restore the natural habitat, and I looked into the available volunteer opportunities. Being older and not particularly healthy, I thought that I would be best suited to species assessment. This involved counting invasive species in designated sampling areas, a method I had learned to use in a marine biology course in college.

When I read the details, I discovered that the volunteer didn't do a little careful weeding: he or she would identify a possible weed and an 'expert' would come and decide whether and when to pull it. My nonsense detectors went off. I felt nostalgic for the days when children were cash-poor and would retrieve weeds—with roots—in exchange for cash. If they made mistakes, they didn't get to do it again. A group of streetwise—parkwise, in this case—kids could have finished the park in a week. But the goal didn't seem to be to remove the unwanted plants, it was to perpetuate the kinds of processes that tend to proliferate around research institutions. I didn't participate for fear of wasting my time and enabling their lack of common sense. The group proved me wrong. The restoration advanced rapidly and successfully in harmony with its community, and I am grateful to those whose patient trust saw it through.

KS Wild

While in Ashland on a writing retreat that included inspiration by the Oregon Shakespeare Festival and support from a strong cooperative that supplies safe local food, I looked into local groups that were restoring habitats. I found a few non-profit groups that were raising awareness of one or another species or habitat or that provided educational opportunities for local children. One was raising funds for a good-faith effort in what some call care of creation, but this yielded only enough funding to hire a staff to raise more funds to do the actual work of habitat protection and restoration. As is often the case with such groups, they ended up having little time to do—or to organize—effective action in the outdoors.

When I returned the following fall, I was thrilled to discover—amid the smoke of local forest fires—a group called the Klamath-Siskiyou Wildlands Center (KS Wild). This group was gathering a large volunteer corps rich in elders who had moved to the area to enjoy their post-employment years. The group was also partnering with the Forest Service as it worked to reverse the worst consequences of late modern policies that turned forests into tree farms—à la Gifford Pinchot—and delayed fires until they became catastrophic; introduced habitat-eroding roads; and impoverished vast reservoirs of biodiversity. The group was also supporting what we herein call eden lands—that is, those self-sustaining living habitats that support communities of interrelated species, including habitat-integrated humans, that coevolved over millennia. By the time of my next visit, another habitat-restoration group, Lomakatsi, was working intensively to protect habitats for fees, with grants available to those in need. I hope someday to be one of many doctors who join in groups that take direct action to 'protect the best and restore the rest.'

Scallops

The Seattle area is rich in individuals, groups, and organizations working actively to transition from the late modern economy to a local, living one. A few include: the Living Futures Institute; Yes! Magazine; Earth Ministries; Green Drinks; Business Alliance for Local Living Economies; Bainbridge Graduate Institute; Compassionate Seattle; the Bullitt Foundation; and a variety of Coastal Salish communities. Alongside these stand the grassrootsiest of all: Sustainable Communities All Over Puget Sound, or SCALLOPS. This loose organization of volunteers includes neighborhood groups that are implementing aspects of the Transition Towns movement sponsored by Prince Charles and rooted in the permaculture movement. These draw together neighbors from across social spectra—from well-coiffed master gardeners to wild-haired goat-milkers.

These groups are whatever the current neighborhood activists make them. Members thus participate in a variety of community efforts such as serving the homeless, sustaining local habitat-integrated businesses, and restoring and enriching artificial and natural habitats. As with Oriental medicine, in which the patient is viewed as new at each visit, the group of activists is new—and reconstitutes—at each meeting, and so waxes and wanes in effectiveness with the mood of locals who step up to lead. If there are any doctors among these, I have not heard of them.

The localist movement is spreading fast in the Cascadia bioregion, and includes all kinds of social containers that support motivated individuals to cooperate with their neighbors or to catalyze an incipient group of volunteers. These organizations tend by nature to be amorphous, unpredictable, uncontrollable, and best-suited to easy-going people lovers whose primary aim is to create community. For doctors accustomed to highly-controlled, highly productive group activities, this kind of near-spontaneous congregal action can seem like a child's playdate: a chance to make nice and have fun without accomplishing anything in particular.

It would therefore be easier to gather doctors who are passionate about habitat restoration and wish to transition to the post-employment years with colleagues. As your lifework and legacy become less kinetic and frenetic and you contemplate how best to mentor and elder your juniors, you can negotiate a steep learning curve and share ideas more easily in company. You can discover how to transform the productivity of your career—which may have been high with respect to tangible deliverables and low with respect to the ineffable—into a suitable ethic for the post-employment years. As you transition, you can learn to nurture creativity and undertake adaptive transformation through which to deliver wisdom and lasting leadership.

BETH LOOKS BACK

We are not expecting utopia here on this earth. But God meant things to be much easier than we have made them... Love is indeed a harsh and dreadful thing to ask of us, of each of us, but it is the only answer.

— Dorothy Day via *Christian Mystics* by Matthew Fox

When I first wandered around town trying to go green in the city—and so support my care and cure—I was like Kermit, or maybe Goldilocks and the three little pigs, or a poverty-stricken medieval youth who ran the gantlet in hopes of winning a prize. I went around with childlike naïve trust, heart in hand, looking for someone who might want to receive my peculiar set of abilities and disabilities. Like Aesop—or like most children who read fairy tales—I soon learned many more lessons that I had bargained for. After over a decade of going from group to group and tribe to tribe, remaining the universal outsider who fit in everywhere and nowhere, I realized that I had a tribe, and that the only way to make a difference would be to return to it and appeal to it.

This realization had appalling consequences for me. I had to sympathize with and yet not lie down and be a doormat for close friends who felt an intense urge to punish me for failing to conform to their chosen errors of omission. Perhaps they thought I'd wanted to spend decades of my life in constant pain just to annoy them, or that if they run into some knowledge that isn't in the computer they should whack it with a mental fly-swatter. Many doctors—some primary care specialists excepted—are ugly or ridiculous from outside the system; no one in their right mind would want to work with them. So maybe I am crazy, or a holy fool who is willing to defy norms for your sake.

Anyway, to get a bit more specific: I learned that doctors are essential to the future of life on earth. No one knows our species as doctors do. Our age-old wisdom is real and inescapable, like that of agronomists who retreat behind machines and chemicals but must still face rain or drought and soil depletion or repletion. I learned this by shopping my problems and solutions around, and by seeing for myself that people want their doctors to tell them what to do—and there are good reasons for their desire. Some practitioners in the gray market expect patients to heal themselves in spite of neurotoxins, or to cleanse their bodies of toxins as if they were unstructured bags of chemicals. Like doctors who have no better idea what to do, some of them put on white coats, talk biobabble, and pretend to know—and believe they know—things that are impossible to know or that defy comprehension.

I met many people—some highly sophisticated—who believed that they could study biology as a kind of primitive data processor, or that there had been no toxins until humans produced them. I met doctors who were enmeshed in fatalism and expected to go the way of the species—that is, to accept extinction rather than expect systemic change. None of this is necessary; all of it is unholy foolery. For doctors to abandon our species to the task of ensuring its safety without aid would be demonic; you would not want to live—and die—without noting and amending your part in this error. Nor should you accept self-extinction—or sleep well at night—before figuring out how you can lead your colleagues and patients in restoring and strengthening all bodies as one.

COMMENT

It is said that science demystifies nature, but scientists on the frontier are awed by the elegance and harmony of nature.

— Daniel Matt in *God & the Big Bang*

We late moderns behave as if we can cure our species—and all species—one gene or one toxin at a time. We study ailments in terms of single pathogens, genes, and modifying factors. We allow the limits of reductionism to reduce us to simpletons. We do not have time to pay a lifetime of attention to one pathogen or toxin, one gene, and one modifying factor at a time, or to feed chunks of data from millennia past into mysterious mathematical boxes that seem to magically confirm arbitrary stabs at discovering simplicity in complexity. We humans must live sustainably now—all of us, not excepting those ineffective practitioners who purport to care for individual lives while enabling the destruction of all. We doctors followed our once-heroic efforts down a blind alley in which we try to mend the world one host, one agent of illness, and one environmental factor at a time. We can do better. For practical suggestions, see Jeff Barrie's "Kilowatt Ours" program, sponsored by the Sierra Club, and the project "No Impact Man."

The evolved biosphere is here to aid you. Unimpeded by misguided human acts, it can mend much; our species—re-focused on broader views of care and cure—can do the rest. Doctors, for instance, can begin by evaluating human health in situ, caring for and curing chronic exposure and slowing the contribution of mainstream medicine to humanity's consumptive destruction of the body of life—such as "competing" by proliferating MRIs and hospitals. To live wisely with life requires deep, systemic change that will solve multiple problems at once—what some call solving for pattern.

The textbook for this kind of comprehensive intentional change is the history of habitat-integrated peoples such as the Coastal Salish and Algonquin peoples, the originators of Brooke Farm, and communities of religious dissenters such as Moravians, Mormons, and the Ebenezer colony that continues today as the Amanas. These communities proved possible the vision of forming self-sufficient communities that serve as reservoirs of innovation. These may now take the form of retirement communities whose members have various areas of competency such as medicine—with retirement here defined as living apart with the purpose of evolving better systems. These could emulate the Bullitt Center in Seattle—which had the regulatory autonomy to develop better utility systems such as those for water, waste, and power, and has met the criteria for the Living Building Challenge.

Experimental communities with the autonomy to do better will be most likely to succeed if well-grounded and inclusive of polymaths and members with wide-ranging skills, those who can afford to pay their way—and so to transfer resources to the new economy—and who are passionate about using existing modes of self-governance with minimal shared dogma to join in the practical pursuit of habitat integration and restoration. Such communities can develop syncretic systemic solutions to existing problems that do not foul or weaken the living bodies in which humanity nests. Communities that succeed in devising satisfactory—or better—sustainable lifeways can then form a network for communication, collaboration, inspiration, and education that could synergize the survival and thriving of all in ways that suit individual habitats.

Human society has always has been and will always be an experiment that requires the grounding of each and every human body. With careful attention to actions and consequences, errors can be recognized, defined, and retired as they arise—or very soon after. Letting go of fixed views will allow you to act strategically and efficiently. The latter cannot be done when the species is too systematized and centralized to be receptive to feedback, or to be able to respond to life in real time. New tools could aid and abet this overt plot to survive and thrive. Some to consider include: alternative currencies, organic farming practices, soil restoration and production, living buildings, green burial, and ride and residence sharing.

An experimental clinic that is free to do better could engage those with environmental illnesses in returning to and restoring the habitats on which they depend for personal recovery. This may extend to the unknown number of patients whose fundamental problem is nature deprivation, and who may become able—once living and working in restorative communities—to restore life as it restores them. The development of residential habitat restoration communities and clinics could thus catalyze the transformation of consumptive destruction to sets of practical solutions that others can adapt and develop to suit a variety of locations in life, place and time.

For you, this may begin with contemplating the virtues of aging. You have probably already lost any envy you may have felt towards the young; it takes only the smallest perspective to see how difficult it is to come of age in a time of complex artificial systems. In academic circles, experts who value the long and broad view may assume the role of professor emeritus. No one who has heard Segovia or Rubenstein play in later years can doubt that age offers the chance to distill and express the experience, practice and grace of a lifetime. In Japan, those who reach the pinnacle of an art or craft may be given the role of national treasure. Here and now, you have the chance to step up and define such a role for yourself in which you are able to actively contribute a lifework and legacy that will leave the living world a better—and more lasting—place.

Community Formation for Habitat Restoration and Integration

The more training an individual has the less he is affected by...the condition of prosperity or of adversity...A man acquires this disposition in his soul by considering the truth of things and by knowing the nature of existence.

— Maimonides in *On the Management of Health,* through Weiss and Butterworth

WORKING QUESTIONS

- Which experiences of my past have prepared me to envision a new design for living? Which elements of my knowledge base?
- How can I form the basis of the wisdom of my years so as to prepare the sequence of primed stances, states, strategies, and skills that would enable me to create or contribute successfully to a new experimental community?
- Which of the mistakes of my past—or the human past—would I regard as cautionary tales useful in avoiding the pitfalls of haphazard or dysfunctional community formation?
- What medical communities of the past—such as tuberculosis sanitaria for the mentally ill, or long-term care facilities for the demented—can I learn from now? What communities can I view as exemplary with respect to one or more features?
- How can I develop a new relation to time and risk that will enable me to make the best of my elder years and to create a lifework and legacy that will make the most of my life experience from cradle to grave—or from my most distant ancestor to the generations that extend into the foreseeable future?
- How can I take heart to create and share a sanguine attitude with others? What spiritual, religious or scientific sources of inspiration can I draw on? How can I inspire a community with well-grounded optimism? How can I create and share a possible future?

EXERCISE 1

There are creative manners, there are creative actions, and creative words; manners, actions, words, that is, indicative of no custom or authority, but springing spontaneous from the mind's own sense of good and fair.

— Ralph Waldo Emerson in The American Scholar speech at Cambridge, 1837

Choose and read up on two or more of the following planned communities: Plymouth or Dorchester Colonies; Rhode Island; Shaker communities; the Oneida colony; Hygiene, Colorado; the colony of Pennsylvania; Canberra, Australia; the Ebenezer Colony; Salt Lake City; Salem, Massachusetts; Brook Farm; Jamestown; Saccidinanda Ashram; New York City; Kalaupapa; Chicago; Shoshoni Yoga Retreat; the Amanas; or any indigenous, monastic, or restorative group that formed by design and that you have visited—or can visit now—in person. Extract from its formative years five rules of thumb useful in guiding the formation of a medical residential community designed to restore life as a whole.

EXERCISE 2

Take your journal to another habitat and record your impression of the flora and fauna, including the human species and its consumption, destruction, and poisoning as well as its alterations—including any support for wild species or re-wilding.

EXERCISE 3

Travel to the nearest or dearest area of habitat restoration that you can find out about through a local action-oriented group or through the Society for Ecological Restoration. Research what they did and how it's coming along. What would you do the same way? What would you do differently? Record everything that your detective work can teach you now that primes you for your legacy in some way.

Engaging All of Your Body

Let us accept the world is a mystery. Nature is neither solely material nor entirely spiritual. Man, too, is more than flesh and blood; otherwise, no religions would have been possible.

— Albert Einstein

All new forms of apprehension and comprehension begin with curiosity that is followed up with desire or necessity. You may have suppressed these qualities in you when the group dynamics and ways of thinking of your profession imposed uniformity designed to 'bring up the bottom'—e.g. assure minimum standards—by imposing conformity to selected practices. This unfortunately 'brings down the top' by squelching curiosity and perspicacity and creativity, dividing doctors from their own life experience and their ability to learn from it. This top-down management—and the imposition of complex systems that require obedience to questionable authorities—teach you to regard your embodied experience as irrelevant. The consequent virtuality supports systems that seem to function best when you keep your head down, keep your mouth shut, and disregard anything edited out of virtuality—such as the sixth extinction. This may have been enabled by instilling screen addiction that may respond to an Internet AA program like reSTART in Bellevue, Washington.

Your loss of independent thought will likely have made it difficult for you to take note of your body, to read and interpret it, and to use what it has to teach you to improve your self-care—or to enhance any kind of care or cure. The good news is that your body is still waiting for you to unlock and read its vast store of experience and to use your highest cortical functions—your knowledge and wisdom—to unlock its vast teaching potential. While you were using your evolutionary potential to adhere to a grab-bag of fixed expectations—many provisional or outdated—your body was automatically gathering all of the data and information that you will need to contribute substantively to the care of life on earth.

With the transition to elderhood, you are free to recover the attention that you were spending on algorithms designed to enforce selected metrics. You are free to rediscover, revive, and engage the fertile curiosity of your youth. As you do this, you can revel in childlike wonder, which will return to you when you explore the body that countless generations have come to know before you and to know it from the inside by virtue of the best possible tool—itself. When you glean your embodied life lessons, you will encounter phenomena that are new to you and that have been forgotten or ignored by moderns. These will support you in undertaking the slow and halting process of 'putting it all together' as you explore—perhaps for the first time—the body's capabilities for creating movement, music, and sequences of being and doing that you may formalize for personal and shared self-patterning.

ANECDOTES FROM MEDICAL LIVES

I tell him of the amazing plant drawings that I have seen by autistic savants—drawings based purely on perception without any botanical knowledge. Dick, however, insists that knowledge and understanding only sharpen his perceptions... and he can convey this... in a way... impossible without knowledge and intention.

— Oliver Sacks in *Oaxaca Journal*

What do you see and know of the immanent universe in which we are immersed? Far too little. To survive, you must see more, and fast. You must see through the eyes of pilgrims, voyageurs, and travelers. You must—for your descendants to survive—be as self-sacrificing and venturesome as Howard Ricketts and his ilk, who left the herd to explore the body of life with open eyes and minds and who deciphered the causes of epidemic infectious diseases. That work required the kind of courage that moderns recognize and admire as physical bravery in the face of hazard. The work ahead calls for a different kind of courage: that of the prisoner, monk, or mendicant who endures privation and emerges prepared to see the worst and best of life and yet also to love the whole of it, and so to be able to hope and dream and to do what seems impossible.

Late moderns have had a glimpse of aspects of the body that cannot be gauged against the corpse that has, in the modern era, served as your profession's gold standard. One of these is the microbiome, the inner habitat comprised of the non-pathogenic organisms on which you rely for life, such as those that live in the colon and synthesize vitamin B12. And yet, the relation of this inner habitat to the body of life has been ignored. Fortunately, biomedical scientists who study the infinitesimal are able to study some of the hordes of tiny protectors that coat each and every one of us inside and out, and to recognize—by using methods borrowed from soil chemists—that they may have some living

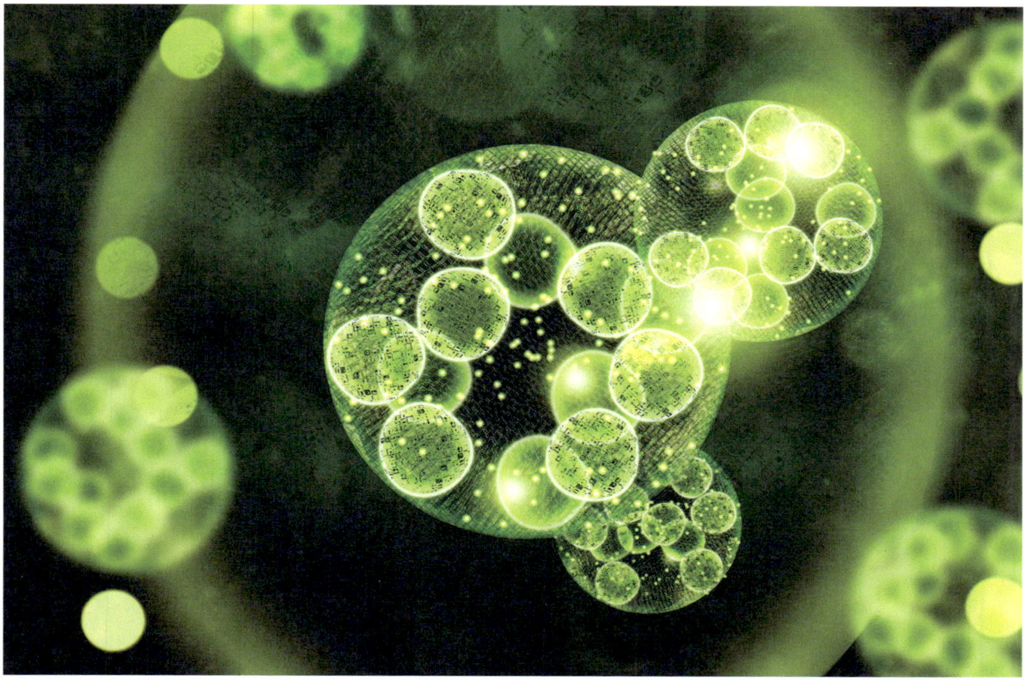

relation to the soil and its habitats and so—materially at the microbiological level—with the larger bodies in which we nest.

Late modern biomedical researchers have already recognized that humans rely on essential minerals that come from the crust of the earth, and on nutritive gases that are produced by the body of life and sustained as the earth's atmosphere. As we form the new basic science of macrobiology, we can take heart and explore our bodies and their relation to our living milieu from the inside out. Fortunately, our species long ago developed sophisticated arts that enable seekers to do this, and these have been engaged by those of your peers who are enlivening the fertile periphery of medicine with ancient forms of wisdom perpetuated through spiritual and religious vocations. One that more doctors are using now is body mindfulness.

Isaac

In college, Isaac majored in the arts. He relived the collective social disillusionment with romantics who had sought to be carried away by feeling, and who inadvertently fed the idolatry and demagoguery that enabled late moderns to take the human history of slavery, empire, and mass murder to new lows. He enjoyed the sardonic humor of surrealists whose strange new filters shattered the old stereotypes and freed humans to invent new perceptions.

Having attended a large urban university influenced by Freudian thinking, it was only natural that Isaac should choose to go into medicine and to pursue the specialty of psychiatry. Like Dr. Viktor Frankl before him, he went to the wards well-grounded and able to see through the layers of social pretense offered by patients and by those who treated them. Unlike Dr. Frankl, Isaac was more conditioned by media than by community. His dark sense of humor did not enliven, relieve, or connect him with patients. It prepared him to laugh at them.

When patients told him stories of travel in outer space and made strange helmets out of aluminum foil, the communication that he received was comedy, to which he responded with an irrepressible urge to laugh. Not unlike his young female peers who ran into the bathroom to cry, he ran into the next room to laugh. If the room's interface with the ward was a two-way mirror, he had the opportunity to observe 'thought disorders' and to enjoy hilarity without restraint.

If Isaac had known of Dr. Viktor Frankl, he might have been able to put his perceptions and his humor to good therapeutic purpose. He might have learned to calm his own fears—and those of his patients—or to create shared therapeutic narratives to replace idiosyncratic or destructive ones. In other words, he could have helped to write the stories of human restoration or redemption that sustain the consensus of the real *in situ* and allow patients to gain and regain an agreed-upon normality. Or he could—like some of his peers—have chosen to specialize in drugging such toxic states, thereby protecting society in the short run at the cost of failing to find the cause. As it was, he chose another specialty.

Hugo

While dropping in on a rock-and-roll Christmas party held in a nearby clinic for integrative medicine, I met a physician who belonged to a small group of family practitioners who were part of a large, radically inclusive, experimental, and rapidly evolving practice. The physician was tall, lively, and gregarious, a man with an expansive mind and manner. As his bright eyes and wide gestures filled the space in a side hall, he spoke effusively of the energies around him and of the new practitioner who was revealing them to him.

The new practitioner was a strikingly attractive, well-dressed therapist whose new brand of personal transformation was inspiring the clinic and its collaborative clientele. Her therapy involved a patented gismo that lent itself to single or continuing consultations, short-term residential healing retreats, and efficient certifications. While her philosophy was too thin and her abilities too specific to add to what I had already learned through the gray markets in religion and medicine, I was immediately drawn to her. The closer I got to her, the better I felt—and I was not feeling very well. I felt an impulse to corner her and keep her to myself. But I let her go and took away an important realization: her state of being and her ability to share it represented an ancient form of interpersonal care modernized as energy medicine.

As I opened my perceptions to her and the physician beside her, I sensed that his energy—like the energy of some transvestites—was subject to powerful, rapid upward fluctuations. To be near her was healing; to be near him was discombobulating. He was ungrounded. Absent the community held by the clinic, he could have become lost in inner space. He had yet to structure the new world of energy that she was revealing to him, and yet to incorporate into the whole of his body and his practice. He was like me, I supposed: opening his perceptions to the intangible and exploring, mapping, and discovering the limits of the energy body from the inside out.

Tara

While attending a spiritual conference outside Boulder in the front range of the Rocky Mountains, I paused near one of the three elderly men leading the conference. Each represented a different religious tradition. While regarding his being, I had the odd thought—not far from the topic of the conference but disembodied and out of context—that he and the other two in the aggregate were a kind of fountain of yan. They were powerfully and essentially masculine—and complementary to the feminine. In other words, they embodied what some might call the male principle or the divine male.

A woman paused beside me, regarding the teacher carefully. She said, "It's like a fountain of yan." This was too improbable. I had to believe that she—like others I had met in this alternative world—had abilities that I did not. When we got to talking, she said that she was a physician, and told me that early on in her career she had found to her shock and dismay that she had the ability to hear the thoughts of her patients. The ability supported her development of sensitivity and empathy, but it was one-sided. Her patients could not hear her thoughts, and she could not discuss this with her peers for fear of being committed to a mental institution.

This unwanted gift isolated her even as it exposed her to naked psyches

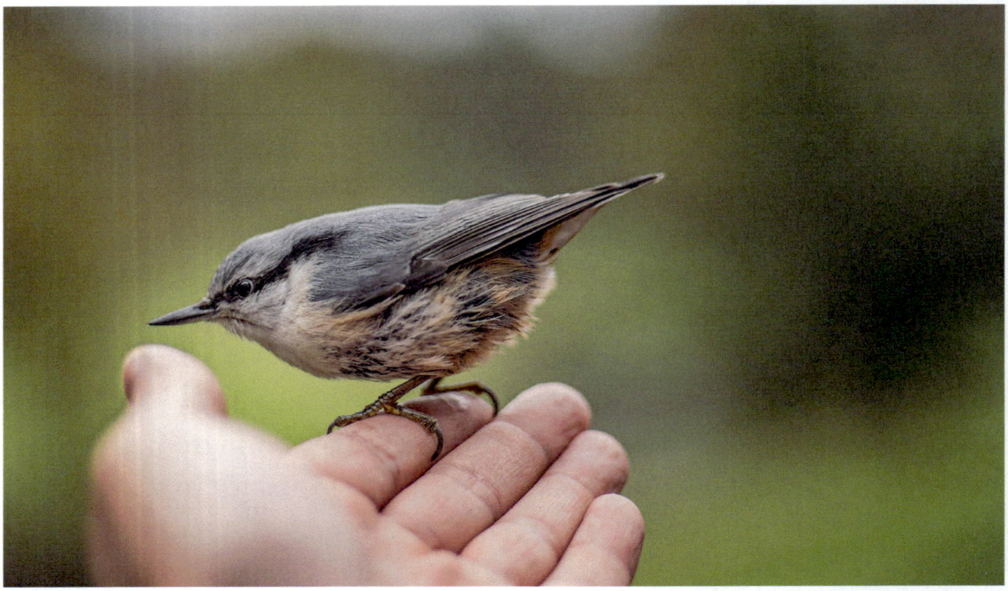

filled with pain and suffering. The inner darkness and complaints of others became a burden that isolated her further by interfering with her peace of mind, her enjoyment of friendship, and her obligation to meet the expectations of self and others. Her medical ego was gutted, along with the habits that had protected her from the inner struggles of others and that were beginning to work against her.

I felt a pang of guilt. I would have wanted to befriend her, but my own inner pain and suffering were like a nest of snakes; I had as yet to bear witness to my experience in a meaningful way as a medical detective and creative. To put this in Hippocratic terms, I had yet to turn its poison into medicine. Only individuals and groups with intense prayer or meditation practices could tolerate my presence with equanimity. I didn't want to expose anyone to the added burden of my inner struggles—however much I might be able to abstract them—or myself to someone I couldn't comprehend.

I was also reluctant to expose myself to a dose of a type of 'interbeing' that I might not be able to tolerate. I had little ability to use my five senses or sense awarenesses to mediate the give and take of ethereal interbeing—that is, the intangible phenomena of being that extend beyond the skin and interpenetrate those of others. For me, the phenomena of interbeing were mediated by the whole body. The challenge of managing my relation to it was, like Tara's, deepened by the lack of a partner like Frank Herbert, who was pleased with his wife's unusual abilities, and by the lack of a social container such as a religious community that could structure interbeing productively so as to fill it with faith in life and good works. In not exploring that aspect of the human experience, I could get on with my intellectual work and let those who could observe and intervene constructively to do so. Tara and I imbibed the blessings offered by our wise religious elders and went our separate ways.

BETH LOOKS BACK

Human beings have an enormous capacity for taking things for granted...If there is to be genuine human progress, happiness, goodness, and creativeness must be maintained by the individuals of successive generations throughout the whole span of lives that are by nature nonprogressive and in the teeth of circumstances that must often be unfavorable.

— Aldous Huxley in "Reflections on Progress" in *Huxley and God*

When I became disabled, I was actively and continually neurotoxic Luckly, I had had the unusual advantage of having worked with investigators who studied cognitive psychology and group behavior in physicians and who had encountered and pushed the limits of medical epistemology. And, having been exposed to conflicting forms of brainwashing from my earliest years, I escaped—if only just—those which came with medical training. I was prepared and able to engage my conscience in the role of detached observer. Unexpectedly, while neurotoxicity spoiled my states of being, it also impelled me to improve them and at the same time turn to direct experience and to 'go meta'—used here to mean going toward higher-level abstraction. After a time of confusion, I undertook an odyssey through the brave new world of social experimentation initiated by others who—for reasons of their own—were earning a living in the gray markets of religion and spirituality. Most experienced the body in ways that were pre-modern, and strange to those of us whose raw childhood experiences were formed by sports or by the performing arts, and who had learned to conceive of these experiences in terms of anatomical ideas derived from corpses.

What I discovered was well-encapsulated by the parable of the blind men and the elephant—that is, by an image of various sages, each of whom can access and conceive of only one aspect the living body. For students of medicine, this aspect was the corpse and selected functions measurable through modern means. For students of religious science, mind-only Buddhism, or black magic. The flesh was generated and controlled by consciousness; most who were not

MDs viewed the body in ways that drew on ancient Biblical teachings; the Daoist model of body, mind, and spirit; or the tantric model of the subtle body. These constructs were held together by teachings rooted in one or more ancient or innovative lifeways inclusive of what Quakers call faith and practice.

The upshot of my search was the recognition that ancient sages learned how to care for and sometimes cure the body from the inside out, and moderns learned to do the same from the outside in. The trick was to put them together, which was nearly impossible within the systems that embedded late modern medicine—even for psychiatrists. Physicians leading the integration of medicine were too bound to their social responsibilities to free themselves for this task, and those who did medical research were too bound to economic forces to think freely or creatively. The only way I could make fundamental progress would be to work alone and use a pen and paper in pursuit of syncretic, connective, renascence thinking. This is exactly the kind of work that wise elders have always done, and that work is essential now.

Fortunately, our species is not depending on medicine to devise new ways of life that will enable our species to survive and thrive. Emergence is well under way, and well able to support the evolving—and soon to be continuous—renascence of Hippocratic medicine. And, though medicine is as slow as religion to change at the fundamental level, wise elders set examples millennia and centuries ago; we have only to follow their lead. To read Maimonides now is to realize both how much we have gained and also how much we have lost. To bring forward the best of the recent and distant past is therefore the task before you; you can jumpstart this process by coming to know and love and care for your body from the inside out.

COMMENT

It is this Breath that fills us with the vitality needed to work forth—not toward our inevitable death, but toward that silent repose in the midst of action, where individual being is finally open to the Oneness of Lover and Beloved.

—Jean-Yves LeLoup in The Gospel of Mary Magdalene

When anatomy galvanized the Scottish Enlightenment, clergy refused to leave their comfort zones. Doctors comprehended the body as best they could on their own. Their comprehension turned concrete; that is, the modern forebears of the profession grabbed the cadaver and clung to it, admitting to their minds lessons elaborated by gross anatomy and then newer ones discovered by microscopes or in home laboratories. With social engineering and diffusion of responsibility in complex systems, doctors have been losing the art of the physical exam, the confidence to comprehend patients in situ, and the will to develop common sense. We put on white coats and retreated into glass and metal temples to read EEG's and EKG's and to pooh-pooh the bodily production of energies. But for the 'happy few' protecting public or occupational health, modern physicians ignored the dissemination of toxic waste; missed ground-breaking work in ecology, agriculture, and theology; and missed the deconstruction of modernity that helped to make way for the new.

For the purposes of this book, we let go of the cadaver, the microscope, and all the modern advances that have revealed so much about so little. We don't pooh-pooh them; they saved countless lives and we are grateful for them. We only set them aside so as to be able to move beyond them and to decide what to take with us as we head into the unknown—and hopefully not too brief—future of life on earth. We look back at the wisdom that derived from Hippocrates' recognition of the humors and the nature of the flesh, and at the wisdom that came of seeing the flesh as *adama* or elements animated by spirit that lives on via yogis, doctors of Asian medicine, and feminine and indigenous traditions from around the globe. We trust the body to reveal itself, and ourselves to learn to comprehend the whole of it.

This, of course, begins with learning to say, as the writers of Canada's classic Red Green show put it: "the three little words that men find so hard to say: 'I don't know'." In other words, we make free to use the safety of the post-employment years to release the heavy burden of being a late modern know-it-all and take pleasure in exploring the body that we presumed to know but in fact failed to comprehend or contextualize. We begin with a model of the body that integrates and accommodates previous constructs created by the species. Integrative medicine clinics cannot do this because various practitioners take different views of the body and miss the big picture that includes the flesh as well as its being.

To learn more and more about the body, and to comprehend and contextualize it as we go, we use a new provisional model that supports personal, particular, and subjective knowledge of the body. In other words, we learn to fearlessly experience our own bodies and to get to know them from the inside out. We do this in the context of the late modern base of knowledge that has given us the greatest—and therefore most dangerous—control of the body and its ailments. We do this to undertake the care of all lives as one in situ—that is, in each and all of the habitats that together comprise the biosphere as a whole.

As you saw in the sevenfold construct earlier in the book, this provisional model views the human body as comprising seven levels or facets: awareness, understanding, perceptions, sensations, energy, flesh, and interbeing. The level of flesh includes fourteen nested levels or aspects useful to doctors, one for each part of the review of systems. We here assume that you comprehend the flesh and its fourteen levels but may be unfamiliar with part or all of the other six. Keep in mind that these can exist in the same place at the same time because flesh is the only aspect that is matter; therefore, only flesh displaces other matter inside the bounds of the largest organ, the skin.

You will have become aware of some of the electrical signals emitted by the energy body when you learned to analyze clinical recordings of the electrical activities of the brain, heart, and muscles. As with the general public, you will have seen infra-red images that reveal the bodily emanation of heat. You will not have encountered the energy body as a whole because it has no anatomical correlate; rather, it is electromagnetic, a time-varying integral of protean vectors, a fluid summation of resultant dynamic fields. In other words, it is intangible, ethereal, alive, and complex—so complex as to make artificial complex systems seem child's play in comparison. And yet this aspect of the body was investigated, mapped, and put to good use during the classical period of Indian history, and you can feel it and learn to comprehend it through the perennial knowledge and wisdom of the Himalayas. If your flesh is damaged and requires your conscious assistance, you will find the energy body invaluable for its capacity to restore and reconstitute abilities again and again.

You may tend to think of sensations as phenomena related to anatomical correlates such as the organs of the five senses, the cranial nerves, and their related cortical processing centers. All these are necessary but not sufficient to comprehend the facet of the body that we call sensations. This facet is inclusive of somatic and visceral nerves that detect phenomena; sense awarenesses that construct phenomena like pleasure, the gourmet palate, the musical ear, and the global sensory milieu that we know as states of being like joy or compassion; and the ability to create time-based sensory experiences such as the pooling of fluctuating states to share the energies of prayer or to enhance states of sexual arousal that may lead to ecstatic release of energy. For most

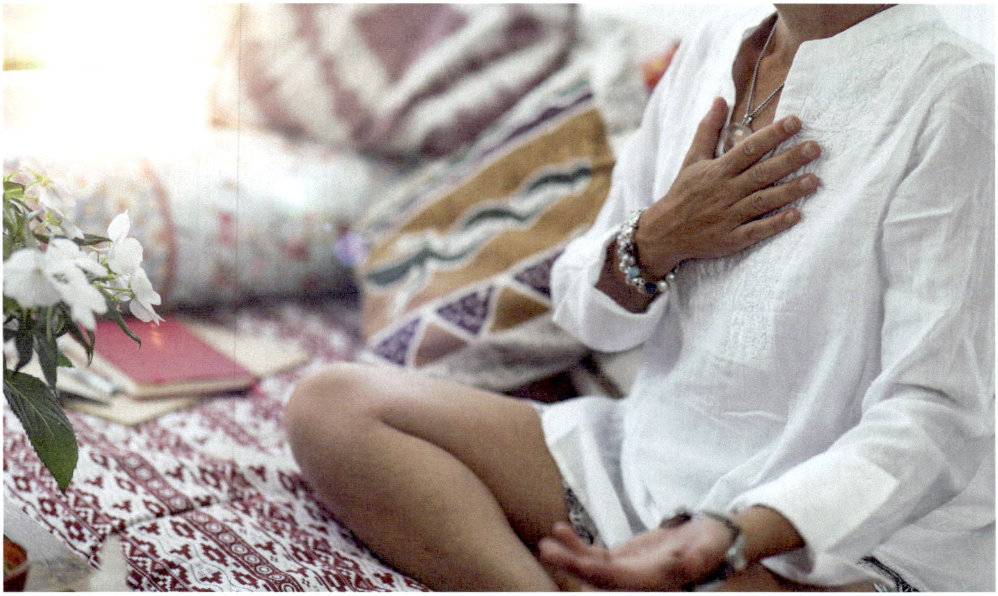

of us, sensations are so familiar that they recede into the background of our lives, where we take them for granted until reminded of them in relation to the upward transcendence called spirituality or the downward transcendence labeled materialism.

As with sensations, the facet of the body we call perceptions exceeds the cortical processing centers and related neural circuitry. These are necessary but insufficient to comprehend the faculty of perceptions that we get to know from the inside out. Perceptions include all of the conditioned responses that connect incoming data with pre-programmed behaviors customized to flesh and being. These conditioned responses free your understanding and awareness to focus on new or odd experiences that require attention and that are not amenable to a typical response or to offhand dismissal. These may arise from any location in the body and may prompt a proximal or global response. Examples include your spinal nerve reflexes and your responses to this text, which may be provisional and amenable to rapid and evolving alteration. As you know, most perceptions quickly become so automatic as to be inaccessible to attention or intention; this is their purpose and the challenge they pose to new learning.

Of understanding we need say little that is new except that we include apprehension as well as comprehension. That is, we include recognition of non-literal and poorly localized phenomena that you—or anyone—may have yet to comprehend, and that invite comprehension. In you, with your education and experience, this facet of the body is very strong—sometimes too much so as you seek to broaden the scope of your understanding to admit new phenomena and develop new wisdom. Of awareness we also need say very little. We use it here to refer mainly to a spacious and unstructured view of time, life, and its substrates, and a strong ability to pay attention to phenomena and to concentrate on them at will.

Interbeing is a term coined by Buddhist monk Thich Nhat Hanh to update existing spiritual terms such as collective consciousness and scientific terms such as ecology. As formulated here, interbeing possesses a material aspect that includes resources exchanged within the body of life. For instance, it includes the exchange of oxygen and carbon dioxide through the lungs; the exchange of moisture and salt through the skin; and the ingestion and excretion of minerals and nutrients that cycle through aggregated bodies such as species and habitats.

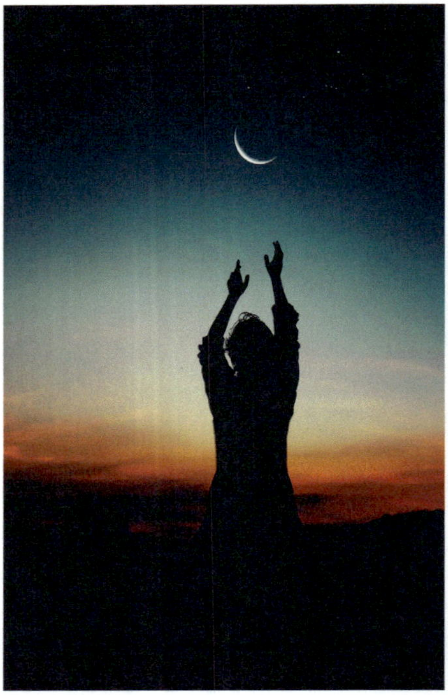

Interbeing also includes myriads of intangible phenomena such as: the atmospheric or interpersonal energies known as chi or ki in Asian traditions; the energy of attention, as when you feel someone staring at you; the communication—at a distance—of presence, anger, love through means that we here provisionally call entanglement in reference to the scientific recognition of pairings of particles sustained across time and distance. For the purposes of this book, we use interbeing to refer to any aspect of your body that interfaces with the outside.

Body: Flesh and Being

Everything should be made as simple possible, but no simpler.

— Albert Einstein

EXERCISE

The diffusion of information is not necessarily the diffusion of knowledge,' she explained, and 'the triumph over matter does not always or often lead to the triumph of Soul.' And, 'when it is made over easy for men to communicate with one another, they learn less from one another.

— Margaret Fuller through Megan Marshall in *Margaret Fuller: A New American Life*

In this body-mindfulness exercise, you have the opportunity to become familiar with a way of localizing each facet of the body in the energy centers so well-described—eventually to the point of baroque decadence—by classical Hindu adepts. Note that your body is your gold standard, that the experiences and embodiments of others may vary substantially, and that it falls to you to know yourself and to respond to your flesh and being as they are and not according to an abstract notion. Be appreciative of ancient wisdom and yet ready to go where no one has gone, to engage that which you have yet to know, and to learn and apply lessons that no human may know.

Set aside a period of twenty minutes during which you will be undisturbed and free to lie down in a comfortable place. If this is difficult, try waking up early and doing the exercise quietly in bed as you relax and extend your rest. Be sure that the place in which you relax is free of electronic devices.

Be aware that as your body opens to interbeing, you may have experiences that are unpleasant. If you have had a very strong prayer or meditation practice, or you can enter into and abide in strong care states, your centers may open easily and your energy may flow. If you sense a hell state, release it and enter into and hold a strong care state as an antidote that you can learn to share with others. Learning these skills requires calm, fearless patience and is easy and safe for anyone with clinic-or street-smarts who has learned to relax and yet remain prepared for the odd unexpected and potentially unpleasant encounter.

Now, begin with the flesh. Rest both palms on the midline of your abdomen between your pubis and navel. Bring your awareness to your palms. Allow your focus to sink toward the front of your spine. Contemplate your miraculous flesh and offer it well wishes or bless it as suits you. If you like, try affirming silently in your mind, *May my flesh be restored and revived,* or devise a well-wish of your own. Allow your being to enter into a care state and let your body relax into kind wishes or loving blessing.

After several minutes, slip your palms up to your navel and rest them there. Offer a phrase such as *May my energy body be strong and centered,* and take a few moments to enjoy your care state. If you are prone to excess stomach acid, you may find that you are obliged to keep this step very brief, or that you can modify it acceptably by resting one palm on either side of your navel.

When you are ready, slip your palms up and rest them on your epigastrium, offering a phrase such as *May my sensations aid me in caring for my flesh,* or *May my sensations support my perceptions in easing my loving care of life.* If and when you feel ready, or if you experience any unwanted gastric responses, move on to the next step.

Slip your palms upward to the physical heart and rest them there as you allow your care state to intensify in response to a phrase such as *May my perceptions support my reconciliation with love and my restoration of life.* Allow your focus to move into the chambers of your dynamic heart. If you are distracted by your heart's motion, shift your palms to your breastbone and allow your focus to sink into your lower heart center, which is in front of the spine at the level of the xiphisternum or so. If your field of vision fills with white heart light, enjoy it as long as you like. [Caution: do not open your heart if you expect to soon be called to respond to heartbreaking suffering or to heart-hardening trauma or violence.]

Now slip your palms upward to the space at the center of your brow. If you like, rest your hands on your upper body and use one fingertip or your inner eye—that is, your third eye or mind's eye—to focus on the point on the inner surface of the skull between your eyebrows. Offer a phrase such as *May my understanding be clear enough to support the best care of life.* If you enjoy the state that arises, allow your focus to remain there as long as you like—but take care to avoid or interrupt distasteful experiences that originate in interbeing.

Now slip your palms to the crown of your head, that is, to the place in your skull where your fontanelle used to be. Once again, if you find it awkward to use your palms, use a fingertip or your mind's eye to guide your focus. Offer a phrase such as *May my awareness be free of obstacles or boundaries.* If you see white crown light, allow your focus to remain in your crown as long as you wish, taking care to sustain your care state and to remain grounded through your pelvic bones. If you like, allow your focus to rise a few inches above your crown.

When you have finished, move your hands down from your crown—sweeping your arms outward and downward in semicircles if you are alone—and allow your palms to rest for a few minutes on your thighs as you offer a phrase such as *May my part of interbeing be a source of strength, light, and love.*

When you have finished encountering and nurturing all of the facets of your body, relax as long as you like, sustaining and deepening your care state so long as it continues to restore you. Be prepared to enjoy yourself until your focus begins to fade or you feel fatigue overtaking any facet of your body. Allow yourself as much recovery time as you like. If you notice anything new about your body as a result of the exercise, write it in your journal.

Writing Prompts

Choose from among the following those questions that capture your curiosity and may sustain your interest for several days or more. Dwell on those that reveal the facets of the body you have disregarded or bullied, and learn to treat them tenderly with loving solicitude. Make a note of any surprises in your journal. Continue using prompts like these until you are able to examine your embodied experiences, with the aim of gradually leaving behind those that are unnecessary or harmful, and nurturing those that promise to catalyze your restoration and rebirth.

- What part of this experience belongs to my flesh? My sensations? My perceptions?
- What parts of my flesh are most robust and vital? Which need my tender, loving care?
- How strongly centered is my energy body now? How stable is the core channel that runs in the front of my spine? How low or high is my center of energy? Can I center it several finger-widths below the navel and so optimize its strength and stability?
- What sensory phenomena are most familiar to me? What data do I tend to register from the outside? From the inside? What stimuli do I track so as to actively amplify and alter them for duty? For pleasure?

- Which habits are most useful to me? Which are most in the way? Which do I recognize in the course of the day and find amusing, or take as outdated and ready for dismissal? What is it that I am sick and tired of pretending to respond to in the usual or prescribed way when in fact I am already responding to it in a completely different way?
- Where are the blind spots in my recognition of the phenomena that are taking place in and around my body? In my state of being and the shifts in the baseline state that track my becoming? Where are the blind spots in my comprehension of my life? My work?
- What am I most curious to see that seems to exist just outside my worldview? What aspect of the unknown is calling to me, or intrigues me most? What am I aware of now that I wasn't aware of last week? Last year? How can I engage it constructively? To what that I have been ignoring up to now am I inclined to pay attention? What would I like to contemplate and concentrate on so as to resolve an inner or outer conflict? What do I enjoy concentrating on? What objects of my focus do I dislike? Can I resolve the dislike or ignore them or otherwise find a strategy—or form the skills—to move on?
- What things in the milieu trigger hell states? Can I remove the triggers or strengthen my heavenly states of being? How can I engage and enrich my artificial habitats and the natural ones on which my body relies for life? How can I find out more about the species that are indigenous and essential to my habitat? What are the major sources of toxicity and lasting damage in my area? If my work is contributing to the poisoning or consumptive destruction of the habitat or biosphere, what can I do to turn that source of death into a source of life? Can I do likewise in my life outside work?

Defining Macrobiology

Looked at from the point of view of other organisms, humankind…resembles an acute epidemic disease, whose occasional lapses into less virulent forms of behavior have never yet sufficed to permit any really stable, chronic relationship to establish itself.

— William H. McNeill in *Plagues and Peoples*

The advent of macrobiology as a basic science of clinical medicine is long overdue. Since the early modern invention of the microscope, physicians have focused more and more on infinitesimal organisms and their control. As late modern social crusaders sought to impose basic laboratory science on medical practice, to pursue blind faith in technology, and to rely on social science methods and fields like law and economics, doctors have become more database-dependent and clustered in referral hospitals and clinics that offer intensive interventions. We have delved so deeply into molecular and cellular biology as to disregard the big picture—and clinical observation and study.

From ancient times to this epoch, popular narratives that continue to shape us tell tales in which the social status quo is disrupted, a scapegoat is found and punished, and order is restored. In almost all cases, the status quo—however unsatisfactory—is seen as far better than change, which is imposed by outside forces. There are few tales of problem-solving—except in the context of outside rescue or hitting it rich. There are tales of rebirth—some of which left the popular realm to become scriptures that guide transformation from within. It is time for new ways of thinking that support self-guided initiative and personal responsibility.

To leave modernity behind is to think in new currencies such as time and love. If you behave as if time is money—when in fact it is priceless—or as if modern constructs of efficiency are more important than life itself, you lose the chance to make good use of your most precious resource: the time on earth that remains to you. Likewise, if you treat medicine as a social machine, you lose the chance to follow the lead of architects, designers, organic farmers, and others at the periphery who are creating the new living and increasingly local and sustainable economies that are arising as the machinery of mass over-consumption winds down. Similarly, if you view the body as matter and its being and becoming as belonging to clergy or habitat restorers, you lose the chance to synthesize solutions to the late modern medical problems of our species and its habitats.

To leave modernity behind, you put analytic thinking and reductionism into perspective. Hegel framed this process in terms of thesis, antithesis, and synthesis. As an emerging expert in care and cure who takes the body of life as the patient that holds all patients, you may be inspired by the image that NASA called the blue marble, the image of earth from space. This reveals as nothing else can the truth of continuity that underlies the human projections of borders and ownership and rights to use evolved life as if it were a product. The sight of the globe gives us a view in which it is not only practical but mandatory to treat the biosphere first and work inward to care for each species and all as one. To break this down so that we can quantitate problems and solutions will requires us to think finitely, and deterministically. Assumptions of infinity and chance are of little use in treating any body, indvidual or aggregated. We must therefore create new tools that will allow us to solve our present problems. One possible source of apt methods is category theory, which has applications in information science. If you have strengths in the three M's—medicine, math, and music—you may wish to discovery any utility it may have in relation to this month's exercises.

The methods for modeling nested bodies that are finite and dependent begin, like all new approaches, as acts of imagination held by a few minds until they are developed enough to be tested against reality—in this case, the reality that illnesses rarely belong to the human species alone.

To embrace the future in this way—by defining actionable problems and solving them—is to affirm that the practice of medicine is—like all human ailments and their causes and consequences—forever dynamic and mysterious, and in need of new solutions to previously unseen problems. This requires courage, love, and honor as well as attention to the acute observations by which Hippocrates formed the profession, the virtues by which Maimonides transformed the medieval world, and the determination and sacrifice of Vesalius that enabled us to study the dead and so to develop the capacity to rescue the living.

ANECDOTES FROM MEDICAL LIVES

On his six-acre Port Townsend farm, Frank Herbert finally established his 'Ecological Demonstration Project' to explore the application of alternative energy sources, such as wind, solar, and methane gas. [This] was a Frank Herbert Story in and of itself, one in which he 'learned by doing,' as he liked to say—the best way of learning anything.

— Brian Herbert in *Dreamer of Dune: The Biography of Frank Herbert*

Late modern doctors—and all professionals who work for the public good—are now dangerously over-managed and under-led. This is because late modern managers have formed social machines in the images of those industrial and technological ones that use humans as functions. Doing so put humans in the position of serving their tools. For a while, you will have been able to interface between the tools and your patients and society. This capability ended with the invasion of information systems that impose excessive centralized control and so put virtual reality first. Such systems attack the rare targeted error at the cost of imposing pervasive neglect of the real. They prevent evolution from the periphery and preclude the use of life experience for 'spontaneous' improvement. Worse, they work against conscience, personal responsibility, personal and interpersonal agency, ethics, and all other positive human skills and virtues on which the species must rely. They will have coopted your narrative and thus your growth and development. If you have remained fully human, your spirit is strong. You have become a superhero.

Compared to that ordeal, your transformation of medicine will be easy and good fun for the elder years, when it is natural for the tangible aspects of the body to decline and the rest to come into their own. If you have a pension or other means of support, you will be free—for the first time in memory—to do the right thing according to the conscience derived from your life experience. This is essential. Each doctor has gathered a unique series of observations and created a particular personal narrative that is—as Buckminster Fuller pointed out—essential to the whole. The species learns—you and we learn—as do each and all.

By turning outward and becoming aware of how you interface with the environment—consciously or automatically, with or without exchanging explicit consent—you prepare your awareness for macrobiology. This will ultimately prepare you to be able to scan the full spectrum of care across time (from the beginning of biological time to the end of your life and of life on earth) and across scale (from the level of an atom or prion to the level of the forest and biosphere). You will—for the first time—be able to care for human life in its living context, as needs must.

If you have been participating in the awakening to the biosphere that is underway around the globe, you will have engaged the realities of the environment and our human degradation of it. This will have opened your eyes to the consequences of your species' reckless behavior and to the manifestations of those consequences in patients. Having seen those, you will be truly ready to abstract and comprehend macrobiology—that is, the comprehension of evolved life on the human scale and above—and to use what you learn to grow into the role of medical elder and to help turn this end time into a time of rebirth.

Gil's Ethics

During his neurology fellowship in the 1970s, Gil worked at a local natural foods cooperative in a university church. He appeared as a bearded, fierce-seeming creature who resembled a member of the Chicago Seven. He was one of the radical new foodies who consumed whole-grain breads, cheesy vegetarian enchiladas, and lentil soups that had been promoted from poor food to trendy food by Frances Moore Lappe's *Diet for a Small Planet.*

Gil had been born in the east and was moving steadily west. After his training, he continued from one university position to the next until reaching the west coast. There, while on a house call to a young man dying of brain cancer, he met a former hippie who was a self-proclaimed doctor-hater but who could not resist Gil's passionate and compassionate heart.

Gil married her, started a family, and got involved in his community. His family joined a synagogue that followed orthodox as well as reconstructionist Jewish practices. They then joined a group dedicated to community supported agriculture with the aim of catalyzing the growth of a local sustainable economy in which farmers could transition to natural and then to organic methods for raising crops. The family aimed to cook the safest possible family meals, to promote health and prevent disease, and to protect the land. They did this in the context of a big picture and an evolving ethos that was rooted in ancient traditions and in forward-thinking change.

In other words, they were way ahead of their time. They were walking the walk of their faith decades before the phrase came into wide use; acting from a love of life in professions that laid claim to such love but could be slow to act on it; and by example led their peers and juniors in creating a better world. They continued to do this well into the retirement years and so inspire the rest of us to step up and to continue their work of devising and championing more life-affirming ways of becoming and doing.

Max's Explorations

Some years ago, Max, a trauma surgeon at a large regional hospital, moved to the outskirts of his metropolitan area. Like most medical specialists, he focused on his work and earned sufficient income and status to give his family the best that society had to offer. He had a large lot and home, a fine car, and everything that he thought he should want. He worked hard, played hard, encouraged his children to do the same, and let the zeitgeist take them where it may. One of the places that it took them was the world of competitive sports. His children competed in regional events that took the family to indoor arenas and also into the outdoors. They participated in excursions organized by non-profit associations or that were packaged and sold to the public as outdoor adventures.

As they followed their bliss into the wild forests that seemed abundant in the region around their home, they became increasingly familiar with their habitats and more and more aware of human encroachments on them. They saw the ravages of forest fires and discussed the controversies surrounding fire control. As they fell in love with nature and became aware of the responsibilities of caring for it, they began to question social processes that they had taken for granted. They became aware of their habits of consumption.

Like Frank Herbert before him, Max began to experiment with energy production. He put in a windmill that powered home batteries. He told his children, who told everyone they knew—including my son, who had met his children at climbing events. What we heard was vague enough to suggest that Max might have gone off the grid. We had already met—and still hoped to work with—builders who produced single- or multi-family dwellings that were net-zero or better; that is, that produced as much or more power than they consumed. This trend had begun with survivalists who lived in the mountains off the grid, and was finally spreading to the local, living economies that were forming to solve systemic problems through creative new ways of living that supported self-sufficiency and that used new tools such as alternative currencies.

Knowing that he, too, was a physician, I called Max and asked him about his experiment. He hastened to say that his home was not even close to self-sufficient,

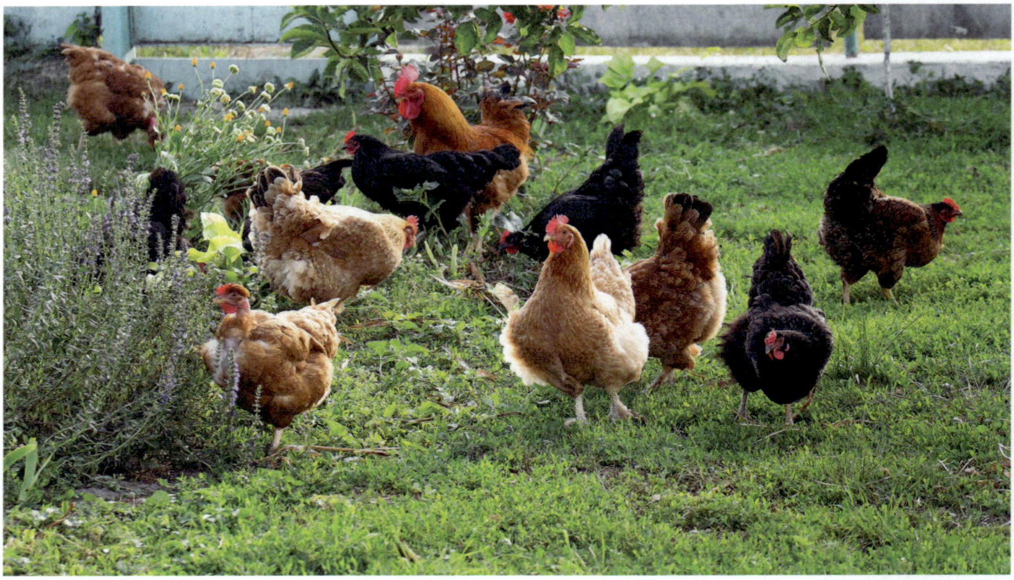

that his project had provided them with a little extra power but that they were by and large living like the majority of late modern urbanites. It was not clear to him that replicating infrastructure would be better for the environment in the long run. He was still thinking things through, working things out. Half a century after Frank Herbert turned his Cascadian home into an ecological demonstration project, the pioneering work done by him and other visionaries of the Cascadia bioregion is catalyzing innovation and change.

Dan's Yard

Dan grew up in California and then studied, trained, and worked in various parts of the west and southwest before finally returning to his home state to start his career and to raise a family in a sunny, low-density neighborhood that was developing rapidly. As his children were born and his medical career intensified, his free time slipped away; he began to feel disappointed and discouraged. He was working full-out all the time. He used up his store of motivation. His health began to deteriorate. He put on weight. He was on track to follow the pre-modern and modern pattern of a medical life that ended in early death or burn-out.

To restore balance in the expected way, Dan put himself on anti-depressants and used his free time to putter around the house and yard with the dogs and children. He had many skills and was good with a budget, so he refreshed himself by updating the bathrooms and kitchens of his home and re-landscaping his yard. Over time, he installed stone walks, built and put up wood fences, and put in native, drought-resistant plants appropriate to the surrounding habitat. He created an artificial environment that would substitute for the natural world that he missed. His dream for retirement is to spend all of his time caring for his patch of the body of life.

BETH LOOKS BACK: Taking off the Blinders

The nature of any cutting-edge science is that most of our current ideas are wrong. That's not a denigration of science; it's the way science progresses... It becomes downright dangerous, then, if we rush to apply every incremental insight or technique within a theoretical framework that is probably wrong."

— David Suzuki in *The Autobiography*

Family legend has it that my Yankee ancestors were Puritans who emigrated from England to American in 1640. In those days, the journals of John Winthrop and others reveal that while in the context of the English way of life at the time the immigrants were radical protestants, they kept hoping to wake up and find themselves back in the English countryside, which was the product of roughly 10,000 years of radical habitat destruction. They couldn't wait to get rid of the wilderness that terrified them.

Sometime in the next four hundred years, their descendants adapted; they came to love the forest, and kept following its edge westward. More recent family lore has it that Pa Wilson, one of my great-grandfathers who was respected for the farming skills he had used to move back the frontier a few acres, loved to camp out in the forest. He was skilled in farm and forest life, and could make a delicious apple pie in his frying pan over a campfire. He sustained good relations with forest-integrated peoples, who stayed at his farm every fall on the way east but left just before the harvest. He said he paid them to work the fields; his neighbors poked fun at him for that. When he sold his farm, the new owner paved it over. Pa lost heart. Like all of his modern ancestors—perhaps all of his ancestors since the Druids—he had destroyed his place in the body of life and watched the destruction accelerate and alienate him from the disappearing wild.

With the advent of ecology, population biologists began to use mathematical modeling that belied the difficulty of grappling with large-scale biological systems. Then an advocate of disease control—McDonald—put in his oar and developed some deterministic equations on the dynamics of malaria in East Africa, thereby opening the door to grassroots prevention of malaria through the removal of discarded, water-filled, mosquito-breeding cans and tires. Dr. Mervyn Susser put this and other model-driven medical interventions together with ecological thinking and medical history in his 1973 book *Causal Thinking in the Health Sciences*. More recently, habitat-integrated peoples have been reappearing in long non-fiction narratives such as M. Wylie Blanchet's *The Curve of Time* and Laura Dassow Walls' *Henry David Thoreau: A Life*. Even scientists are taking other species seriously, as Peter Wohlleben discusses in his charming book *The Inner Life of Animals*. Hope Jahren, author of *Lab Girl*, is working on hundred-year studies of trees. Our species is meeting life where it is, and applying the wisdom of the globe to learning to abide in the womb of nature.

Medical thinking is ready for the next great leap: leaving behind the human exceptionalism that has been justified by applying the worldview of desert theology to all habitats. Almost all of the assumptions that underlie modern thinking have the same fatal flaw: they enslave, exclude, or destroy the body of life that can no longer hide from the brave new world of consumption that exploded in medieval times, accelerated alarmingly with mass production, and is now about to make or break our evolution. Now that biological reality has our attention and biocentric thinking is under construction, we have the chance to comprehend life on earth and our impact on it. This will take the development of macrobiological thinking, which must use abstractions that allow our minds to grasp our problems and to craft the solutions that lie ahead of us.

COMMENT

The Universe of Life and the Complete Dependence of Nested Bodies

I've left out a final feature of stories, the coda, a retrospective evaluation of what it all might mean, a feature that also returns the hearer or reader from there and then of the narrative to the here and now of the telling. In conversations I've had about what makes a story, few people mention this...

— Jerome Bruner in *Making Stories: Law, Literature and Life*

The old narratives we love led our species to become what it is— a 'paragon of animals' on the brink of inadvertent self-extinction, a species so divided from its living context that it is not content to suicide: it must take the fruits of three hundred million years of evolution with it. We know that the body of our species is on a collision course with the body of life on which it depends, and yet our learned helplessness is so convincing to us that we are willing to accept a catastrophic loss of faith in what we can and must do to make good on the history of life. We simply don't know what to do. We need new narratives, long macrobiological and emerging medical novels that imagine plausible ways forward into a living future.

We have outgrown ancient tales that warn against perturbations in the social order that endanger the tribe and call on a micromanaging God to set things right. We have likewise outgrown modern narratives that idolize our tools—e.g. late modern technologies and complex systems. We have also outgrown scapegoating; when our idols tarnish, we cannot make the usual suspects pay the price. More and more of us are seeing the consequences of our actions and recognizing that we are each and all responsible. More and more of us are changing. To go further requires new narratives for urgent change.

We have already begun them. New non-fiction narratives enable us to comprehend life and to care for it. Old nursery tales of trolls, giants, and angry gods have given way to tales of floods, ice ages, and lava flows. The past century showed us what comes of tales of supermen—e.g. the archetype of the Nazi übermensch—and we have relegated them to comic books. We have seen that running away to another planet with our old habits intact is a fantasy, and a dark one at that. Many of us grasp that failure is not an option.

As doctors, it is our responsibility to relinquish the late modern fantasies that divide our species from the body of life and its future. These include molecular narratives that we try to transfer to events that are unfolding on the human scale and above. To focus on the urgent task of sorting through the mix of truth and falsehood that we inherited, we can stop working hard to create a virtual reality that makes it nearly impossible to learn from life experience. As Henry Ford put it, if we keep doing what we've been doing, we'll keep getting what we've got. For the sake of the young who face the task of surviving and thriving in spite of us, or dying in the trying, we must tell well-grounded tales of success—real or plausible and worth essaying.

A speculative non-fiction narrative that we are ready to create is this month's topic: macrobiology. This field—if developed—would offer abstractions that fit biological realities that are finite, deterministic, complex, and completely

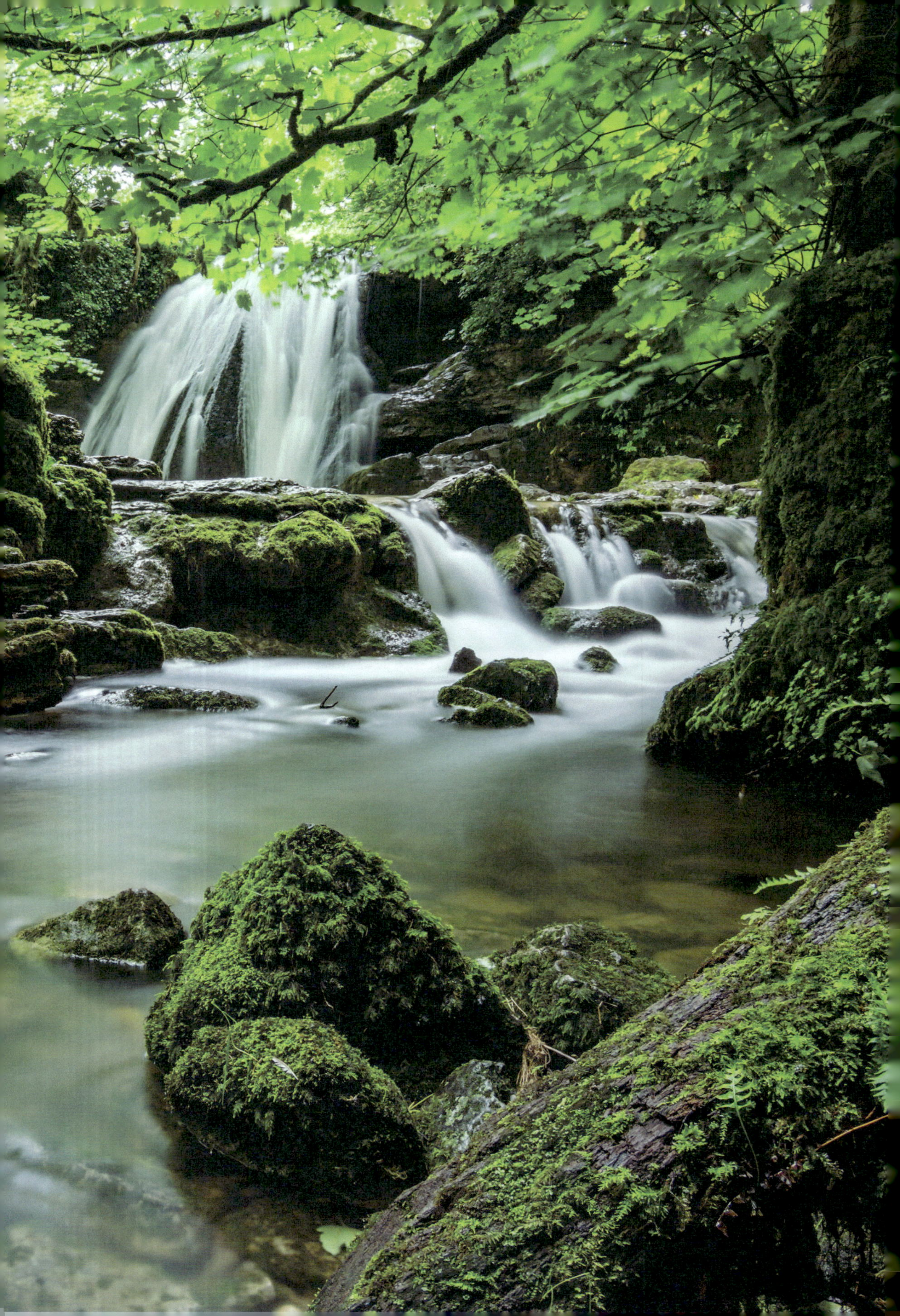

interdependent. Our present methods focus on one or two popular molecules amongst millions that may matter, assume that they are independent—an untenable assumption in biology—and then assemble them into easy to interpret but simplistic, contextless, and ungrounded models that we accept as valid if they merely do not fall apart. Doctors, field biologists, theologians, and habitat restorers could instead use macrobiological ideas and methods to express relations in and between species and habitats, and to comprehend the flow of emerging epidemics, such as chronic ambient poisoning, that affect the body of life as a whole. Symbolic, deterministic abstractions that are as complicated as biochemical pathways like the Krebs cycle could provide a far better fit to medical ecology than do statistics.

Set and category theory may lack the necessary time functions to create these abstractions, but topology or representation theory may enable us to look at the universe of life—the thin green and blue skin of the earth—and to see how we as a species fit into and interact with our habitats. We can then use scenarios incorporating these interactions in the way of sensitivity analyses in decision analysis, and so discover what is important and how we may develop a reasonable methodology suitable for the scale under study—and then question our assumptions. In other words, these narratives can allow us to see and manipulate our ideas and push the envelope of epistemology while never forgetting that it may give way again at any time—if we are lucky.

Good narratives for the future would model character arcs in which doctors move from fatalistic acceptance of chronic illness and the end of life on earth to self-talk like: I don't know but I can find out; I never thought of that but I will think about it now—and from now on; I came, I saw, I cared; and doctor, cure thyself. In doing so, doctors can partake of the fruits of the history of social dissidence that gave rise to the radical reformation and that evolved into the great rights movements of the past century—especially human rights—as well as the movement toward personal agency and responsibility that has been evolving in evolutionary time. This means taking part once again in the kind of epochal changes that arise at the grassroots level and spread through pervasive, intentional, congregal paradigm change.

Drawing on Embodied Experience

The emotions and the passions exert a powerful influence over the physical organism. It is important, therefore, that they be held under restraint by the reasoning faculties. This rule applies equally to joy, fear and grief; to avarice, anger, and hatred; and, above all, to the sexual passion. They are a prolific source of disease of the nervous system, and have caused the dethronement of some of the most gifted intellects.

— Dr. R.V. Pierce in *The People's Medical Adviser*

EXERCISE 1: ABSTRACTING YOUR NESTED BODIES

Consider the habitat categories below (from the IUCN 2015 Red List of Threatened Species). Find and mark your present habitat(s).

1. Forest
2. Savanna
3. Shrubland
4. Grassland
5. Wetland-inland
6. Rocky areas
7. Caves/subterranean
8. Desert
9. Neritic-marine pelagic
10. Marine oceania
11. Marine deep ocean floor
12. Marine intertidal
13. Marine coastal supratidal
14. Artificial – terrestrial
15. Artificial – aquatic
16. Introduced vegetation
17. Other
18. Unknown

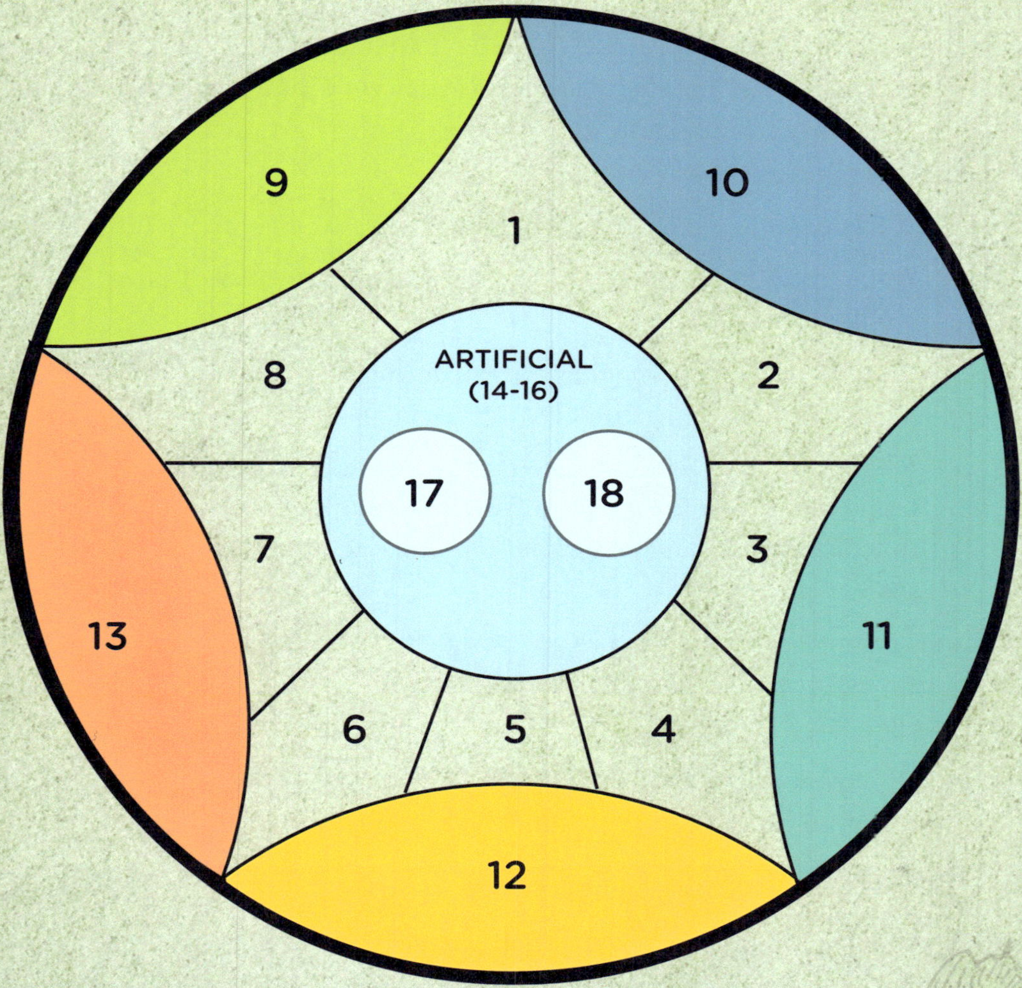

ABIOTIC CONTEXT
(air, water, rock, gravity, topography, etc.)

EXERCISE 2: Writing Your Body into its Living Context

This month, use cues to inspire your imagination and write out what you imagine in your journal. Write as many spontaneous responses as you like over the course of the month. Let them be fictional or non-fictional in accord with your inclination. Let them develop as your views and ideas percolate and evolve. If you wish to integrate your responses into a narrative, write it in your journal—or wherever you like.

- When I think of biomedical narratives inclusive of ecology, I think of...
- When I think of biomedical narratives inclusive of spirituality or theology, I think of...
- When I think of biomedical narratives inclusive of field biology or habitat restoration, I think of...
- When I think of melding views and constructs from all areas of human endeavor for the purposes of envisioning a sustainable future in which our profession enables the body of humanity to act as a system of the body of life, I see...
- When I envision myself as a wise elder who is able to turn the experience of a lifetime into wisdom that I can use for mentoring and eldering, I think of....
- When I think of sources of inspiration for my own personal rebirth through the transition to medical eldering, I think of...

EXERCISE 3: Living Heritage as Identity

Formulate identity statements that place you in the aggregated bodies in which you nest and in which your ancestry unfolded. Some prompts may help you to start:

1. Thinking back to my eight great-grandparents, I have roots in the body of humanity as it was 100, 200, 500, 1000, and 2000 years ago in places such as...
2. The habitat there at that time was...
3. The biome at that time was...
4. In my life, I have lived in habitat types that include...
5. Who, when, and where am I in the local area (200 mi radius) of the

> body of humanity? Of my habitat(s)? Of my bioregion? Right now, how healthy are the bodies of my species in this place? My habitats? Other species (pollinators, insects)? Life on earth?

In your journal, write a question and hold it in your mind. When a response coheres, express it in symbols or images, a group of symbols or images, or as an outline of a long narrative—real or speculative. Maximize your relational ideas and minimize the fragmentation introduced by information overload.

EXERCISE 4: Revisiting Your Formative Experiences

Write a list of the ten life experiences that were most important in forming your character.

Compare this list to the one you made in June. How and why do they differ? Have your efforts during this winter and spring of transition led to any signs of new wisdom? To the beginnings of emergence? Reflect on your efforts and write about any gains (and losses) in your journal.

EXERCISE 5: Emerging Abstractions

If you are fond of math or logic, you may enjoy wrestling with these optional exercises.

Optional Exercise A

Examine the equation below, which represents the body of life (L) as the union across habitats types (18) of the union of human (H) and non-human (NH) species in each.

$$L = \bigcup_{X=1}^{X=N} (H \cup NH)$$

> [Note that the equation is species-ist; if human behavior does not change, and humans continue to replace non-humans at a high rate of speed, the equation—and the body of life itself—will soon break down.]

Thinking of set theory, which allows for complete sampling and assumptions of dependence and thereby avoids the limitations of social science methods that exclude life and provide a poor fit to biological systems, you can plausibly visualize finite and nested processes. The symbolism of set theory avoids reductionism that is incompatible with life and thus with survival. State the meaning and potential utility of this formulation in your own words in your journal.

Optional Exercise B

Attempt to formulate an equation that would allow a hospital to estimate the harm done to patients and staff and their habitats by the production (soil to soil) of an MRI machine and the treatment of false positives and the risks of Alderman syndrome and to weigh it against the risks to patients of any failures of early detection that might improve quality of life for five years or more.

What information would we need in order to show whether MRI use is or isn't spending the future of life and risking the health of today's grandchildren?

EPILOGUE

Putting it All Together

In his autobiography, The Making of Mind, *A. F. Luria traces his own intellectual development in relation to the changing moods of neurology throughout his long lifetime; his chapter on "Romantic Science" particularly brings out his sense of the indispensability of case histories, and how the narrative is crucial to medicine.*

— Oliver Sacks in *An Anthropologist on Mars*

Review your year of transition by reviewing your journal. If you made the mistake of powering through the book rather than using it to marinate on reflection and repatterning, start over again and create a resource worthy of your past and your future.

If your journal is already a rich source of documented views, realizations, integrations, and transformations, use it to outline your medical life story to date. Include the whole of your life story if you are ready to do so, and if it catalyzes your narrative formation.

Essay

Write 5,000 words or more on whether or how you wish to complete your adult career by doing a capstone project that you define.

Essay

Write 5,000 words or more on whether or how you wish to formulate your legacy.

Narratives

Write a memoir of 5,000 words or more, and a speculative narrative of 5,000 words or more on the completion of your life.

If or when you have completed the online Discovery curriculum, consider joining the Doctors of Life International discussion group and sharing your plans.

If you go on to write a memoir, you are invited to submit it to Future Medicine. Kindly include the "[By] for" series label in your cover letter.

Have a wonderful Elderhood!

Acknowledgements

I owe my faith in humanity to those peers and mentors who engage the unknown as a source of sacred and inchoate new knowledge to be perceived and brought to light for the betterment of the world: particularly Michael Goodman, Ronald Perline, Professor Peter Meier, and Professor Monte Lloyd. I owe my patterning for discovery to those teachers who shared ideas and methods for inviting or embodying new knowledge: Rev. Cynthia Bourgeault, Imam Jamal Rahman, Rabbi Zalman Schachter-Shalomi, Rev. Matthew Fox, Geshe Kelsang Gyatso, Mantak Chia, Phabongkha Rinpoche, Sakya Monastery, and most of all Rabbi Ted Falcon.

I owe a deep debt of gratitude to: the University of Chicago method of free and open exchange of ideas; investigators who mentored me in laboratory sciences including C.N. Yang and Lucia Rothman-Denes; past physicians who gave their lives to advance the profession, especially Semmelweis and Dr. Howard Taylor Ricketts, whose portrait hung at the end of a hallway in the Pritzker School of Medicine; those mentors who taught me about medical detection and population medicine, especially Dr. Pierce Gardner, Drs. Tom Vernon and Ellen Mangione, Drs. Jose Cordero and David Swanson; Bill Foege and his colleagues for showing that humans can cure the species; and most of all Dr. Buchanan, master of the teaching anecdote, and his lineage of Edinburgh-trained doctors that trace back to the Scottish Enlightenment, when inspired physicians intervened and began to try for cure.

I am similarly indebted to those who are leading the present sea change in other fields, and who taught me about the emerging paradigm, especially: field biologists Joe Hutto and Janine Benyus through their TED talks; the New Hassids and New Monastics in religion and theology, and other unitive thinkers presently doing retreats; the developers of the seven petal living building paradigm and the Bullitt Center, especially Bob Hull and Mike Jobes, as well as Hammer-in-Hand, TC Legend Homes, and Anne Raab.

A number of teachers and colleagues helped me to see medicine from a psychological or anthropologic perspective, to see the errors and arbitrary constructs that limit and warp medical judgement, and to avoid mindless conformity to the herd mentality: Arthur Elstern; Amos Tversky and David Kahneman; the society for Medical Decision Making; Dr. Alvan Feinstein; Ron LaPorte; Lorna Moore; in the clinic setting, Drs. Mond and Shapiro; and student Nancy Gegen.

Equally instrumental in the development of my perspective as a physician were those who acquainted me with medicine in various populations: Dr. Joel Mason and his father, who arranged a summer externship at St. Vincent's Hospital in New York; Dr. Joel Silversten and colleagues in Nairobi for the medical student rotation at Kenyatta National Hospital; Dr. Pekka Puska of the International Epidemiology Association meetings in Helsinki and Joensuu; and to my husband for taking me to many national and international diabetes meetings. I would also like to thank Howard Nagatani and my other Sansei friends and the Holocaust survivors who inspired me to go on when I thought I couldn't, especially the Sperlings, Jellineks, and Frankels, as well as Philip Maisel and also Victor and Elly Frankl.

Last but not least I thank my parents for teaching me to respect all people and to value education and culture over money and possessions, and thank Chansonette Beck, Ann DiSalvo, Deidre Krupp, and Deborah Mokma for book development and editing; and Chris Molé for book design.

More About the Author

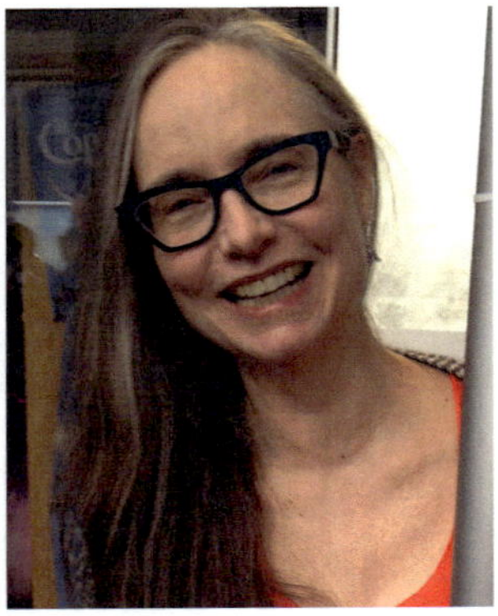

Beth Alderman, MD, MPH earned her AB and MD degrees from the University of Chicago and her MPH from the University of Washington. After Board Certification in Preventive Medicine and Public Health, she took a faculty position in the University of Colorado Medical School Department of Preventive Medicine, Biometrics, and Medical Informatics, where she did population-based epidemiological studies of adverse reproductive outcomes and methodological studies in clinical epidemiology. In her next faculty position at the University of Washington School of Public Health, she focused on risk factors for birth defects. In 1996, she fell ill with the mysterious new plague and was given the provisional diagnosis "chronic fatigue syndrome". She has spent her time since studying her own case and pondering the reasons that her beloved profession failed her so completely. Fortunately, she discovered her cure, which may be of use to others suffering from one or more of the emerging epidemics affecting humans, their habitats, and life on earth.

Medical Detective

Discerning Chronic Ambient Poisoning

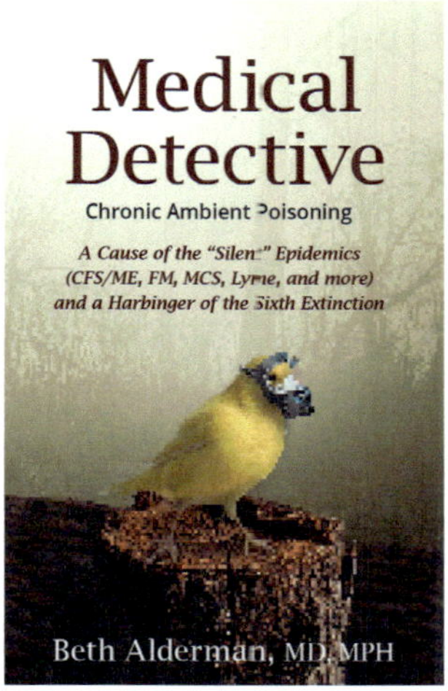

ISBN: 978-1-7321110-7-3

One day in December of 1996, the author (a physician, medical detective, and academic epidemiologist), developed disabling brain fog as part of a decade-long descent into painful and pervasive chronic illness. Having studied the causes of birth defects through population-based studies, and the limitations of modern medicine through methodological studies, she had inadvertently prepared to investigate the causes of her illness—a mysterious new plague provisionally labeled "chronic fatigue."

After a fifteen-year search, she found a doctor whose elimination diet relieved her brain fog and enabled her to self-diagnose chronic ambient poisoning, the human-caused plague that is overtaking our own species along with birds, bees, and habitats, and presaging the sixth extinction.

Available through Amazon.com.
See our publishing website: www.FutureMedicine.us
and educational website: www.EvolveMedicine.us

The Chronic Illness Owner's Manual

Volumes I and II

The Chronic Illness Owner's Manual series is for patients with chronic illness, and for the people who care for them. Suitable for individual or small group use, it offers a comprehensive, systematic, step-by-step approach to engaging modern medical systems, and to healing from the inside out.

The books comprise anecdotes, excercises and quotes that address recovery through seven aspects of the body: awareness, understanding, perceptions, sensations, energy, flesh and interbeing. The frames, constructs, patterns and processes employed by the series are drawn from traditions of medicine, field biology, theology and psychology from around the globe. Their synthesis offers an emerging, sustainable, biocentric, contextual and customizable approach to creating a new and better life that continues to evolve in keeping with your unique meaning, purpose, and vision of abundant life.

The Chronic Illness Owner's Manual series complements care and cure courses available online through our nonprofit partner at www.EvolveMedicine.us.

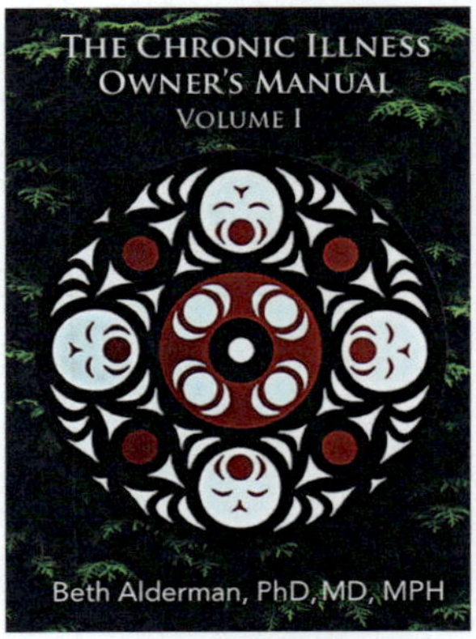

ISBN: 978-1-7321110-8-0

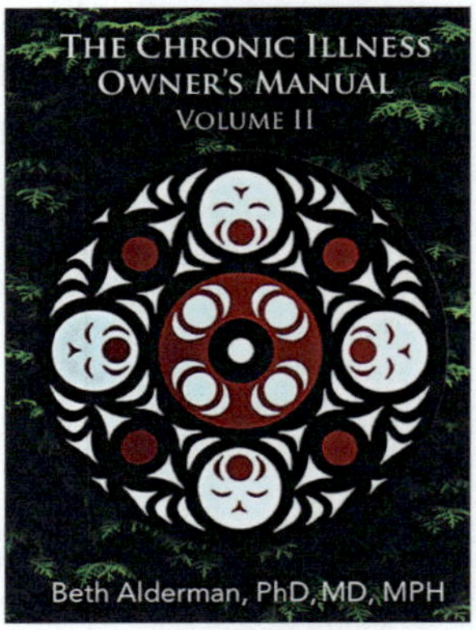

ISBN: 978-1-7321110-9-7

Made in the USA
Monee, IL
03 May 2026

49396330R00178